Living Donor Kidney Transplantation

Current Practices, Emerging Trends and
Evolving Challenges

Edited by

Robert S Gaston, MD
Jonas Wadström, MD

Living Donor Kidney Transplantation

Current Practices, Emerging Trends and Evolving Challenges

Edited by

Robert S Gaston, MD

Division of Nephrology
University of Alabama at Birmingham
Birmingham, Alabama, USA

Jonas Wadström, MD

Division of Transplantation Surgery
University Hospital
Uppsala, Sweden

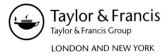

Taylor & Francis
Taylor & Francis Group

LONDON AND NEW YORK

© 2005 Taylor & Francis, an imprint of the Taylor & Francis Group

Cover based on a design created by Suzanne Lundqvist Tengzelius

First published in the United Kingdom in 2005
by Taylor & Francis, an imprint of the Taylor & Francis Group,
2 Park Square, Milton Park, Abingdon, Oxon OX14 4RN

Tel.:   +44 (0) 207 017 6000
Fax.:   +44 (0) 207 017 6699
E-mail: info.medicine@tandf.co.uk
Website: http://www.tandf.co.uk/medicine

Although every effort has been made to ensure that all owners of copyright material have been acknowledged in this publication, we would be glad to acknowledge in subsequent reprints or editions any omissions brought to our attention.

Although every effort has been made to ensure that drug doses and other information are presented accurately in this publication, the ultimate responsibility rests with the prescribing physician. Neither the publishers nor the authors can be held responsible for errors or for any consequences arising from the use of information contained herein. For detailed prescribing information or instructions on the use of any product or procedure discussed herein, please consult the prescribing information or instructional material issued by the manufacturer.

A CIP record for this book is available from the British Library.

Library of Congress Cataloging-in-Publication Data

Data available on application

ISBN 1-84184-316-4

Distributed in North and South America by
Taylor & Francis
2000 NW Corporate Blvd
Boca Raton, FL 33431, USA

Within Continental USA
Tel.: 800 272 7737; Fax.: 800 374 3401
Outside Continental USA
Tel.: 561 994 0555; Fax.: 561 361 6018
E-mail: orders@crcpress.com

Distributed in the rest of the world by
Thomson Publishing Services
Cheriton House
North Way
Andover, Hampshire SP10 5BE, UK
Tel.: +44 (0) 1264 332424
E-mail: salesorder.tandf@thomsonpublishingservices.co.uk

Composition by Wearset Ltd, Boldon, Tyne and Wear

Printed and bound in Great Britain by CPI, Bath

Contents

    Kiil Park, Jong Hoon Lee

12. Nondirected living donors   151
    Arthur J Matas, Cheryl L Jacobs, Catherine A Garvey, Deborah D Roman

13. Legal and ethical dilemmas in living donor kidney transplantation   157
    David PT Price

14. Financial and insurance considerations for living donors   165
    Jürg Steiger, Thomas R McCune

15. Is it desirable to legitimize paid living donor kidney transplantation programmes?

    Part 1: Evidence in favour   171
    Janet Radcliffe Richards

    Part 2: Evidence against   181
    William D Plant

    Index   191

Preface

Living donor kidney (LDK) transplantation has become the definitive approach to the treatment of end-stage renal failure, providing a better quality of life and the best opportunity for survival when compared with dialysis or transplantation from a deceased donor. The number of live kidney donors is increasing rapidly worldwide and, since 2001, has surpassed the number of deceased donors in the USA. Several factors have influenced this change. The advent of laparoscopic nephrectomy has reduced the morbidity of the nephrectomy procedure, making more donors receptive to an interruption of the healthy course of their lives. Just as importantly, seminal outcome data reported by Terasaki and Cecka enabled an expansion of LDK transplantation irrespective of the human leukocyte antigen (HLA) match or the donor–recipient relationship. Now, even blood type disparity or a positive crossmatch between the donor and the recipient is no longer the insurmountable biological obstacle to successful transplantation that it was just a decade ago. Any person who is well and willing to donate may now be a live kidney donor.

This year marks the fiftieth anniversary of the first successful kidney transplantation between identical twins. In a relatively brief period, LDK transplantation has progressed from an experimental modality to standard treatment. Francis Moore recognized early on that LDK transplantation would challenge the medical dictum to 'first do no harm', but also predicted that it would persevere: 'the living human donor provides by far the best tissue'. Indeed, the advantages of LDK transplantation are now readily apparent and the procedure is increasingly accepted even as our understanding of donor risk is becoming better defined.

This compendium brings a timely reflection of the modern day practice of LDK transplantation, assembled by an outstanding group of experts. The authors convey the nuances of the current situation, the responsibility of the medical community to the live kidney donor as a patient and the potential for complacency regarding donor risk. Their perspective is consistent with principles highlighted at a recent international forum on the care of the live kidney donor (Amsterdam, 2004) that emphasized ethical principles of voluntarism, informed consent and medical follow-up. These principles must dictate medical practice in LDK transplantation for the foreseeable future.

Perhaps future generations of physicians will understand the profound dilemma that permeates our current experience. There is an insufficient supply of organs and a demanding remedy that rationalizes potential harm to a well individual. Human live donor transplantation cannot be the ultimate solution to the ever-increasing need for organs. Nevertheless, there is a visionary sensibility to be underscored. Until *primum non nocere* can be restored to the pedestal of medical care by the use of an alternative source of organs (not derived from humans), this book comprehensively records the best practices currently available.

Francis L Delmonico, MD
Harvard Medical School
Massachusetts General Hospital
Boston, Massachusetts, USA

Introduction and acknowledgements

Successful solid organ transplantation originated with the living kidney donor. It has always been the desire of many involved to move beyond utilizing healthy persons as a source for transplantable organs. Nevertheless, a half-century later, we find ourselves, in many ways, more dependent on living donors than ever. This circumstance incorporates the impact of numerous changes in the field, not least of which is the dramatic improvement in outcomes for kidney transplant recipients and the resulting unprecedented demand for the procedure. In many countries, living donors now provide the majority of transplantable kidneys. Despite substantial efforts to address medical and ethical questions that have accompanied utilization of live donors since inception in 1954, new challenges continue to arise, often in almost rapid-fire sequence: laparoscopic donor nephrectomy, ABO- and MHC-incompatible transplantation, unrelated donors, non-directed donation and, somewhat ominously, paid donors. All these developments have maintained issues surrounding the living donor at the forefront of kidney transplantation.

Living Donor Kidney Transplantation: Current Practices, Emerging Trends and Evolving Challenges is an attempt to summarize, for the first time, the changing face of this field in a single, readily accessible volume. Its focus is clinical, and we anticipate its greatest utility to be among all categories of healthcare professionals involved in, or intending to begin, a living donor kidney programme. While each chapter stands alone as an informative examination of a specific issue, we hope those seeking a comprehensive, state-of-the-art overview of living donor transplantation will find the entire volume eminently approachable.

This work originated in a series of international symposia devoted to the topic of living donor kidney transplantation. Proceedings of these meetings, convened in Lisbon, Miami, Berlin and Venice between 2001 and 2003, remain accessible (at the time of publication) at www.livekidney.com. The content reflects the input of an intuitive steering committee (John Forsythe, Arthur Matas, Kiil Park, Kazunari Tanabe and Gilbert Thiel) as well as the collective insights of a renowned group of contributors from Asia, Europe and the Americas. We are indebted to them for their labours without which neither the symposia nor the textbook could have succeeded.

Likewise, this effort would not have been possible without the ongoing support of two entities: Fujisawa* and Thomson ACUMED. The idea for a project to address issues associated with living donor kidney transplantation originated with Fujisawa Healthcare, Incorporated. Fujisawa's generous funding for the project, with no restrictions on content or contributors, is extraordinary and gratefully appreciated. The consummate professionals at Thomson ACUMED (especially Sharon Smalley, Rachel Ramsay, Andrea King and Jo Jackson) provided outstanding organizational and editorial support. Our gratitude to these two special groups of people cannot be overstated.

Given the time commitment inherent in an effort like this, we are indebted to colleagues in Uppsala and Birmingham for their assistance with clinical duties. We are also blessed with supportive, understanding

*On 1 April 2005, Fujisawa ceased to exist following a merger with Yamanouchi to create Astellas Pharma

families, and express our gratitude to them (especially our wives, Eva and Susie) for their ongoing support.

Finally, we dedicate this book to those who have made transplantation a successful option for so many, namely, those brave souls whose faith in our judgement and skills has enabled them to contribute so significantly to the lives of others: living donors. Perhaps one day, such sacrifices will no longer be necessary. For now, however, we can only offer our humble thanks.

Jonas Wadström, MD
Robert S Gaston, MD

List of contributors

David M Briscoe, MB, MRCP
Division of Nephrology
Children's Hospital Boston
Boston, Massachusetts
USA

Arnold G Diethelm, MD
Department of Surgery
University of Alabama at Birmingham
Birmingham, Alabama
USA

Ingela Fehrman-Ekholm, MD, PhD
Karolinska University Hospital
Stockholm
Sweden

Jesse A Flaxenburg, MD
Division of Nephrology
Children's Hospital Boston
and
Division of Nephrology
Brigham and Women's Hospital and Harvard
Medical School
Boston, Massachusetts
USA

John LR Forsythe, MD, FRCS
Transplant Unit
Royal Infirmary of Edinburgh
Edinburgh
UK

Catherine A Garvey, RN, BA, CCTC
Department of Surgery
University of Minnesota
Minneapolis
Minnesota
USA

Robert S Gaston, MD
Division of Nephrology
University of Alabama at Birmingham
Birmingham, Alabama
USA

Anders Hartmann, MD
Medical Department
Rikshospitalet University Hospital
Oslo
Norway

Cheryl L Jacobs, LICSW
Department of Surgery
University of Minnesota
Minneapolis
Minnesota
USA

Bruce Kaplan, MD
Department of Medicine
University of Florida
Gainesville, Florida
USA

Jong Hoon Lee, MD
Transplantation Center
Myongji Hospital
Kwandong University College of Medicine
Goyang
Korea

Jennifer A Lumsdaine
Transplant Unit
Royal Infirmary of Edinburgh
Edinburgh
UK

Lorna P Marson, MD, FRCS
Transplant Unit
Royal Infirmary of Edinburgh
Edinburgh
UK

Arthur J Matas, MD
Department of Surgery
University of Minnesota
Minneapolis
Minnesota
USA

Thomas R McCune, MD, FACP
Nephrology Associates of Tidewater, Ltd
Eastern Virginia Medical School
Norfolk
Virginia
USA

Herwig-Ulf Meier-Kriesche, MD
Department of Medicine
University of Florida
Gainesville, Florida
USA

Robert A Montgomery, MD, DPhil
Department of Surgery
Johns Hopkins University School of Medicine
Baltimore
Maryland
USA

Christa Nolte
Division of Nephrology
University Hospital Basel
Basel
Switzerland

Kiil Park, MD, PhD
Transplantation Center
Myongji Hospital
Kwandong University College of Medicine
Goyang
Korea

William D Plant, FRCPE
Department of Renal Medicine
Cork University Hospital
Cork
Ireland

David PT Price, LLB (Hons), PGCE, ILTM
Department of Law
De Montfort University
Leicester
UK

Dr Janet Radcliffe Richards
Centre for Bioethics and Philosophy of
    Medicine
University College London
London
UK

Stuart W Robertson, MB, ChB
Division of Nephrology
Children's Hospital Boston
Boston, Massachusetts
USA

Deborah D Roman, PsyD
Department of Surgery
University of Minnesota
Minneapolis
Minnesota
USA

Christopher E Simpkins, MD
Department of Surgery
Johns Hopkins University School of Medicine
Baltimore
Maryland
USA

Jürg Steiger, MD
Clinic for Transplantation Immunology and
Nephrology
University Hospital Basel
Basel
Switzerland

Kazunari Tanabe, MD
Department of Urology
Tokyo Women's Medical University
Tokyo
Japan

Gilbert T Thiel, MD
Division of Nephrology
University Hospital Basel
Basel
Switzerland

Dimitrios Tsinalis, MD
Division of Nephrology
Kantonsspital St Gallen
Switzerland

Gunnar Tydén, MD
Department of Transplantation Surgery
Huddinge University Hospital
Stockholm
Sweden

Jonas Wadström, MD, PhD, Dr HC
Division of Transplantation Surgery
University Hospital
Uppsala
Sweden

Daniel S Warren, PhD
Department of Surgery
Johns Hopkins University School of Medicine
Baltimore
Maryland
USA

A brief history of living donor kidney transplantation

Robert S Gaston, Arnold G Diethelm

INTRODUCTION

The concept of organ transplantation to cure illness in afflicted humans dates back almost to the beginning of recorded history. It permeated Greek and Roman mythology, contributed to the canonization of saints in early Christian tradition and provided the conceptual basis for innumerable failed and ignoble surgical procedures over the centuries. Yet, in treating patients with no options other than certain demise, surgeons and physicians continued to pursue the dream of achieving cure by replacing diseased organs with healthy ones. Progress was painfully slow, and in agonizing increments, as has been well documented elsewhere.[1–5] However, ultimately organ transplantation succeeded because of a fortuitous confluence of several factors: the kidney as a paired organ, an identical twin with chronic kidney failure, and the willingness of a healthy person (the unaffected twin) to participate in the process by donating a kidney. Although rapid advances in transplantation immunology have generated enormous insights into the relationship between graft and host, it is difficult to envision how the clinical enterprise could have been sustained without the success enabled by those early living donors.

EARLY EVENTS IN RENAL TRANSPLANTATION

Major advances in anaesthesia and antiseptic technique in the late nineteenth century paved the way for vascular surgery, pioneered by Alexis Carrel in the early years of the twentieth century.[6] Carrel also recognized that the kidney, as a paired organ, might prove amenable to transplantation. His work with canine autografts demonstrated that a kidney could be removed from its retroperitoneal home, grafted into a distant location and revascularized, and it would resume production of urine. Denervation of the kidney appeared to have no adverse impact on renal function, and its histological appearance remained relatively unchanged.[7] Carrel's observations that similar outcomes could not be achieved when a kidney from one dog was transplanted into another signalled the frustration that would plague the field for many years to follow.

The end of the Second World War heralded a flurry of interest in human renal transplantation. For a century before, understanding of kidney disease had progressed only incrementally beyond Bright's description of uraemic death in 1836.[8] The concept of acute renal failure as a consequence of severe injury and hypotension emerged during the War as surgeons were able to save the lives of severely injured patients, thus forestalling immediate death and allowing other sequelae to ensue. It was found that patients could recover from trauma-induced 'acute renal failure' if they could be kept alive long enough to allow the healing process to occur. However, in others, there was progressive deterioration in kidney function over time that appeared to be irreversible, and for these individuals with 'chronic renal failure', no lifesaving options were apparent.

The earliest benefit of a kidney transplant in a human was as a 'bridge' which functioned for 48 hours, allowing enough time for the native kidneys to recover.[9] Several years later, in Chicago, a surgeon performed a similar 'bridge' procedure, which involved placing an allograft orthotopically, in a retroperitoneal location.[10] The allograft was obtained from a deceased donor, and the recipient lived for five years after the operation (despite the fact that 10 months postoperatively, surgical re-exploration revealed a non-functioning, shrunken allograft). Further experience with cadaveric kidneys in the late 1940s and early 1950s in the Ukraine, Paris and Boston resulted almost uniformly in allograft failure and the demise of the patient.[5,11,12] Even if the transplants functioned initially, the newly described phenomenon of immunological rejection ultimately destroyed the kidney.[13]

THE EMERGENCE OF THE LIVE DONOR

The first known living donor kidney transplantations were performed in Paris in 1951 but without notable success. In 1952 at Hôpital Necker, a 16-year-old boy underwent surgical removal of a grievously injured solitary kidney. Within the following several days, a kidney from his mother (the first living related donor) was implanted into his body. Function was maintained with resolution of uraemic symptoms until rejection and death ensued three weeks later. During the same era, several other renal transplantations were undertaken in Paris using organs from relatives, but none lasted more than a few months.[4] Towards the end of 1953 it appeared that the immunological obstacles associated with kidney transplantation might be insurmountable.

During the late 1940s, what might now be called a 'renal unit' was established at the Peter Bent Brigham Hospital in Boston under the supervision of George Thorn and John Merrill.[9,12] This was fashioned around the early surgical experience of David Hume and the availability of a modified Kolff dialyser (the Kolff–Brigham kidney). By 1954, Hume had entered military service and a young

plastic surgeon, Joseph E Murray, assumed surgical leadership of the unit (Figure 1-1). Unlike Hume, whose operative technique involved anastomosing the renal allograft to the femoral vasculature and externalizing the ureter on the thigh, Murray had extensive experience placing kidneys in the iliac fossa in dogs. This procedure used a ureteroneocystostomy to provide urinary drainage into the bladder using a technique pioneered by Rene Kuss in Paris.[2,11] Murray's experiments confirmed the earlier findings of Carrel that denervation and transplantation had little impact upon renal function.[3]

A 23-year-old man, Richard Herrick, was referred to the Brigham unit by his internist in Brighton, Massachusetts, on 26 October 1954. Previously healthy, Herrick had developed advanced renal insufficiency and fortuitously, had an identical twin brother, Ronald (Figure 1-2). Pioneering work had previously shown that skin grafts were readily accepted between identical twins, and it was

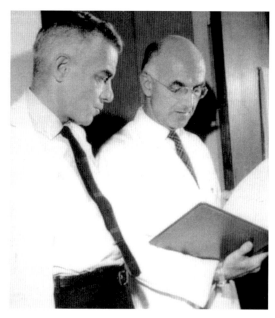

Figure 1-1 John Merrill (left) and Joseph Murray in 1958. Reprinted with permission from *A Miracle and a Privilege: Recounting a Half Century of Surgical Advance.* © (1995) by the National Academy of Sciences, courtesy of the National Academy Press, Washington, DC.[9]

suspected, but not known, that a kidney would likewise be accepted. After stabilizing the patient with dialysis, a successful exchange of skin grafts between the brothers confirmed their genetic identity. Substantial ethical debate ensued among doctors and family members about the advisability of unilateral nephrectomy in a healthy person, following which the Brigham team elected to proceed. Both operations were successfully performed on 23 December 1954, and the transplanted kidney functioned immediately. Richard subsequently led a full life, with marriage and two children, until his death from recurrent renal disease eight years later.[3] The donor, Ronald, remains alive, and was

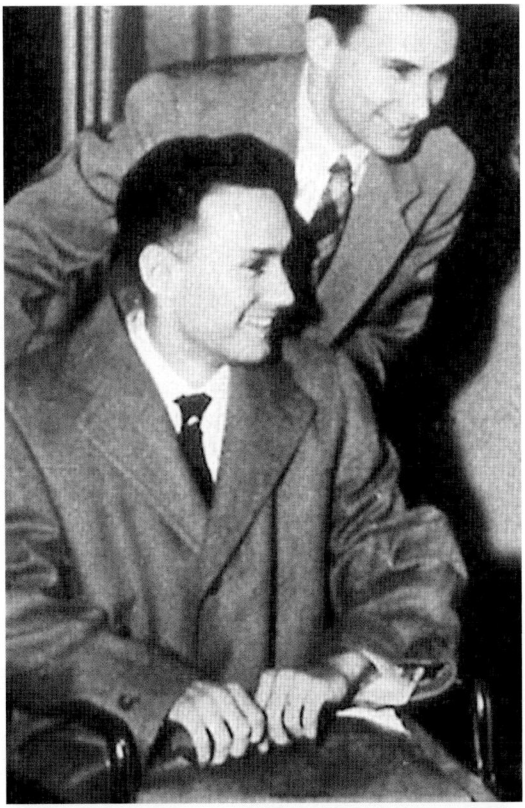

Figure 1-2 Richard (seated) and Ronald Herrick leaving the Brigham in 1956. Reprinted with permission from *A Miracle and a Privilege: Recounting a Half Century of Surgical Advance.* © (1995) by the National Academy of Sciences, courtesy of the National Academy Press, Washington, DC.[9]

recently honoured (50 years later) by the American Transplant Congress. Another twin transplant, performed in 1956 between two sisters, resulted in survival of both donor and recipient to this present day. In his memoir, Murray notes:[3]

There were those who dismissed the event as a one-in-a-million occurrence, and not something that would add greatly to the store of medical knowledge. They argued, correctly, that there would be very few identical twins like the Herrick brothers, so this advance would not benefit the majority of patients with renal failure. But in my view they failed to understand that this was just the first step.

Although the first successful transplant occurred against a backdrop of repeated failures, it undoubtedly laid the cornerstone for modern transplantation. More than 30 twin transplants were subsequently performed, establishing the paradigm that kidney transplantation could successfully treat the previously fatal condition of chronic renal failure.[4,14] These transplants contributed to the standardization of operative technique and perioperative management, as well as providing insight into the physiology of a transplanted kidney, all of which were of supreme importance in future developments. In addition, much attention was focused on issues surrounding the donor, including initial attempts to understand risks associated with donor nephrectomy and to communicate them openly to the donor, thereby promoting autonomy in decision making. The donor's role, even in 1954, was paramount to the process.[2,14,15]

In the years that followed, efforts to enable renal transplantation between non-twin pairs (allografts) were pursued with renewed vigour. In 1959, the first long-term success (27 years) was achieved using radiation to suppress the immune response to a living donor transplant.[16] As vividly described below, the selflessness of the donor was evident throughout the process:[3]

John and I never conversed in a donor-donee context. We were brothers and each other's best friend, and there simply seemed no reason to discuss our personal contributions, if indeed they were such, to the history of kidney transplantation. I always believed, and still do, that the contribution of a donor is not an unusual one. It is nothing more than the rare chance, or fortune, to be a Good Samaritan to one's kin.

However, the overall experience in Boston and elsewhere remained humbling, with little success, and significant morbidity and mortality being the norm.

By 1960, it was evident that an alternative approach to control rejection might be possible. In the previous year, Schwartz and Dameshek reported the immunosuppressive effects of 6-mercaptopurine (6-MP) in rabbits, with 'drug-induced immunological tolerance' to foreign protein.[17] Additional experiments documented the efficacy of 6-MP in canine kidney transplantation.[18] Using Hitchings and Elion's modification of 6-MP into an orally administrable form (azathioprine), several groups began to perform successful kidney transplantations with 'chemical immunosuppression'.[19,20] The Boston unit again led the way, as azathioprine enabled the first successful kidney transplantations to be undertaken using cadaveric kidneys.[21] Nonetheless, in their initial reports of 13 'homografts', Murray and colleagues noted that the most successful and longest surviving transplants were the three undertaken using organs from voluntary living donors.[22] However the authors cautioned: 'in the present state of knowledge it seems advisable to continue a study with the use of expendable kidneys, concentrating on efforts to overcome the logistical problem in obtaining and preserving cadaveric kidneys'. Thus, over the next two decades, the focus remained on development of transplantation using kidneys from deceased donors.

GROWTH IN DIALYSIS AND DECEASED DONOR TRANSPLANTATION

The availability of azathioprine and corticosteroid-based immunosuppression in the 1960s and 1970s fostered enough success to promote further growth in the area of renal transplantation. Those years also witnessed rapid advances in availability and outcomes of chronic dialysis. Long-term vascular access via Cimino arteriovenous fistulae and improved dialysis membranes, along with development of cuffed peritoneal catheters that facilitated chronic peritoneal dialysis, enabled broader application of dialytic approaches to renal replacement therapy. With 1-year graft survival rates of 50–75% the norm, the unpredictable availability of cadaveric kidneys, and substantial morbidity associated with long-term immunosuppression, Rennie's 1978 editorial reflected contemporary standards regarding therapy for end-stage renal disease (ESRD):[23] 'a transplant . . . can be considered only a temporary respite from the basic form of treatment, which is dialysis'.

Nevertheless, significant advances in transplantation occurred during this period. Tissue typing, with identification of human leukocyte antigens (HLA), allowed greater predictability of successful transplantation between donor and recipient pairs. Availability of antilymphocyte antibody (ALS) reduced reliance on large doses of corticosteroids, while cimetidine and effective antimicrobials improved the ability to cope with morbidity after transplantation.[24] Outcomes for recipients of kidneys from well-matched live donors became quite good, even with the availability of relatively primitive immunosuppression (ALS, azathioprine, prednisone). Although uncertainty about outcomes and concerns over the short- and long-term risks to donors tended to keep the focus on cadaveric transplantation (in the USA, living donors accounted for only 16% of renal transplantation performed between 1976 and 1980[25]), in some countries (e.g. Japan and Norway) living donors remained the primary source of transplantable kidneys.

RENEWED EMPHASIS ON THE LIVING DONOR

It is difficult to assign a precise date to the re-emergence of the live donor, but it occurred around 1990. In the USA, the Social Security amendments of 1972 had provided financial support for the care of patients with ESRD. However, access to dialysis remained restricted, not only because of limited numbers of dialysis facilities and transplantable kidneys, but also due to the multidisciplinary groups in some medical centres (so-called 'life or death' committees) that evaluated which patients should and should not be offered chronic dialysis or transplantation.[26] By the mid-1980s, it was no longer considered ethical to deny ESRD care to patients, and the committees were disbanded. Dialysis units proliferated, and the number of patients referred for transplantation grew rapidly. The National Organ Transplant Act of 1984 established a network of organ procurement organizations, and Medicare responded by initiating payments for immunosuppressive medications while mandating evaluation of all ESRD patients as potential transplant candidates.[27]

Against this backdrop of policy evolution there were equally significant advances in transplant therapeutics, with the introduction of several potent, and less toxic, immunosuppressant therapies: ciclosporin was followed by mycophenolate mofetil, tacrolimus, daclizumab, basiliximab and sirolimus.[28] Recipients of kidneys from deceased donors could now reasonably expect a 90% chance of keeping an allograft for at least a year, with the expectation of 10–15 years off dialysis. The outcomes were even better for recipients of kidneys from living donors. These therapeutic advances culminated in the revolutionary finding by Wolfe and colleagues, published in 1999, that, on average, a patient with ESRD receiving a transplant from a deceased donor could expect their life expectancy to double when compared with remaining on dialysis (Figure 1-3).[29]

The net impact of these developments has been a dramatic growth in the number of patients desiring transplantation. Even in countries with well-developed organ procurement systems, supply has failed to keep pace with growing demand. In the USA, where the waiting list grew from 20 000 to 50 000

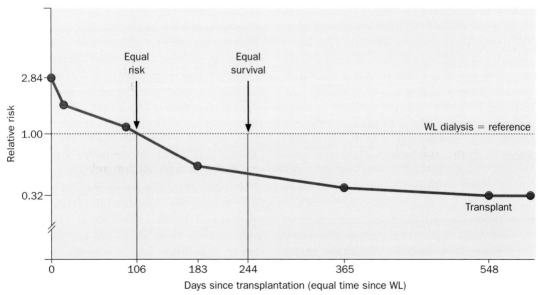

Figure 1-3 Adjusted relative risk of death among 23 275 recipients of a first cadaveric transplant, compared with remaining on dialysis and the waiting list (1.00). Redrawn from Wolfe RA et al[29], with permission from the Massachusetts Medical Society.

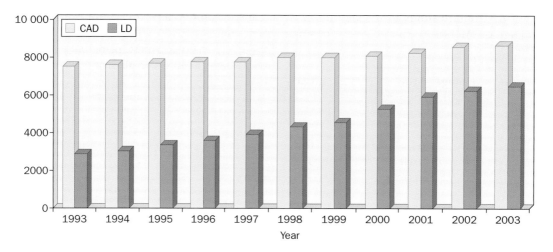

Figure 1-4   Kidney transplants performed in the USA, 1993–2003, by donor source. CAD, deceased donor; LD, living donor.[35]

between 1992 and 2001, the number of available kidneys from deceased donors grew by only 1% per year.[30] In line with these statistics, a recent study indicates that even major alterations in the organ procurement process cannot reasonably be expected to meet demand for transplantable kidneys from deceased donors.[31]

Living donor kidney (LDK) transplantation has continued to evolve throughout the present era. Currently, there remains an identifiable survival benefit associated with LDK transplantation, as 95% of recipients now achieve 1-year graft survival, with significantly less morbidity and mortality than with deceased donor kidneys.[30] Additionally, the expected longevity of these kidneys is superior with a graft half-life of almost 20 years. Indeed, the availability of a living donor kidney is the surest way to undergo pre-emptive transplantation, affording the patient with advanced chronic kidney disease the best possible outcome.[32,33] While these developments in many ways parallel progress that has occurred in deceased donor transplantation, two additional major changes peculiar to the live kidney donor have directly contributed to the near tripling of the annual number of LDK transplants undertaken in the USA over the past decade (Figure 1-4).

The relative inadequacy of azathioprine-based immunosuppression was reflected in the need for HLA similarity between donor and recipient to produce a desirable outcome. The availability of more effective immunosuppression with ciclosporin-based regimens allowed the first widespread challenges to this presumption. HLA similarity no longer seemed a prerequisite, as good outcomes accrued even for poorly matched donor–recipient pairs. Would it now be advisable to move beyond genetically related individuals as donors? Concerns about donor safety and uncertainty regarding whether an unrelated person might have sufficient investment in the recipient's outcome to justify the risk of donation meant that the first forays into genetically unrelated transplants were confined to spouses or very close friends. These 'emotionally related' persons were highly motivated to donate to a specific individual with ESRD.

In 1995, a landmark report by Terasaki and colleagues documented that HLA-mismatched spousal transplants resulted in graft survival superior to all but identically matched kidneys from deceased donors.[34] Recent years have seen this concept evolve into a growing number of living-unrelated donors. In 2003, over 2100 such individuals accounted for almost a third of LDK transplants performed in the USA.[35]

Further modifications to the definition of acceptable donor–recipient relationships include:[36,37]

- paired exchange – two donors incompatible with their intended recipients mutually donate to each other's originally designated recipient
- list-paired exchange, where a kidney from a compatible deceased donor becomes part of a similar transaction.

In fact, in some countries, the current acceptable terminology of 'directed donor' (a person donating a kidney to a specified recipient) exists as a counterpoint to the new term of 'non-directed donor', applied to an individual motivated to donate a kidney to an unknown recipient, who is usually selected from a waiting list by the transplant centre.[38,39]

The other major advance in LDK transplantation is more technical in nature. Surgical approaches to donor nephrectomy had evolved little since the days of Murray and Kuss. Of late, another new term, minimally invasive donor nephrectomy, has emerged to describe novel approaches to surgical removal of a kidney for transplantation.[40] These procedures, most commonly utilizing laparoscopy, have become widely accepted in the USA and Europe. A recent multicentre survey confirmed previous reports of a low incidence of morbidity and mortality associated with laparoscopic surgery.[41] Arguably, reduction in perioperative morbidity and recovery time after surgery has, in some instances, stimulated once-reluctant potential donors to proceed.[42]

CONCLUSION

Over the past five decades, kidney transplantation has emerged as the treatment of choice for ESRD in most patients, with organs from living donors being at the forefront. Early successes were possible only because of their commitment and sacrifice. Now, with improving outcomes and increasing demand for transplantation, dependency on living donors is greater than ever before. Although some of the old questions persist, principally ongoing concern regarding the physical risks taken by living kidney donors,[43–45] as yet no universally accepted answers are available. In fact, new questions are emerging. For example, we need to ascertain whether the benefits of LDK transplantation can be routinely extended to patients with positive crossmatches or ABO incompatibility. Likewise, it is becoming necessary to decide if it is advisable to use donors with isolated medical abnormalities, such as hyperlipidaemia or easily controlled hypertension. The ethical issues surrounding compensation of donors for their time or financial outlays are also an important topic of debate. Historical accounts of renal transplantation during the next half-century will doubtless document our ongoing enlightened struggle with these issues.

REFERENCES

1. Starzl TE. *The Puzzle People: Memoirs of a Transplant Surgeon*. Pittsburgh: University of Pittsburgh Press, 1993.
2. Tilney NL. *Transplant: From Myth to Reality*. New Haven: Yale University Press, 2003.
3. Murray JM. *Surgery of the Soul: Reflections of a Curious Mind*. Canton, MA: Science History Publications, 2001.
4. Richet G. Hamburger's achievement with early renal transplants. *Am J Nephrol* 1997; **17**: 315–317.
5. Hamilton DN, Reid WA. Yu Yu Voronoy and the first human kidney allograft. *Surg Gynecol Obstet* 1984; **159**: 289–294.
6. Carrel A, Guthrie CC. Anastomosis of blood vessels by the patching method and transplantation of the kidney. *JAMA* 1906; **47**: 1647–1651.
7. Carrel A. Transplantation in mass of the kidneys. *J Exp Med* 1908; **10**: 98–140.
8. Bright R. Cases and observations illustrative of renal disease accompanied with the secretion of albuminous urine. *Guys Hosp Rep* 1836; **I**: 338.
9. Moore FD, *A Miracle and A Privilege: Recounting a Half Century of Surgical Advance*. Washington, DC: Joseph Henry Press, 1995.
10. Lawler RH, West JW, McNulty PH, Clancy EJ, Murphy RP. Homotransplantation of the kidney in the human. *JAMA* 1950; **144**: 844–845.
11. Hamburger J, Vaysse J, Crosnier J, Auvert J, Dormont J. Kidney homotransplantation in man. *Ann N Y Acad Sci* 1962; **99**: 808–820.

12. Hume DM, Merrill JP, Miller BF, Thorn GW. Experiences with renal homotransplantation in the human: report of nine cases. *J Clin Invest* 1955; **34**: 327–382.

13. Medawar PB. The behavior and fate of skin autografts and skin homografts in rabbits. *J Anat* 1944; **78**: 176–199.

14. Murray JE, Merrill JP, Harrison JH. Renal homotransplantation in identical twins. *Surg Forum* 1955; **6**: 432–436.

15. Harrison JH, Bennett AH. The familial living donor in renal transplantation. *J Urology* 1977; **118**: 166–168.

16. Merrill JP, Murray JE, Harrison JH et al. Successful homotransplantation of the kidney between non-identical twins. *N Engl J Med* 1960; **262**: 1251–1260.

17. Schwartz R, Dameshek W. Drug-induced immunologic tolerance. *Nature* 1959; **183**: 1682–1683.

18. Calne RY. Rejection of renal homografts: inhibition in dogs by 6-mercaptopurine. *Lancet* 1960; **1**: 417.

19. Calne RY, Alexandre GP, Murray JE. A study of the effects of drugs in prolonging survival of homologous renal transplants in dogs. *Ann N Y Acad Sci* 1962; **99**: 743–761.

20. Zukoski CF, Lee HM, Hume DM. The prolongation of functional survival of canine renal homografts by 6-mercaptopurine. *Surg Forum* 1960; **11**: 470–472.

21. Merrill JP, Murray JE, Takacs FJ et al. Successful transplantation of a kidney from a human cadaver. *JAMA* 1963; **185**: 347–353.

22. Murray JE, Merrill JP. Prolonged survival of human kidney homografts by immunosuppressive drug therapy. *N Engl J Med* 1963; **268**: 1315.

23. Rennie D. Home dialysis and the costs of uremia. *N Engl J Med* 1978; **298**: 399–400.

24. Huntley RT, Taylor PD, Iwasaki Y et al. Use of anti-lymphocyte serum to prolong dog homograft survival. *Surg Forum* 1966; **17**: 230–233.

25. Cook DJ. Long-term survival of kidney allografts. In: Terasaki P (ed) *Clinical Transplants 1987* Los Angeles: UCLA Tissue Typing Laboratory, 1987; 277–285.

26. Alexander S. They decide who lives, who dies. *Life Magazine*, 7 November 1962; 102–125.

27. Institute of Medicine (US). *Kidney Failure and the Federal Government* Washington, DC: National Academy Press, 1991.

28. Gaston RS. Evolution of medicare policy involving transplantation and immunosuppressive medications: past developments and future directions. In: Field MJ, Lawrence RL, Zwanziger L (eds) *Extending Medicare Coverage for Preventive and Other Services*. Washington, DC: National Academy Press, 2000; D23–38.

29. Wolfe RA, Ashby VB, Milford EL et al. Comparison of mortality in all patients on dialysis, patients on dialysis awaiting transplantation, and recipients of a first cadaveric transplant. *N Engl J Med* 1999; **341**: 1725–1730.

30. Gaston RS, Alveranga DY, Becker BN et al. Kidney and pancreas transplantation. *Am J Transplant* 2003; **3**(suppl 4): 64–77.

31. Sheehy E, Conrad SL, Brigham LE et al. Estimating the number of potential organ donors in the United States. *N Engl J Med* 2003; **349**: 667–674.

32. Hariharan S, Johnson CP, Bresnahan BA et al. Improved graft survival after renal transplantation in the United States, 1988 to 1996. *N Engl J Med* 2000; **342**: 605–612.

33. Meier-Kriesche HU, Port FK, Ojo AO et al. Effect of waiting time on renal transplant outcome. *Kidney Int* 2000; **58**: 1311–1317.

34. Terasaki PI, Cecka JM, Gjertson DW, Takemoto S. High survival rates of kidney transplants from spousal and living unrelated donors. *N Engl J Med* 1995; **333**: 333–336.

35. United Network for Organ Sharing. http://www.unos.org. (data retrieved 10 May 2004).

36. Delmonico FL, Morrissey PE, Lipkowitz GS et al. Donor kidney exchanges. *Am J Transplant* 2004; **4**: 1628–1634.

37. Park K, Moon JI, Kim SI, Kim YS. Exchange donor program in kidney transplantation. *Transplantation* 1999; **67**: 336–338.

38. Matas AJ, Garvey CA, Jacobs CL, Kahn JP. Nondirected donation of kidneys from living donors. *N Engl J Med* 2000; **343**: 433–436.

39. Adams PL, Cohen DJ, Danovitch GM et al. The nondirected live-kidney donor: ethical considerations and practice guidelines. A National Conference Report. *Transplantation* 2002; **74**: 582–589.

40. Ratner LE, Ciseck LJ, Moore RG et al. Laparoscopic live donor nephrectomy. *Transplantation* 1995; **60**: 1047–1049.

41. Matas AJ, Bartlett ST, Leichtman AB, Delmonico FL. Morbidity and mortality after living kidney donation, 1999–2001: survey of United States transplant centers. *Am J Transplant* 2003; **3**: 830–834.

42. Pradel FG, Limcangco MR, Mullins CD, Bartlett ST. Patients' attitudes about living donor transplantation and living donor nephrectomy. *Am J Kidney Dis* 2003; **41**: 849–858.

43. Abecassis M, Adams M, Adams P et al. Consensus statement on the live organ donor. *JAMA* 2000; **284**: 2919–2926.

44. Ellison MD, McBride MA, Taranto SE, Delmonico FL, Kauffman HM. Living kidney donors in need of kidney transplants: a report from the organ procurement and transplantation network. *Transplantation* 2002; **74**: 1349–1351.

45. Fehrman-Ekholm I, Duner F, Brink B, et al. No evidence of accelerated loss of kidney function in living kidney donors: results from a cross-sectional follow-up. *Transplantation* 2001; **72**: 444–449.

Advantages of living donor kidney transplantation in the current era

2

Herwig-Ulf Meier-Kriesche, Bruce Kaplan

INTRODUCTION

It is widely accepted that kidney transplantation is associated with a survival advantage over maintenance dialysis, and therefore it has become the standard of care for patients with end-stage renal disease (ESRD). While the mortality advantage is undisputed, the exact mechanism by which this benefit accrues is the subject of much speculation and study. In this chapter we discuss possible reasons for the survival benefit associated with transplantation and, in particular, the association between chronic renal insufficiency and the incidence and progression of heart disease.

It is generally acknowledged that chronic renal failure is associated with acceleration of the progression of heart disease.[1] It also appears that acceleration of cardiac disease is related to the severity of renal dysfunction, with the greatest risk occurring once patients begin maintenance dialysis. The rates of cardiovascular morbidity and mortality are higher among those with chronic renal failure than in the general population. It has been estimated that cardiovascular disease mortality is increased approximately 10-fold among patients with ESRD, even after accounting for patient age, sex, race and the presence of diabetes.[2,3] Ischaemic heart disease and heart failure are prevalent in approximately 50% of patients beginning dialysis,[2] and case fatality from these diseases among patients with ESRD is extremely high.[3] Successful kidney transplantation progressively reduces the incidence of cardiac mortality, and it is therefore associated with an overall survival benefit in subjects undergoing kidney transplantation.[4]

Currently over 60 000 patients are awaiting kidney transplantation in the USA. As about 10 000 deceased donor kidney transplantations are undertaken each year, waiting times are progressively increasing and are projected to approach an average of 10 years by 2010.[5] Worldwide, many other countries face the same challenges. Consequently, utilization of kidneys from living donors has become the only practical option for patients with ESRD to avoid maintenance dialysis and optimize outcomes after transplantation.

SURVIVAL BENEFIT OF RENAL TRANSPLANTATION

Patients with ESRD who receive a kidney transplant live longer than those who continue on long-term dialysis.[6] Candidates for transplantation are a highly selected subgroup of those with ESRD; on average they are younger, healthier and of higher socioeconomic status than those remaining on dialysis.[6] However, these factors only partially account for the survival advantage associated with transplantation. Wolfe et al[6] examined mortality in transplant recipients using data from the US Renal Data System (USRDS), which included more than 46 000 patients placed on the waiting list after first undergoing dialysis. Patients receiving a deceased donor transplant, including those in whom transplantation was unsuccessful, were compared with patients on the waiting list with an equivalent length of follow-up. This was considered to be a more appropriate comparator group than the total population of patients with ESRD. Transplant recipients experienced an initial increase in mortality, with nearly a three-fold higher death rate than controls during the first few weeks following transplantation. Mortality remained elevated in transplant recipients until day 106 post-transplantation, after which it fell until it was below the mortality of those patients on the waiting list (Figure 2-1). By day 244, average life expectancy in the two groups was equal. The analysis also showed that over three to four years, the estimated mortality among transplant recipients was 68% lower than among patients who remained on dialysis. On the basis of these findings it was concluded that there was a substantial cumulative survival benefit in patients receiving a deceased donor transplant despite the risks associated with transplant surgery. Across all age groups this translated into an approximate doubling in the life expectancy among patients receiving a transplant.

Although this study did not directly examine cardiovascular mortality, it can be speculated that, because of its high co-existence among patients with ESRD, a reduction in cardiovascular death might underlie a major portion of the accrued survival advantage. In fact, a more recent study described a steep increase in the prevalence of cardiac death by dialysis vintage among patients waiting for a transplant and a progressive decease in cardiac death rates by transplant vintage (Figure 2-2).[4] The study showed that there was a reduction in the prevalence of cardiac-related deaths among recipients who retained a functioning transplant, suggesting that transplantation halts or possibly even reverses the progression of cardiovascular disease. This positive trend was observed in a setting where many of the traditional cardiac risk factors, such as hypertension, dyslipidaemia and diabetes, are exacerbated by the immunosuppressive regimens used for renal transplantation. As a result, it seems likely that restoration of renal clearance alone plays a dominant role in providing cardiovascular benefit.

Established survival benefits associated with kidney transplantation have been extrapolated from patients deemed healthy enough

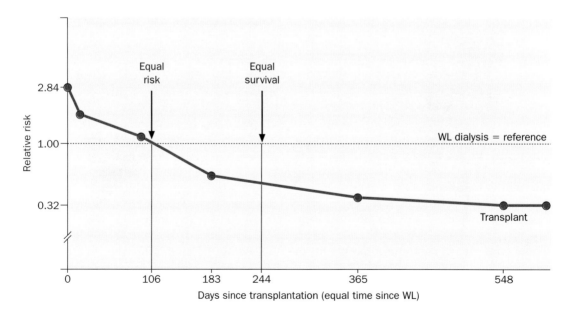

Figure 2-1 Relative risk of mortality among first cadaveric transplant recipients (n = 23 275) compared with wait-listed (WL) dialysis patients (n = 46 164). Relative risk adjusted for age, sex, race, end-stage renal disease cause, WL year and time to WL. Redrawn from Wolfe RA et al[6] with kind permission from the Massachusetts Medical Society.

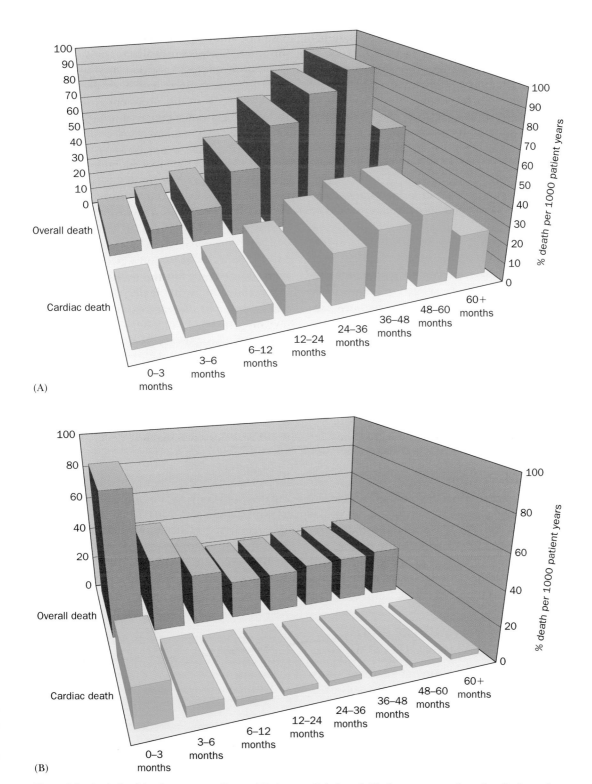

Figure 2-2   Analysis of death rates according to (A) time on dialysis and (B) time post-transplantation. Redrawn from Meier Kriesche HU et al[4] with kind permission from Blackwell Publishing.

to be placed on the transplant waiting list. However, in the USA only about 25% of all patients with ESRD are wait-listed for transplants.[7] The measurable survival benefit in kidney transplantation in the USA indicates that the selection algorithm is working fairly well. Whether the same results could be achieved by being more inclusive in the selection of prospective transplantation candidates is not known.

The survival benefit of kidney transplantation over dialysis has been demonstrated in several high-risk groups. Wolfe et al showed that the survival benefits held true in the oldest transplant recipients, across race groups and even in patients with ESRD secondary to diabetes,[6] a subgroup known to be at particularly high risk for perioperative cardiovascular complications. It has subsequently been shown that other high-risk groups including obese patients, as well as those who have undergone extensive periods of maintenance dialysis, also accrue significant survival benefits from kidney transplantation when compared to maintenance dialysis.[8,9]

Based on the current evaluation practice for kidney transplantation, even those patients who were deemed as too high risk for transplantation in the past can now safely receive transplants with the benefit of an improved life expectancy. Furthermore, transplanting kidneys from living donors can minimize the risks. In fact, risk reduction is one of the principal benefits of living donor kidney (LDK) transplantation.

IMPACT OF DIALYSIS ON POST-TRANSPLANTATION OUTCOME

Given the improved survival of renal transplant patients, it is reasonable to speculate that patients on dialysis may experience adverse effects that predispose them to poorer outcomes (i.e. higher mortality) after they have received a transplant. This hypothesis is supported by an analysis of USRDS data that demonstrated that survival with a functioning graft was inversely related to the amount of time patients awaiting a renal transplant spent on dialysis.[10] The relation was 'dose-dependent', which means that each increment in dialysis time was associated with an increase in mortality. The consistency of this observation in subgroups of patients with kidney disease (e.g. glomerulonephritis) or systemic diseases (e.g. hypertension or diabetes) suggests that poorer outcomes are unlikely to be due to longer exposure to a systemic disease process (Figure 2-3).

The data presented thus far are consistent with the hypothesis that lengthening time on dialysis represents ongoing exposure to the adverse effects of chronic kidney disease, such that patients are in a relatively disadvantaged state by the time they undergo transplantation. The effects may include altered concentrations of homocysteine, lipids and advanced glycosylation end products, as well as a generalized inflammatory state. These biochemical changes may predispose patients to cardiovascular damage and the allograft to vascular damage. Patients on dialysis also suffer poor nutrition and may be less tolerant of immunosuppressive agents after transplantation (Table 2-1).[11]

Examination of the impact of duration of pretransplant dialysis as a predictor of cardiovascular mortality has demonstrated a similar trend. Analysis of USRDS data on patients who received a transplant between 1990 and 2000 showed that age-adjusted cardiovascular death free survival over 10 years post-transplantation was related to time spent on

Table 2-1   Proposed uraemia-related cardiovascular risk factors[11]

- Albuminuria
- Hyperhomocysteinaemia
- Anaemia
- Abnormal calcium/phosphate metabolism
- Extracellular fluid volume overload and electrolyte imbalance
- Oxidative stress
- Inflammation
- Malnutrition
- Thrombogenic factors
- Sleep disturbances
- Altered nitric oxide/endothelin balance

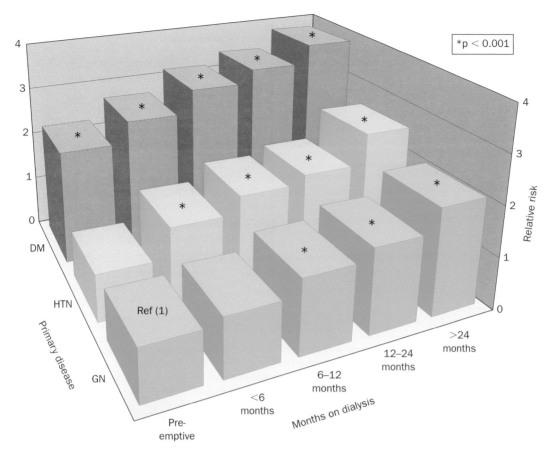

Figure 2-3 Relative risk of death with a functioning graft in patients with underlying diabetes mellitus (DM), hypertension (HTN) and glomerulonephritis (GN). Redrawn from Meier Kriesche HU et al[10] with kind permission from Blackwell Publishing.

dialysis in a stepwise negative manner.[4] This relation was observed in separate analyses of both deceased and living donor transplants.

The negative effects of prolonged dialysis could possibly be also in part due to allocation of poorer kidney grafts to patients who have been on the waiting list for a long period of time. If, on the other hand as we believe, waiting time is a donor-independent risk factor, it would have to be considered modifiable. A study was undertaken using USRDS registry data on 2405 kidney pairs harvested from the same cadaveric donor and transplanted into recipients on dialysis with different waiting times: 0–6 months and more than 24 months (Figure 2-4).[8] The overall

non-adjusted graft survival at five and 10 years was higher among patients with the short waiting time (78% and 63%, respectively) than among those who received their transplant from the same donor after waiting two or more years on dialysis (58% and 29%, respectively). Similar results were found in a multivariate analysis correcting as best possible for potential recipient bias.

A separate analysis of all recipients of deceased and living donor kidneys showed that graft survival in cadaveric renal transplant recipients with a waiting time of less than six months was equivalent to that in LDK recipients who had waited for a transplant while on dialysis for more than two

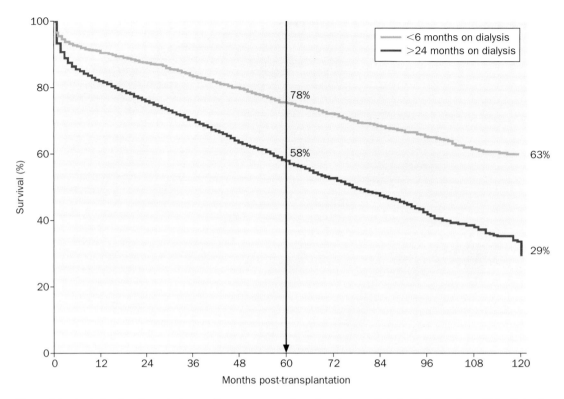

Figure 2-4 Analysis of graft survival according to pretransplant duration on dialysis. Redrawn from Meier-Kriesche HU et al[8] with kind permission from the Transplantation Society and Lippincott Williams & Wilkins.

years (Figure 2-5).[8] This study identified waiting time on dialysis as one of the strongest independent modifiable risk factors for poor renal transplant outcome. However, even after a prolonged wait, patients who eventually received a deceased donor transplant had lower mortality than those who continued on dialysis. After almost five years, the mortality risk among patients who received a transplant after prolonged dialysis was 56% lower than in patients who continued on dialysis for the same amount of time. This observation suggests that it is possible to halt whatever ongoing damage occurs during dialysis by renal transplantation. Importantly, prolonged periods of maintenance dialysis do not appear to prevent patients from benefiting from transplantation.

Life expectancy, on the other hand, is strongly affected by dialysis time, and, in order to have the best life expectancy, patients with ESRD should receive a renal transplant as quickly as possible after onset of the disease. Early discussion of the options for patients with chronic kidney disease allows patients and families to make plans for potential living donation or timely wait listing in an attempt to avoid prolongation of the waiting time for a transplant. In the USA, the average 3-year plus period on the waiting list continues to increase.[5]

Although the data presented above indicate that maintenance dialysis is harmful for patients, it is important to remember that only a fraction of the dialysis population will be eligible for transplantation. For those patients who are deemed unsuitable for transplantation, maintenance dialysis is obviously life saving.

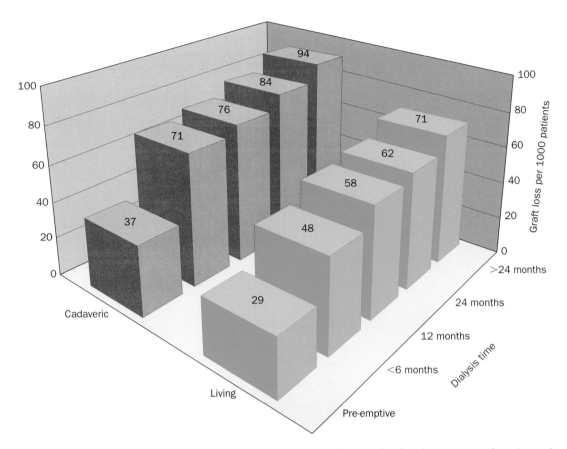

Figure 2-5 Comparison of rates of graft loss associated with living donor and cadaveric organ transplantation and according to time on dialysis prior to transplantation.[8]

MORTALITY FOLLOWING RENAL ALLOGRAFT LOSS

Death rates are markedly increased after loss of a renal allograft (Figure 2-6). Factors that increase mortality after return to dialysis were studied using USRDS data. Mortality among patients who lost a primary renal allograft was compared with that in patients with a functioning transplant.[12] Based on 10 years of follow-up, the annual death rates adjusted for multiple risk factors were increased more than three-fold in patients who lost their grafts, and cardiovascular mortality was increased more than seven-fold after graft loss. Multivariate Cox proportional hazard regression analysis demonstrated that the length of time spent on dialysis before the primary transplant was among the strongest

predictors of overall as well as cardiovascular mortality after graft loss. On the other hand, the amount of time patients spent with a functioning graft did not show a dose-related effect with regard to mortality, indicating again that cardiovascular disease progression occurs on dialysis and is slowed, or even halted, by kidney transplantation.

Comparison of death rates for the different ESRD subgroups (i.e. those on dialysis, on the waiting list, after transplantation and after graft loss) shows mortality to be high in unselected patients on dialysis but considerably lower in those placed on the waiting list for a renal transplant. Mortality then declines considerably after renal transplantation, but increases to pre-transplant levels in those patients who lose their grafts. These estimates suggest that the clock of cardiovascular and

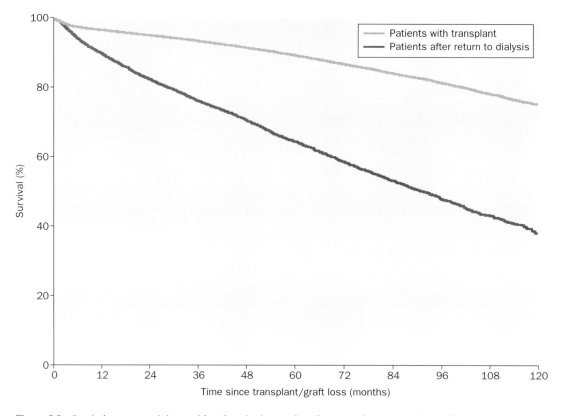

Figure 2-6   Survival among recipients with a functioning graft and among those returning to dialysis after graft loss. Redrawn from Kaplan B et al[12] with kind permission from Blackwell Publishing.

general disease progression may stop ticking when patients with ESRD receive a transplant only to resume at an accelerated rate when the protective effect of the transplanted kidney is lost.

RENAL FUNCTION AND CARDIOVASCULAR PROTECTION

The association between renal failure and cardiovascular disease is explained in part by predisposing factors shared by the two illnesses, such as hypertension, dyslipidaemia and diabetes. As mentioned previously, there is also strong evidence that renal insufficiency itself may predispose to the development and progression of cardiovascular disease. Indeed, decreased renal function at one year is a known risk factor for allograft loss.[13]

An analysis of USRDS data was undertaken to determine whether impaired renal function is also a risk factor for death, in particular for death from cardiovascular causes, with or without a functioning graft.[14] The analysis included 48 832 adults who had received a first renal transplant between 1988 and 1998 and had a functioning graft one year post-transplantation. Patients were divided into seven groups on the basis of serum creatinine measurements at one year post-transplantation until June 1999. The analysis showed that cardiovascular mortality accounted for 30.1% of the nearly 6 000 deaths that occurred during follow-up among patients with a functioning graft. Cardiovascular events were the most frequent cause of death with a functioning graft, followed by infectious complications (11.7%) and malignancy (10.1%). Univariate analysis revealed a strong, graded relation

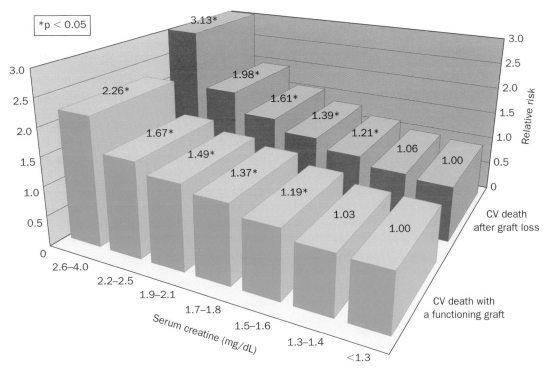

Figure 2-7   Relation between serum creatinine levels and relative risk of cardiovascular (CV) death among patients with a functioning graft and among those with graft loss. The creatinine is at one year post transplant. The endpoint is cardiovascular mortality that either includes or excludes death after graft loss. The statistical significance refers to the difference from baseline. Redrawn from Meier-Kriesche HU et al[14] with kind permission from the Transplantation Society and Lippincott Williams & Wilkins, Inc.

between 1-year serum creatinine and cardio-vascular mortality. Two aspects of this relation, its dose-dependency and the time lag between measured differences in renal function and differences in cardiovascular mortality, support a causal link between decreased renal clearance and cardiovascular mortality. The mortality differences first appeared two to three years post-transplantation and widened throughout the 10-year follow-up period.

As part of the same study, separate multivariate Cox proportional hazards analyses were undertaken for cardiovascular mortality in patients with and without a functioning graft. The analyses included covariates for all risk factors with the potential to influence cardiovascular mortality recorded by USRDS, including demographic descriptors, cause of ESRD, length of dialysis before transplantation, year of transplantation, immunosuppressive therapy and many other risk factors.

The effect of renal function on cardiovascular disease was found to be independent of the other traditional risk factors included in the multivariate model. After adjustment for these factors, 1-year serum creatinine demonstrated a stepwise association with cardiovascular mortality in patients with a functioning graft and in those with graft loss (Figure 2-7). In the subset of patients with a functioning graft, several factors in addition to 1-year serum creatinine were associated with cardiovascular mortality. The analysis showed that mortality increased with recipient age and, as in previous studies, with time spent waiting for a transplant on dialysis versus receiving a pre-emptive transplant. Cardiovascular mortality was also higher in ESRD caused by hypertension or diabetes than in ESRD due to glomerulonephritis. However, mortality was lower in African-American recipients, recipients of a living donation and those who had received transplants most recently.

Epidemiological studies in the general (non-ESRD) population provide additional support for a protective cardiovascular effect of renal function. Cardiovascular mortality is disproportionately high in patients with renal insufficiency even before the onset of ESRD and it increases as a function of worsening renal function in this population.[15] The excess risk even extends to patients with early signs of renal insufficiency.[16,17] The Framingham Heart Study supports these findings. In patients with mild renal insufficiency, cardiovascular mortality was associated with traditional risk factors such as hypertension, diabetes and unfavourable lipid profiles.[18] However, after allowing for higher rates of traditional risk factors, poor renal function was found to act as an independent predictor of cardiovascular mortality in the non-ESRD population.[19,20]

These observations have led to the proposal of a new class of uraemia-related cardiovascular risk factors (Table 2-1). These phenomena occur with increased frequency in patients with uraemia and are either established or at least biologically plausible cardiovascular risk factors. Identification and reduction of uraemia-related risk factors in patients with kidney disease is now recommended, in parallel with targeting of traditional risk factors.[3] It is, therefore, reasonable to presume that many of the uraemia-mediated risk factors cause partial damage and contribute to the elevated risk of cardiovascular complications in patients undergoing kidney transplantation after extended periods of maintenance dialysis.

QUALITY OF THE TRANSPLANTED KIDNEY

In terms of renal function, not only is timely transplantation crucial, but also the quality of the transplanted organ is equally important. It is obvious that living donor kidneys, coming from healthy and extensively screened living persons, on average provide

better renal function than deceased donor kidneys. But this is not the only reason for the better quality of the living donated organs. Other important risk factors associated with deceased donors include the pathophysiological changes associated with brain death of the donor, maintenance in the intensive care unit and possibly extended cold ischaemia times. Hospital stays and recovery times are also significantly longer than with LDK transplantation.

On the basis of the discussion earlier in the chapter, at least some of the survival advantage of LDK transplantation can be ascribed to shorter dialysis times. But, even at equal dialysis times, LDK transplants provide significantly longer graft function, reflecting the benefit of other variables. A corollary is that some of the benefits of LDK transplantation may be lost if the procedure is not executed in a timely manner (see Figure 2-5).

Overall, LDK transplantation has a favourable impact on the waiting list in at least two additional ways. First, for every patient receiving a transplant from a living donor one additional deceased donor kidney is available for another patient on the list. Second, and perhaps more important, is the fact that the longer graft survival associated with LDK transplantation means that fewer patients return to the waiting list after a failed transplant, especially as allograft failure has become one of the major causes of ESRD.

SUMMARY

Renal transplantation in selected patients with ESRD is a life-saving procedure, and the pool of transplantation candidates is therefore growing. Even among high-risk groups, transplantation offers optimal outcomes and measurable benefits in terms of life expectancy. However, the organ supply is static, particularly from deceased donors. In the light of this it seems increasingly inevitable that prolonged waiting times are becoming the norm, obviating some of the potential benefits available with transplantation. Our goals in the years to come are to provide optimal organ quality and minimize waiting times. Until this is accomplished, LDK transplantation provides the best alternative for many patients.

REFERENCES

1. Ruilope LM, van Veldhuisen DJ, Ritz E, Luscher TF. Renal function: the Cinderella of cardiovascular risk profile. *J Am Coll Cardiol* 2001; **38**: 1782–1787.

2. Levin A, Foley RN. Cardiovascular disease in renal insufficiency. *Am J Kidney Dis* 2000; **36**(6 Suppl 3): S24–30.

3. Sarnak MJ, Levey AS. Cardiovascular disease and chronic renal disease: a new paradigm. *Am J Kidney Dis* 2000; **35**(4 Suppl 1): S117–S131.

4. Meier-Kriesche HU, Schold JD, Reed AI, Kaplan B. Kidney transplantation halts cardiovascular disease progression in patients with end-stage renal disease. *Am J Transplant* 2004; **4**: 1662–1668.

5. Xue JL, Ma JZ, Louis TA, Collins AJ. Forecast of the number of patients with end-stage renal disease in the United States to the year 2010. *J Am Soc Nephrol* 2001; **12**: 2753–2758.

6. Wolfe RA, Ashby VB, Milford EL et al. Comparison of mortality in all patients on dialysis, patients on dialysis awaiting transplantation, and recipients of a first cadaveric transplant. *N Engl J Med* 1999; **341**: 1725–1730.

7. US Renal Data System. *USRDS 2003 Annual Data Report: Atlas of End-Stage Renal Disease in the United States.* Bethesda, MD: National Institutes of Health, National Institute of Diabetes and Digestive and Kidney Diseases, 2003.

8. Meier-Kriesche HU, Kaplan B. Waiting time on dialysis as the strongest modifiable risk factor for renal transplant outcomes: a paired donor kidney analysis. *Transplantation* 2002; **74**: 1377–1381.

9. Glanton CW, Kao TC, Cruess D et al. Impact of renal transplantation on survival in end-stage renal disease patients with elevated body mass index. *Kidney Int* 2003; **63**: 647–653.

10. Meier-Kriesche HU, Port FK, Ojo AO et al. Effect of waiting time on renal transplant outcome. *Kidney Int* 2000; **58**: 1311–1317.

11. Sarnak MJ. Cardiovascular complications in chronic kidney disease. *Am J Kidney Dis* 2003; **41**(5 suppl): 11–17.

12. Kaplan B, Meier-Kriesche HU. Death after graft loss: an important late study endpoint in kidney transplantation. *Am J Transplant* 2002; **2**: 970–974.

13. Hariharan S, McBride MA, Cherikh WS et al. Post-transplant renal function in the first year predicts long-term kidney transplant survival. *Kidney Int* 2002; **62**: 311–318.

14. Meier-Kriesche HU, Baliga R, Kaplan B. Decreased renal function is a strong risk factor for cardiovascular death after renal transplantation. *Transplantation* 2003; **75**: 1291–1295.

15. Muntner P, He J, Hamm L, Loria C, Whelton PK. Renal insufficiency and subsequent death resulting from cardiovascular disease in the United States. *J Am Soc Nephrol* 2002; **13**: 745–753.

16. Henry RM, Kostense PJ, Bos G, et al. Mild renal insufficiency is associated with increased cardiovascular mortality: The Hoorn Study. *Kidney Int* 2002; **62**: 1402–1407.

17. Mann JF, Gerstein HC, Pogue J, Bosch J, Yusuf S. Renal insufficiency as a predictor of cardiovascular outcomes and the impact of ramipril: the HOPE randomized trial. *Ann Intern Med* 2001; **134**: 629–636.

18. Culleton BF, Larson MG, Wilson PW et al. Cardiovascular disease and mortality in a community-based cohort with mild renal insufficiency. *Kidney Int* 1999; **56**: 2214–2219.

19. Beddhu S, Allen-Brady K, Cheung AK et al. Impact of renal failure on the risk of myocardial infarction and death. *Kidney Int* 2002; **62**: 1776–1783.

20. Fried LF, Shlipak MG, Crump C et al. Renal insufficiency as a predictor of cardiovascular outcomes and mortality in elderly individuals. *J Am Coll Cardiol* 2003; **41**: 1364–1372.

Immunological advantages of living donor kidney transplantation

Stuart W Robertson, Jesse A Flaxenburg, David M Briscoe

INTRODUCTION

It is well established that tissue typing and the degree of human leukocyte antigen (HLA) matching is a major predictable determinant of graft function and long-term survival following kidney transplantation. Classically, living-related donor (LRD) transplantation has several advantages as regards HLA matching, and these have been proposed as a major mechanism by which LRD transplantation provides the best long-term graft outcome, especially for HLA-identical siblings. Living-unrelated donor (LURD) transplantation, which has no HLA-matching advantage, also results in better outcomes than kidney transplantation from deceased donors, but this is due to other factors.[1,2] In this chapter, we will discuss the relatively under-appreciated concept that access to donor antigen prior to transplantation is also a major advantage of living donor (LD) transplantation and that the pretransplant availability of donor cells can be exploited clinically to manipulate the subsequent immunological response to the transplanted graft.

Over 40 years ago, Brent and Medawar explained that the administration of donor allogeneic cells into a recipient prior to transplantation can result in subsequent immunological hyporesponsiveness to that antigen and, in some circumstances, induces a state of 'tolerance'.[3] Their studies imply that access to and administration of alloantigen prior to transplantation is potentially useful therapeutically. Since the recipient's immunological response to alloantigen is what determines short- and long-term graft outcome, it follows that effective pretransplant manipulation of the recipient's immune system is potentially desirable and should be of clinical benefit.

A wide array of animal studies have clearly demonstrated that it is possible to manipulate the immune response prior to transplantation using donor antigen in such a manner that the post-transplant immunological response can be predicted to be hyporesponsive/tolerogenic.[4–7] Why then has pretransplant administration of donor alloantigen not been advocated or used more widely in humans? Here, we will discuss several ways in which the use of donor antigen has been shown to enhance graft survival, and we will consider proposed mechanisms by which donor alloantigen can predictably induce hyporesponsiveness/tolerance. In addition, we will describe the limited studies in which these manipulations have been successfully used in humans. As a review of every strategy for alloantigen-dependent manipulation of the immune response is beyond the scope of this chapter, the discussion will focus on the manipulations that we predict will soon be used in humans to optimize success following kidney transplantation.

GRAFT SURVIVAL AS A FUNCTION OF TISSUE TYPING

The expression of HLA class I (HLA-A, -B and -C) and class II (HLA-DP, -DQ and -DR) molecules on the surface of donor antigen-presenting cells (APCs) allows the host to identify an allograft as non-self.[8] Recognition of donor allopeptide in the context of donor APCs (the direct response) or on recipient

APCs (the indirect response) has been established to initiate the alloimmune response and to mediate acute and chronic rejection.[9,10] From a basic immunological point of view, it makes sense that the greater the mismatch between donor and recipient, the greater will be the recipient's immunological response to donor antigen. Indeed, multiple reports of kidney transplantation have established this to be the case and that the risk for graft loss following transplantation is highest in patients in whom the mismatch is greatest.[11] As a result of these observations, the intent of pretransplant tissue typing is to minimize the degree of HLA mismatch between the donor (whether living or cadaveric) and the recipient.

Registry data have been used to assess the effect of HLA mismatches on long-term graft outcome. The United Network for Organ Sharing (UNOS) database in the USA indicates that 20% of white Americans with ESRD (end stage renal disease) receive a zero-mismatched kidney; the database also provides data to show that the cumulative number of acute rejection episodes increases with the number of HLA mismatches (21% at one year in matched white recipients compared with 33% in an identical group with five to six mismatches). This translates to a 9% difference in 5-year graft survival between a zero HLA mismatch and a 5–6 HLA mismatch.[11] As immunosuppressive therapy improves, the effect of mismatches on the development of acute rejection may become less obvious, but will likely remain a major factor influencing long-term graft outcome.

It is known that the greater the HLA disparity between the LD and recipient, the poorer the long-term outcome; however, mismatches among LRDs and recipients do not appear to result in as poor an outcome as those following cadaveric transplantation. Thus, as the number of LD renal transplants increases, most will be performed in the presence of one or more HLA mismatches. It follows, therefore, that pretransplant therapies to render the recipient immunologically hyporesponsive (perhaps using donor alloantigen) are potentially advantageous and could help improve long-term outcome following LD transplantation.

DONOR-SPECIFIC TRANSFUSION

The concept of using donor antigen to promote immunological hyporesponsiveness to that antigen is almost as old as the concept of transplantation itself.[3,12,13] Indeed, Brent and Medawar's seminal studies clearly indicated that the administration of allogeneic cells prior to transplantation can induce a state of immune hyporesponsiveness.[3] The injection of fully allogeneic donor cells into a mouse fetus enabled the subsequent acceptance of donor strain skin after birth. In contrast, these same mice rejected skin allografts from a third-party mouse strain. This response, which is unique to transplantation, was termed 'immunological tolerance'. This same response has been studied ever since as a major mechanism by which the immune system learns to recognize self.

Brent and Medawar also demonstrated that there is a window of opportunity for development of neonatal tolerance and that this window varies from animal to animal. Furthermore, it was found that tolerance was not tissue-specific in as much as injections of leukocytes or tumour cells were capable of conferring tolerance to later skin grafts. This, they suggested, may mean that future attempts to produce tolerance in adult animals or in humans may enable use of donor blood as a source of the tolerance-producing antigen. Indeed, it is now well established that donor alloantigen (including HLA class I and II antigens) is expressed at high levels on peripheral blood cells, including APCs (e.g. monocytes and B cells) as well as other cells such as CD34-expressing stem cells.

In the original studies, injection of donor cells after birth often resulted in sensitization to donor antigen. As our understanding of the immune system and mechanisms of sensitization has advanced, it has become clear that the transfer of donor antigen into a recipient can indeed induce hyporesponsiveness; however, the timing, route of administration of antigen and additional immune modulation with immunosuppressive drugs is most important. In addition, the dose of the antigen, HLA matching and the immunodominance of the antigen or epitope have been found to have different effects on the immunological outcome and on tolerance induction.[3–6,13,14]

CLINICAL STUDIES USING DONOR-SPECIFIC TRANSFUSION

As discussed, donor peripheral blood cells are a good source of alloantigen, and it has been proposed that the systemic administration of donor-specific transfusions (DSTs) to recipients is a means of delivery of donor antigen to recipients. In the 1970s, DSTs or third-party blood transfusions were frequently given to patients prior to renal transplantation and, in some centres, they became popular prior to both cadaveric and LD transplantation. Several studies demonstrated that DST prior to LD transplantation was associated with a lower incidence of acute rejection and improved 5- and 10-year graft survival rates, even in the absence of additional immunosuppression.[12,15–17] Furthermore, the acute rejection episodes that did occur were generally milder and more easily reversible, similar to transplants between HLA-identical sibling matches.[15] It was later established that this 'DST effect' occurred in a dose-dependent manner and it was postulated that large amounts of donor antigen were beneficial for improved graft survival.[15,18,19] When DST was originally used, its effect was assessed on the basis of reducing the rate of acute rejection, with little emphasis on the concepts of long-term survival or its effect on the incidence of chronic rejection or tolerance induction.[20,21]

However, increased utilization of DST is limited by the increased risk of sensitization to donor antigen and the potential for graft-versus-host disease (GVHD).[22] For this reason, a few transplant centres advocate the use of DST, and indeed some reports suggested that

the benefit of DST was solely to identify and eliminate potential recipients who were at high risk for poorer outcome (as manifested by susceptibility to sensitization prior to the transplant). Although elimination of these high-risk recipients may have occurred and may have accounted for the DST effect, several studies have suggested that it still could not account for the significant effect of DST on the immunological response and the lack of rejection. Moreover, as we will discuss below, the mechanisms of DST-induced hyporesponsiveness, although complex, imply that real immunological benefit can be achieved. Thus, while it is important to appreciate that sensitization to donor antigen is a real risk of DST, the benefit of true alloantigen-induced immunological hyporesponsiveness is also a real and potentially advantageous phenomenon.

Mechanism of DST-induced immunological hyporesponsiveness

Several research groups, including those of Starzl,[5,23,24] Wood,[6,25] Sachs[26] and Sykes,[4,14] have continued to pioneer the concept that administration of donor alloantigen in the peri-transplantation period can govern the extent to which post-transplant hyporesponsiveness (or tolerance) is achieved. Along with others, these groups have clearly demonstrated that there are three main mechanisms by which a DST can induce allogeneic hyporesponsiveness: (i) the establishment of mixed chimerism; (ii) immune deviation; and (iii) the generation of regulatory (or suppressor) immunological responses.

Mixed chimerism

Mixed chimerism is defined as a state in which donor populations of haematopoietic cells persist in the recipient.[4] Starzl and Sykes have proposed that the presence of donor cells in a transplant recipient may augment immunological tolerance and is a favourable outcome following transplantation.[4,23] It has been suggested that chimerism is initiated by 'passenger leukocytes', which are inevitably transplanted along with a solid-organ allograft. These passenger donor cells, which include stem cells and APCs, migrate from the transplanted organ into the recipient.[5,23,27] It is proposed that the main mechanism by which mixed chimerism can result in allogeneic hyporesponsiveness involves central (or deletional) tolerance[4,28] (Figure 3-1). This occurs when donor-derived APCs take up residence within the recipient thymus and mediate deletion of recipient donor-reactive T cells. Central tolerance has been demonstrated to occur in stringent animal models of tolerance.[25,26,29,30]

It has been suggested that the degree of post-transplant chimerism depends on the numbers of passenger donor leukocytes that are transferred into the recipient from the graft; this can be different among kidney, heart and liver allograft recipients.[23,27] Liver allografts provide significant numbers of donor cells, suggesting that chimerism will be greatest in recipients of liver allografts. However, even following liver transplantation, chimerism is short-lived.[24,31–33] This has led investigators to initiate studies involving the adoptive transfer of donor cells into the recipient at the time of transplant (and/or following transplantation) to promote and enable the persistence of chimerism. If chimerism is a mechanism underlying tolerance, these studies will determine whether chimerism actually causes immunological hyporesponsiveness as opposed simply to being associated with long-term allograft survival. At the time of writing, it is thought that the use of DST and the adoptive transfer of donor bone marrow are the best methods by which mixed chimerism can be enhanced at the time of, or following, solid organ transplantation. Thus, the availability of donor cells for pretransplant manipulation of the

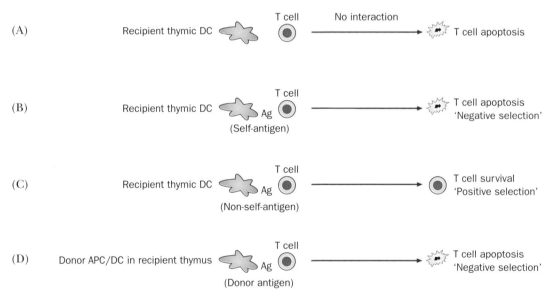

Figure 3-1 Development of central or thymic tolerance. Recipient T cell precursors migrating through the thymus encounter thymic dendritic cells (DC) expressing self-major histocompatibility complex (MHC). (A) In the absence of an encounter with antigen (Ag), the T cell undergoes apoptosis. (B) If self-antigen is presented to the T cell in the context of self-MHC on the recipient thymic DC, the T cell also undergoes apoptosis. This is known as *negative* selection. (C) If foreign antigen is presented to the T cell in the context of self-MHC, the T cell is *positively* selected and will be allowed to mature in the medulla and pass into the periphery. (D) In mixed chimerism, it is proposed that migration of donor antigen-presenting cells (APCs) into the recipient thymic environment facilitates negative selection and deletion of donor-reactive T cells.

alloimmune response, or for subsequent transfer after transplantation (to maintain chimerism), may reflect an advantage of LD transplantation.

Immune deviation

Another process whereby DST can result in immunological hyporesponsiveness is immune deviation. Upon activation, T cells differentiate into two major and distinct subsets characterized by differences in cytokine profiles and effector functions.[34–36] CD4+ T cells differentiate into T helper (Th) type 1 and 2 cells, whereas CD8 T cells differentiate into T cytotoxic (Tc) type 1 and 2 cells. Several studies have evaluated the function of Th1 and Th2 cells in alloimmunity.[37–39] In general, Th1 cells produce interleukin (IL)-2, interferon (IFN)-γ and tumour necrosis factor-α. They participate in cell-mediated immunity promoting delayed-type hypersensitivity reactions. In contrast, Th2 cells preferentially produce IL-4, IL-5 and IL-10 and have anti-inflammatory or tolerogenic properties.[34,35] Several experimental models have demonstrated that Th1 responses are predominant in allograft rejection in association with graft dysfunction, whereas Th2 responses are the prototype associated with hyporesponsiveness/tolerance and are also associated with long-term graft survival.[38] In addition, it has been shown that the Th2 tolerogenic effect can be transferred with Th2 cells from one animal to another;[39–43] and can be reversed by the injection of IL-2.[40] These observations imply that manipulation of the recipient, such that the alloimmune response will be Th2-like and not Th1-like, will result in a more favourable outcome.

Costimulatory blockade is one such therapeutic manipulation which when used in conjunction with DST has been shown to limit Th1 responses and to promote Th2 responses in vivo.[44,45] T cells require at least two major signals for full activation.[46] One signal is the antigen-dependent signal resulting from an interaction between the T cell receptor complex (TCR) and an allogeneic peptide presented to the T cell within the major histocompatibility complex (MHC) molecule on the cell surface of an APC. Additional positive signals, such as those resulting from interactions among T cell CD28 and APC B7-1 and B7-2 or T cell CD154 and APC CD40, have been demonstrated to be an absolute requirement for full T cell activation.[46–48] By definition this costimulatory response results in enhanced IL-2 production and an associated increase in T cell proliferation. Limited costimulation, on the other hand, results in a default activation response involving a Th2 response. When DST is administered at the same time as CTLA4-Ig[49] (a reagent to block B7 interactions) or anti-CD154 (to block CD154–CD40 interactions),[38] subsequent immunological hyporesponsiveness occurs. This treatment protocol results in immune deviation, including an inhibition of Th1 responses and an upregulation of Th2 responses, and is associated with a marked prolongation of rodent cardiac and renal allograft survival.[50] In theory, therefore, it is possible that DST can be administered to humans in combination with CTLA4-Ig (or similar) to facilitate immune deviation and immunological hyporesponsiveness prior to an organ transplant.

Another experimental approach to augment immune deviation is via the manipulation of the dendritic cell (DC), the most important and competent APC present within a DST.[51] DCs are continuously produced from haematopoietic precursors in the bone marrow and are widely distributed in the body. Immature DCs, present in many tissues, fail to induce an immune response but sample self-antigen in peripheral tissues and maintain self-tolerance. They also sample foreign antigens, causing them to mature into immunogenic DCs that have the capacity to initiate primary immune responses.

Recent evidence suggests that DCs may also selectively direct the T-cell-mediated activation response.[52,53] They can initiate either a proinflammatory Th1 immune response or a tolerogenic Th2 immune response. The subset of mature DCs that initiate Th1 responses are called DC1 and are characterized by their ability to produce high levels of IL-12. This cytokine, in turn, stimulates T cells to produce high levels of the Th1 cytokine IFN-γ. In humans, mature DC1s induce strong Th1 responses and also induce cytotoxic T cell activation. In contrast, immature DC1 cells are weak at initiating an immune response but activate both Th1 and Th2 cellular responses. The major stimuli that have been reported to mediate the differentiation of a DC into a DC1 include CD40L–CD40 interactions, IFN-γ, lipopolysaccharide, bacterial CpG and viral RNA. In contrast, other stimuli (including anti-inflammatory IL-10, transforming growth factor-β, prostaglandins and steroids) mediate the differentiation of an immature DC1 cell into a DC that selectively activates T cells to produce Th2 regulatory responses and inhibits Th1 proinflammatory responses. Moreover, there is also a distinct subset of DCs called DC2 cells that are derived from plasmacytoid precursors and promote Th2 cell activation. These cells are produced upon activation with the cytokine IL-3, but can also be produced by many other stimuli, including viruses.

Although this area of immunology is somewhat complex, it has clear implications for transplantation. If it is possible to manipulate a donor DC ex vivo, one could theoretically transfer this cell into a patient to derive a tolerogenic immune response prior to transplantation. Indeed, some researchers believe that this should be the primary issue for consideration in immune modulatory therapy.

Regulation

For some time, it has been recognized that it is possible to transfer transplantation tolerance from one strain of animal to another using T cells.[54–56] For instance, some early studies found that the transfer of T cells from a tolerant recipient rat strain A (that had permanently accepted an allograft from rat strain B) into a naïve rat strain A will allow this naïve rat to permanently accept an allograft from rat strain B without immunosup-

pression.[50,57,58] In contrast, in the absence of T cell transfer, or when T cells from a rejector rat are transferred, no such protection is seen. This regulatory effect on the alloimmune response is quite remarkable and is very potent, at least in animal models.[56,57,59] It has recently been shown to be dependent on the presence of a discrete subpopulation of CD4+ T cells expressing high levels of CD25.[57,60] This observation has advanced our understanding of alloimmunity to the extent that it is currently thought that therapeutic strategies enabling a recipient to mount a regulatory immune response to donor alloantigen is one of the most important issues for the future of transplantation.[57,61,62]

Regulatory immune responses were initially shown to be of importance in the physiological prevention of the occurrence of autoimmunity.[60,62,63] The observation that CD4+CD25+ T cells function in vivo to maintain self-tolerance has proved to be relevant to transplantation. Some recent studies have clearly indicated that this population of regulatory cells are functional in protecting allografts from rejection and in the maintenance of transplant function.[57] Moreover, the generation and maintenance of regulatory cells (in vitro and in vivo) requires constant exposure to alloantigen. In the absence of alloantigen, the numbers of regulatory cells diminish and this is proposed to result in the reactivation of alloimmunity.

CD4+CD25+ regulatory T cells exist in humans post-transplantation and have been shown to suppress immune responses to alloantigen.[64] So, is it possible to generate regulatory immunity to donor alloantigen prior to transplantation? Several animal studies suggest that this mechanism is one of the major immunological effects that occur in response to the administration of donor antigen in a DST. Strom's group has found that CD4+CD25+ cells isolated from mice treated with DST and costimulatory blockade are potent at suppressing the immune response, ensuring long-term survival of skin allografts from the same strain.[65] This was strictly donor-antigen specific, and it is proposed that DST together with anti-CD154 may cause selective expansion of regulatory cell clones which recognize donor MHC and/or may become more efficient in their regulatory function. Taylor et al have shown that regulatory cells can be generated ex vivo by the combination of donor antigen and CD154 blockade.[66] In addition, they found that when these CD4+CD25+ regulatory T cells were transferred back into a naïve mouse, they were able to protect the animal against rejection (GVHD).[67,68] Furthermore, Wood's group demonstrated that regulatory cells generated in vivo by CD154 blockade are capable of preventing not only CD4+ T-cell, but also CD8+ T-cell-mediated rejection.[69] It is, therefore, possible that future therapeutic regimens involving the pretransplant administration of simultaneous DST and costimulatory blockade to induce donor-specific regulation will render the immune system hyporesponsive. Since costimulatory anti-B7 reagents are currently undergoing clinical trials, this is also a real possibility for the future.

THERAPEUTIC USE OF DONOR ALLOANTIGEN TO INDUCE IMMUNOLOGICAL HYPORESPONSIVENESS

As has been discussed above, several studies have demonstrated that administration of donor alloantigen in the form of a DST to transplant recipients can enable mixed chimerism, immune deviation and/or regulatory immune responses, all of which promote subsequent immunological hyporesponsiveness to the specific donor alloantigen. Although no trials are underway using the LD, the use of LD blood cells as a source of alloantigen pretransplantation remains a theoretical advantage to promote one or all of these mechanisms of immunological hyporesponsiveness in the clinical setting.

Over the past 10 years, DST has been used in several studies of human solid-organ transplantation.[70–76] Some of the patients in these trials were sufficiently stable that cortico-steroid immunosuppression was withdrawn post-transplantation. This suggests that at least a small immunological benefit was achieved with this therapy. However, it remains unclear as to what is the optimal therapeutic protocol to test if DST can *actively* promote hyporesponsiveness and augment transplant outcomes. Trivedi et al treated a group of LRD kidney transplant recipients with high numbers of donor peripheral blood mononuclear cells (PBMC), mobilized from LRDs using granulocyte-macrophage colony stimulating factor and harvested using leukopheresis.[77] Compared with controls, the transplant recipients treated with high-dose PBMC had improved graft survival, improved graft function and had corticosteroid immunosuppression withdrawn.[77] Barbari et al examined a series of transplant recipients given DST prior to transplantation while receiving various immunosuppressive agents. They found that the rate of acute rejection was lower in patients who received DST; and proposed that ciclosporin, given before the DST and continued after transplantation, was an optimal regimen.[78]

Furthermore, two recent studies[79,80] have provided clear evidence that it is possible to augment true donor-specific hyporesponsiveness in humans using DST. It was shown that pretransplant 'conditioning' of the recipient was an important therapeutic manoeuvre to facilitate persistent chimerism.[79,80] Cosimi's group carried out transplantations in two patients with end-stage renal disease secondary to multiple myeloma.[79] Both patients received a non-myeloablative conditioning regimen consisting of intravenous cyclophosphamide preoperatively, antithymocyte globulin (ATG) perioperatively and thymic irradiation one day prior to transplantation. On the day of kidney transplant surgery, both recipients also received an infusion of donor bone marrow and were maintained on ciclosporin for approximately 75 days (after which it was withdrawn). Both patients had normal renal function at up to four years post-transplantation in the absence of immunosuppression. Milan et al performed four LRD kidney transplantations and conditioned the recipients with total lymphoid irradiation and ATG.[80] Similar to Trivedi,[77] these investigators administered a DST consisting of CD34+ haematopoietic progenitor stem cells to the recipients. Post-transplantation, maintenance ciclosporin and prednisolone were tapered off. Microchimerism was demonstrated in three of the four patients, none of whom had any episodes of rejection. Immunosuppression was withdrawn successfully in two.

The studies discussed above have shown that administration of donor antigen can improve the outcome following a solid organ transplantation. The potential advantage of having an LD as a source of donor antigen prior to a planned transplantation or following transplantation is most evident. However, it remains to be determined if it is possible to create a stable, mixed chimeric state in the transplant recipient with a non-toxic conditioning regimen prior to organ transplantation. Also, further studies involving larger numbers of patients will be necessary to validate these preliminary studies and assess if augmentation of chimerism leads to the development of hyporesponsiveness/tolerance and improved graft survival.

Costimulatory blockade with a humanized anti-B7 antibody is currently undergoing clinical trials as an immunosuppressive agent to prevent acute rejection. As discussed, several animal studies have identified that pretransplant DST in combination with costimulatory blockade (including anti-B7) can promote hyporesponsiveness, in part a result of immune deviation and regulatory immune responses. Although this is an exciting future possibility for the clinic, we will need to await the results of ongoing trials demonstrating that these agents are immunosuppressive before they can be used for pretransplant manipulation of LD transplant recipients. We suggest that this therapy (if successful) will clearly advantage recipients of LD transplants in the future.

Although not the subject of this chapter, other therapies involving T cell depletion can also be used to augment donor-specific hyporesponsiveness. For instance, Campath 1H is a humanized anti-CD52 monoclonal antibody that profoundly depletes T lymphocytes and transiently depletes B cells and monocytes from the peripheral blood. There have been no completed controlled trials using Campath 1H in renal transplantation, but several pilot studies have suggested that it is effective, promoting excellent graft function and inducing a 'semi' state of tolerance called prope tolerance.[81–84] As discussed, in humans, substantial T cell depletion has been attempted using conditional regimens prior to DST to induce a state of chimerism. Thus, the use of Campath in conditioning regimens along with DST may promote immunological hyporesponsiveness, but this theoretical possibility also awaits further evaluation in controlled clinical trials.

Finally, there are several other observations in animal models that will, no doubt at some point, become feasible for human clinical studies. The ability to use gene therapy to manipulate a donor DC and promote tolerance has been suggested as a possibility.[85,86] For instance, gene transfer ex vivo into a DC can facilitate a DC2 regulatory immune response and immune regulation after subsequent transfer in vivo. If this proves feasible in the setting of transplantation, gene therapy using LD DCs ex vivo may be a feasible approach to facilitate a hyporesponsive recipient immune response to the donor alloantigen. Clearly, if this type of technology becomes a reality for therapy, it will likely again advantage the recipient of the LD transplant. The time it takes to generate immune modulatory dendritic cells ex vivo and their administration pretransplantation would not be feasible with cadaveric donors.

In summary, several lines of investigation suggest that it is possible to promote one of many mechanisms of immunological hyporesponsiveness in the clinical setting. We present evidence that recipients of LD transplants will be advantaged as these studies move forward to the clinic.

CONCLUSION

The availability of donor alloantigen in peripheral blood of LD provides clinicians with an ideal opportunity to manipulate the immune response of a transplant recipient for a period of time prior to, or after transplantation. Administration of donor cells into a recipient in the form of a DST or stem cell transfusion enables analysis of the immunological response prior to the time of the transplantation such that the subsequent response to the transplanted organ can be predicted. When one treats a recipient so that sensitization to the DST does not occur, it is possible to administer donor antigen safely prior to transplantation. Several studies have demonstrated that it is possible to administer donor cells at the time of the transplant and/or afterwards; this therapy results in immunological hyporesponsiveness to the solid-organ transplant. In this chapter, we have discussed a number of methods by which the immune response can be manipulated using donor antigen, and we have discussed mechanisms by which alloantigen may induce a state of hyporesponsiveness in vivo. The ability to manipulate the immune response prior to transplantation using donor antigen is thus a major theoretical immunological advantage of LD transplantation. Clearly the challenge for the future is to translate this understanding to the clinic.

REFERENCES

1. Terasaki PI, Cecka JM, Gjertson DW, Takemoto S. High survival rates of kidney transplants from spousal and living unrelated donors. *N Engl J Med* 1995; **333**: 333–336.
2. Terasaki PI, Cecka JM, Gjertson DW, Cho YW. Spousal and other living renal donor transplants. *Clin Transpl* 1997; 269–284.
3. Billingham RE, Brent L, Medawar PB. Quantitative studies on tissue transplantation immunity. III. Actively acquired tolerance. *Proc R Soc Lond B Biol Sci* 1956; **239**: 357–414.
4. Sykes M. Mixed chimerism and transplant tolerance. *Immunity* 2001; **14**: 417–424.
5. Starzl TE, Demetris AJ, Murase NT et al. The lost chord: microchimerism and allograft survival. *Immunol Today* 1996; **17**: 577–584.
6. Wood KJ. Passenger leukocytes and microchimerism: what role in tolerance induction? *Transplantation* 2003; **75**(9 suppl): 17S–20S.
7. Salama AD, Remuzzi G, Harmon WE, Sayegh MH. Challenges to achieving clinical transplantation tolerance. *J Clin Invest* 2001; **108**: 943–948.
8. Krensky AM, Weiss A, Crabtree G et al. T-lymphocyte-antigen interactions in transplant rejection. *N Engl J Med* 1990; **322**: 510–517.
9. Rogers NJ, Lechler RI. Allorecognition. *Am J Transplant* 2001; **1**: 97–102.
10. Womer KL, Sayegh MH, Auchincloss H Jr. Involvement of the direct and indirect pathways of allorecognition in tolerance induction. *Philos Trans R Soc Lond B Biol Sci* 2001; **356**: 639–647.
11. Cecka J. The UNOS scientific renal transplant registry – 2000. In: Cecka JT, Terasaki PI, (eds), *Clinical Transplants 2000*. Los Angeles: UCLA Immunogenetics Center, 2000.
12. Opelz G, Mickey MR, Terasaki PI. Blood transfusions and unresponsiveness to HL-A. *Transplantation* 1973; **16**: 649–654.
13. Liblau R, Tisch R, Bercovici N, McDevitt HO. Systemic antigen in the treatment of T-cell-mediated autoimmune diseases. *Immunol Today* 1997; **18**: 599–604.
14. Wekerle T, Sykes M. Induction of tolerance. *Surgery* 2004; **135**: 359–364.
15. Salvatierra O Jr, Vincenti F, Amend W et al. Deliberate donor-specific blood transfusions prior to living related renal transplantation. A new approach. *Ann Surg* 1980; **192**: 543–552.
16. Opelz G, Sengar DP, Mickey MR, Terasaki PI. Effect of blood transfusions on subsequent kidney transplants. *Transplant Proc* 1973; **5**: 253–259.
17. Potter DE, Portale AA, Melzer JS et al. Are blood transfusions beneficial in the cyclosporine era? *Pediatr Nephrol* 1991; **5**: 168–172.
18. Opelz G, Graver B, Terasaki PI. Induction of high kidney graft survival rate by multiple transfusion. *Lancet* 1981; **1**: 1223–1225.
19. Mendez R, Mendez RG, Iwaki YI et al. Improved allograft survival in nonidentical living related donor transplants using donor-specific blood transfusions. *J Urol* 1985; **133**: 383–385.
20. Burlingham WJ, Grailer A, Sparks-Mackety EM et al. Improved renal allograft survival following donor-specific transfusions. II. In vitro correlates of early (DST-type) rejection episodes. *Transplantation* 1987; **43**: 41–46.
21. Salvatierra O Jr. Donor-specific transfusions in living-related transplantation. *World J Surg* 1986; **10**: 361–368.
22. Burlingham WJ, Stratta R, Mason B et al. Risk factors for sensitization by blood transfusions. Comparison of the UW/Madison and UC/San Francisco donor-specific transfusion experience. *Transplantation* 1989; **47**: 140–144.
23. Starzl TE, Zinkernagel RM. Antigen localization and

migration in immunity and tolerance. *N Engl J Med* 1998; **339**: 1905–1913.

24. Starzl TE, Murase N, Thomson A, Demetris AJ. Liver transplants contribute to their own success. *Nat Med* 1996; **2**: 163–165.

25. Karim M, Steger U, Bushell AR, Wood KJ. The role of the graft in establishing tolerance. *Front Biosci* 2002; **7**: e129–e154.

26. Cosimi AB, Sachs DH. Mixed chimerism and transplantation tolerance. *Transplantation* 2004; **77**: 943–946.

27. Starzl TE, Demetris AJ, Trucco M et al. Cell migration and chimerism after whole-organ transplantation: the basis of graft acceptance. *Hepatology* 1993; **17**: 1127–1152.

28. Khan A, Tomita Y, Sykes M. Thymic dependence of loss of tolerance in mixed allogeneic bone marrow chimeras after depletion of donor antigen. Peripheral mechanisms do not contribute to maintenance of tolerance. *Transplantation* 1996; **62**: 380–387.

29. Ali A, Garrovillo M, Oluwole OO et al. Mechanisms of acquired thymic tolerance: induction of transplant tolerance by adoptive transfer of in vivo alloMHC peptide activated syngeneic T cells. *Transplantation* 2001; **71**: 1442–1448.

30. Gopinathan R, DePaz HA, Oluwole OO et al. Role of reentry of in vivo alloMHC peptide-activated T cells into the adult thymus in acquired systemic tolerance. *Transplantation* 2001; **72**: 1533–1541.

31. Caillat-Zucman S, Legendre C, Suberbielle C et al. Microchimerism frequency two to thirty years after cadaveric kidney transplantation. *Hum Immunol* 1994; **41**: 91–95.

32. Schlitt HJ, Raddatz G, Steinhoff G et al. Passenger lymphocytes in human liver allografts and their potential role after transplantation. *Transplantation* 1993; **56**: 951–955.

33. Starzl TE, Demetris AJ, Trucco M et al. Systemic chimerism in human female recipients of male livers. *Lancet* 1992; **340**: 876–877.

34. Mosmann TR, Cherwinski H, Bond MW et al. Two types of murine helper T cell clone. I. Definition according to profiles of lymphokine activities and secreted proteins. *J Immunol* 1986; **136**: 2348–2357.

35. Mosmann TR, Coffman RL. TH1 and TH2 cells: different patterns of lymphokine secretion lead to different functional properties. *Annu Rev Immunol* 1989; **7**: 145–173.

36. Abbas AK, Murphy KM, Sher A. Functional diversity of helper T lymphocytes. *Nature* 1996; **383**: 787–793.

37. Kishimoto K, Dong VM, Issazadeh S et al. The role of CD154-CD40 versus CD28-B7 costimulatory pathways in regulating allogeneic Th1 and Th2 responses in vivo. *J Clin Invest* 2000; **106**: 63–72.

38. Hancock WW, Sayegh MH, Zheng X-G et al. Costimulatory function and expression of CD40 ligand, CD80, and CD86 in vascularized murine cardiac allograft rejection. *Proc Natl Acad Sci USA* 1996; **93**: 13967–13972.

39. Sayegh MH, Akalin E, Hancock WW et al. CD28-B7 blockade after alloantigenic challenge in vivo inhibits Th1 cytokines but spares Th2. *J Exp Med* 1995; **181**: 1869–1874.

40. Waaga AM, Gasser M, Kist-van Holthe JE et al. Regulatory functions of self-restricted MHC class II allopeptide-specific Th2 clones in vivo. *J Clin Invest* 2001; **107**: 909–916.

41. Kuchroo VK, Das MP, Brown JA et al. B7-1 and B7-2 costimulatory molecules activate differentially the Th1/Th2 developmental pathways: application to autoimmune disease therapy. *Cell* 1995; **80**: 707–718.

42. McKnight A, Perez V, Shea C et al. Costimulator dependence of lymphokine secretion by naive and activated CD4+ T lymphocytes from TCR transgenic mice. *J Immunol* 1994; **152**: 5220–5225.

43. Perez VL, Lederer JA, Lichtman AH, Abbas AK. Stability of Th1 and Th2 populations. *Int Immunol* 1995; **7**: 869–875.

44. Sayegh MH, Turka LA. T cell costimulatory pathways: promising novel targets for immunosuppression and tolerance induction. *J Am Soc Nephrol* 1995; **6**: 1143–1150.

45. Sayegh MH, Turka LA. The role of T-cell costimulatory activation pathways in transplant rejection. *N Engl J Med* 1998; **338**: 1813–1821.

46. Abbas AK, Sharpe AH. T-cell stimulation: an abundance of B7s. *Nat Med* 1999; **5**: 1345–1346.

47. Sharpe AH, Freeman GJ. The B7-CD28 superfamily. *Nat Rev Immunol* 2002; **2**: 116–126.

48. Judge TA, Wu Z, Zheng XG et al. The role of CD80, CD86, and CTLA4 in alloimmune responses and the induction of long-term allograft survival. *J Immunol* 1999; **162**: 1947–1951.

49. Turka LA, Linsley PS, Lin H et al. T-cell activation by the CD28 ligand B7 is required for cardiac allograft rejection in vivo. *Proc Natl Acad Sci USA* 1992: **89**: 11102–11105.

50. Onodera K, Hancock WW, Graser E et al. Type 2 helper T cell-type cytokines and the development of 'infectious' tolerance in rat cardiac allograft recipients. *J Immunol* 1997; **158**: 1572–1581.

51. Fu F, Li Y, Qian S et al. Costimulatory molecule-deficient dendritic cell progenitors (MHC class II+, CD80dim, CD86-) prolong cardiac allograft survival in nonimmunosuppressed recipients. *Transplantation* 1996; **62**: 659–665.

52. Liu YJ, Kanzler H, Soumelis V, Gilliet M. Dendritic cell lineage, plasticity and cross-regulation. *Nat Immunol* 2001; **2**: 585–589.

53. Kapsenberg ML. Dendritic-cell control of pathogen-driven T-cell polarization. *Nat Rev Immunol* 2003; **3**: 984–993.

54. Lechler RI, Ng WF, Camara NO. Infectious tolerance? Mechanisms and implications. *Transplantation* 2001; **72**(suppl): S29–S31.

55. Hall BM. Mechanisms of induction of tolerance to organ allografts. *Crit Rev Immunol* 2000; **20**: 267–324.

56. Chen J, Huoam C, Plain K et al. CD4(+), CD25(+) T

cells as regulators of alloimmune responses. *Transplant Proc* 2001; **33**: 163–164.

57. Wood KJ, Sakaguchi S. Regulatory T cells in transplantation tolerance. *Nat Rev Immunol* 2003; **3**: 199–210.

58. Qin S, Cobbold SP, Pope H et al. 'Infectious' transplantation tolerance. *Science* 1993; **259**: 974–977.

59. Hara M, Kingsley CI, Niimi M et al. IL-10 is required for regulatory T cells to mediate tolerance to alloantigens in vivo. *J Immunol* 2001; **166**: 3789–3796.

60. Shevach EM, McHugh RS, Piccirillo CA, Thornton AM. Control of T-cell activation by CD4+ CD25+ suppressor T cells. *Immunol Rev* 2001; **182**: 58–67.

61. Abbas AK. The control of T cell activation vs tolerance. *Autoimmun Rev* 2003; **2**: 115–118.

62. Bluestone JA, Abbas AK. Natural versus adaptive regulatory T cells. *Nat Rev Immunol* 2003; **3**: 253–257.

63. Shevach EM. CD4+ CD25+ suppressor T cells: more questions than answers. *Nat Rev Immunol* 2002; **2**: 389–400.

64. Ng WF, Duggan PJ, Ponchel F et al. Human CD4(+)CD25(+) cells: a naturally occurring population of regulatory T cells. *Blood* 2001; **98**: 2736–2744.

65. Zheng XX, Sanchez-Fueyo A, Domenig C, Strom TB. The balance of deletion and regulation in allograft tolerance. *Immunol Rev* 2003; **196**: 75–84.

66. Taylor PA, Noelle RJ, Blazar BR. CD4(+)CD25(+) immune regulatory cells are required for induction of tolerance to alloantigen via costimulatory blockade. *J Exp Med* 2001; **193**: 1311–1318.

67. Taylor PA, Panoskaltsis-Mortari A, Noelle RJ, Blazar BR. Analysis of the requirements for the induction of CD4+ T cell alloantigen hyporesponsiveness by ex vivo anti-CD40 ligand antibody. *J Immunol* 2000; **164**: 612–622.

68. Taylor PA, Friedman TM, Korngold R et al. Tolerance induction of alloreactive T cells via ex vivo blockade of the CD40:CD40L costimulatory pathway results in the generation of a potent immune regulatory cell. *Blood* 2002; **99**: 4601–4609.

69. van Maurik A, Herber M, Wood KJ, Jones ND. Cutting edge: CD4+CD25+ alloantigen-specific immunoregulatory cells that can prevent CD8+ T cell-mediated graft rejection: implications for anti-CD154 immunotherapy. *J Immunol* 2002; **169**: 5401–5404.

70. Rao AS, Fontes P, Iyengar A et al. Augmentation of chimerism with perioperative donor bone marrow infusion in organ transplant recipients: a 44 month follow-up. *Transplant Proc* 1997; **29**: 1184–1185.

71. Rao AS, Fontes P, Iyengar A et al. Perioperative donor bone marrow infusion in recipients of organ allografts. *Transplant Proc* 1997; **29**: 2192–2193.

72. Rao AS, Shapiro R, Corry R et al. Adjuvant bone marrow infusion in clinical organ transplant recipients. *Transplant Proc* 1998; **30**: 1367–1368.

73. Rao AS, Shapiro R, Corry R et al. Immune modulation in organ allograft recipients by single or multiple donor bone marrow infusions. *Transplant Proc* 1999; **31**: 700–701.

74. Zeevi A, Pavlick M, Banas R et al. Three years of follow-up of bone marrow-augmented organ transplant recipients: the impact on donor-specific immune modulation. *Transplant Proc* 1997; **29**: 1205–1206.

75. Otsuka M, Yuzawa K, Takada Y et al. Long-term graft survival of living-related kidneys after donor-specific transfusion. *Transplant Proc* 2000; **32**: 1741–1742.

76. Shapiro R, Rao AS, Corry RJ et al. Kidney transplantation with bone marrow augmentation: five-year outcomes. *Transplant Proc* 2001; **33**: 1134–1135.

77. Trivedi HL, Shah VR, Vanikar AV et al. High-dose peripheral blood stem cell infusion: a strategy to induce donor-specific hyporesponsiveness to allografts in pediatric renal transplant recipients. *Pediatr Transplant* 2002; **6**: 63–68.

78. Barbari A, Stephan A, Masri MA et al. Donor specific transfusion in kidney transplantation: effect of different immunosuppressive protocols on graft outcome. *Transplant Proc* 2001; **33**: 2787–2788.

79. Buhler LH, Spitzer TR, Sykes M et al. Induction of kidney allograft tolerance after transient lymphohematopoietic chimerism in patients with multiple myeloma and end-stage renal disease. *Transplantation* 2002; **74**: 1405–1409.

80. Millan MT, Shizuru JA, Hoffmann P et al. Mixed chimerism and immunosuppressive drug withdrawal after HLA-mismatched kidney and hematopoietic progenitor transplantation. *Transplantation* 2002; **73**: 1386–1391.

81. Calne R, Friend P, Moffatt S et al. Prope tolerance, perioperative campath 1H, and low-dose cyclosporin monotherapy in renal allograft recipients. *Lancet* 1998; **351**: 1701–1702.

82. Calne R, Moffatt SD, Friend PJ et al. Campath IH allows low-dose cyclosporine monotherapy in 31 cadaveric renal allograft recipients. *Transplantation* 1999; **68**: 1613–1616.

83. Kirk AD, Hale DA, Mannon RB et al. Results from a human renal allograft tolerance trial evaluating the humanized CD52-specific monoclonal antibody alemtuzumab (CAMPATH-1H). *Transplantation* 2003; **76**: 120–129.

84. Knechtle SJ, Pirsch JD, Fechner J Jr et al. Campath-1H induction plus rapamycin monotherapy for renal transplantation: results of a pilot study. *Am J Transplant* 2003; **3**: 722–730.

85. Tarner IH, Slavin AJ, McBride J et al. Treatment of autoimmune disease by adoptive cellular gene therapy. *Ann N Y Acad Sci* 2003; **998**: 512–519.

86. Chen D, Sung R, Bromberg JS. Gene therapy in transplantation. *Transpl Immunol* 2002; **9**: 301–314.

Selection and evaluation of potential living kidney donors 4

Lorna P Marson, Jennifer A Lumsdaine, John LR Forsythe, Anders Hartmann

INTRODUCTION

Living donor kidney (LDK) transplantation allows patients with end-stage renal failure the best chance of rehabilitation. However, living donation appears contrary to the most fundamental concept of the medical profession: *primum non nocere* (first do no harm). It exposes a healthy individual to the combined risks of major surgery and life with a single kidney entirely for the benefit of another individual. LDK transplantation should only be undertaken if four essential conditions are met,[1] and these form the basis of the evaluation process of the living donor:

- The risk to the donor must be low.
- The donor must be fully informed.
- The decision to donate must be entirely voluntary and not due to coercion.
- The transplant must have a good chance of providing a successful outcome for the recipient.

There is a steady increase in LDK transplantation worldwide,[2,3] and with the severe shortfall in the number of cadaveric kidneys available for transplantation, it is likely and appropriate that this trend should continue. However, there is significant variation in the practice of living donor assessment,[4] and thus the recent International Forum on the Care of the Live Donor was timely.[5]

This chapter will discuss the different aspects of evaluation of the potential living donor, summarizing current standards and practices,[1,6,7] while seeking areas of controversy and future developments.

The Amsterdam consensus statement emphasises that the purpose of the evaluation process is to ensure the overall health and well-being of the donor, minimizing unnecessary medical risk to both donor and recipient. It should quantify any potential technical difficulties that might compromise the success of nephrectomy and subsequent transplantation. The evaluation should also address safety issues for the recipient, including risks for transmission of infections or malignancies as well as ensuring adequacy of kidney function in both donor and recipient after the operations.[8,9]

The donor must be fully informed of the risks of surgery: donor nephrectomy is associated with a very low perioperative risk, mortality of 0.03% being commonly reported.[7,10] It has been suggested that the risk can be compared with the risk of dying in a car accident during the next year, for potential donors to grasp the practical meaning of such an incidence rate.[7] In addition, clinicians involved in the evaluation process must be certain that the donor is making a voluntary decision to donate without coercion.[5]

IDENTIFYING POTENTIAL LIVE DONORS

The commonest scenario leading to LDK transplantation is that a family member contacts the transplant centre with a wish to donate. A recent report from Scandinavia showed that 77% of donors initiated the process and 13% were solicited by the recipient.[11] Changing circumstances and definitions of acceptable donor–recipient relationships may soon alter this dynamic.

Who are the donors?

The optimal donor, by general consensus, is an adult member of the immediate family of a patient with end-stage renal disease.[1,6,7] However, the use of emotionally related, but genetically unrelated, living donors has become increasingly common worldwide,[12–15] and this practice is supported by different guidelines.[1,6,7] On the other hand, extending acceptable relationships to include, for example, altruistic strangers as donors is generally not supported, primarily because of fears of commercial incentive or psychological coercion.[6,7]

In the majority of centres, the recipient is provided with information about living donation early during the assessment process, and it is left to the discretion of the family to contact the centre should they wish to pursue living donation. An alternative strategy has been adopted in Norway, whereby the family is contacted directly by a member of the transplant team to discuss the issue. Such a strategy serves several purposes: the potential donor has access to the correct information and can discuss concerns directly with a transplant professional; the transplant candidate is not forced to confront a loved one seeking favours; and the potential donor who is unwilling to proceed further can opt out at any stage without having to provide an explanation to their relative.

INFORMED CONSENT

Written documentation of informed consent is mandatory in most countries, with the understanding that consent can be withdrawn at any time.[1] It has been recommended that donor evaluation should be under the direction of an individual who is not directly involved with the proposed transplantation or the recipient's care (an independent 'donor advocate') to avoid bias in the process.[1,6] UK guidelines advocate the use of a third party to be a spokesman for the potential donor to avoid coercion, and the British Transplantation Society also has an ethics committee for advising on difficult donor issues.[1] Likewise, a recent consensus conference in the USA recommended that an independent donor advocate should be involved in the evaluation process.[16]

Socioeconomic aspects

A disincentive to living donation is the financial burden experienced by the donor through expenses and loss of income during the evaluation and the perioperative periods. In a US survey, 23% of kidney donors reported unrecovered expenses associated with donation; similar experiences were reported in Norway.[17,18] It is very important to discuss the financial implications with the potential donor at an early stage. In some countries, including Norway and individual states in the USA, documented expenses and loss of income are potentially reimbursable. In the future, efforts should be made to minimize any financial hardship to the donor, particularly as LDK transplantation is such a cost-effective intervention for management of patients with end-stage renal failure.

SELECTION PROCESS AND PRELIMINARY MEDICAL ASSESSMENT

The ideal donor is young with no previous medical history or current illness. However, many potential donors may manifest medical conditions or risk factors that must be taken into account when evaluating candidacy for donor nephrectomy. When a potential donor is identified, a preliminary assessment should be made to identify any obvious medical or psychosocial contraindication to donation to avoid unnecessary further investigations. The assessment should include:

- Brief medical history
  - age
  - past history of diabetes, malignancy, hypertension or renal disease
  - body habitus, weight (body mass index)
  - smoking.

- Preliminary clinical and laboratory evaluation
  - blood pressure measurement
  - urine dipstick
  - ABO and human leukocyte antigen (HLA) typing
  - lymphocytotoxic crossmatching.

Contraindications to living donation arising from the preliminary assessment include extremes of age, obesity, known diabetes and significant hypertension. These are discussed in more detail later in the chapter and in Chapter 5. In many centres, ABO incompatibility is also a contraindication; this is discussed in Chapter 9.

The preliminary visit also provides an opportunity to supply the donor and recipient with written information that they can take away with them and peruse at their leisure. It is important that this information is sufficient for the donor to understand fully the risks and consequences of the donation procedure, as well as the advantages for the recipient, before consent is obtained.[1,6,7] Unfortunately, evidence from current practice suggests that written information is not reliably given to all potential donors and that the disseminated information is not uniform.[19,20] Standardization of the topics to be covered in donor brochures and further implementation of their use would be valuable to ensure minimum standards of donor understanding. Suggested topics for inclusion in such brochures are outlined in Table 4-1.

COMPLETE DONOR MEDICAL EVALUATION

Assuming no contraindications have arisen from the preliminary visit, the potential donor will undergo a complete medical evaluation. The assessment process can be organized by a dedicated transplant coordinator or specialist nurse.[1] The donor evaluation comprises a full clinical examination to assess general health as well as to look for specific issues that are relevant as part of the anaesthetic and surgical assessment. These are summarized in Table 4-2. Assessment must also include a thorough psychosocial evaluation, with the primary purpose of determining the competence of the donor in understanding the risks and implications of donor nephrectomy and thus granting consent. In the presence of overt psychiatric illness, the doctor in charge must determine adequacy of treatment and whether or not the psychiatric diagnosis compromises the consent process.[21]

On completion of the clinical examination, initial investigations are instigated as outlined in Table 4-3. Full assessment of renal function of the donor is made at this stage, providing that there are no medical contraindications to proceed. Assessment of renal anatomy is made on completion of the evaluation process as it provides essential information for surgery.

Table 4-1 Important topics for information for potential donors[19]

Recipient issues	Donor issues
Advantages of living donor transplantation:	Voluntarism versus coercion
Reduced waiting time	Medical fitness and health required
Improved graft outcome	Socioeconomic consequences
Pre-emptive transplantation	Relevant laws and regulations
Potential complications:	Time schedule for assessment
Risk of graft failure	Length of hospital stay
	Surgical technique and options
	Perioperative risk
	Postoperative course
	Sick leave
	Long-term adverse effects: medical and psychological

Table 4-2 Summary of full clinical assessment of potential living donors

History
- General health: obesity, hypertension, diabetes
- Cardiovascular risk: past medical history, family history, smoking, obesity
- History of thromboembolic events or bleeding disorders
- Respiratory risk (for anaesthesia): past medical history of asthma, chronic obstructive pulmonary disease, smoking
- Risk of renal disease: family history, (particularly if disease in recipient is familial), past history of renal infections, haematuria
- Psychiatric history

Examination
- General
- Cardiovascular
- Respiratory
- Abdominal

Table 4-3 Initial investigations for living donor assessment

Immunology screen	Blood group; HLA type; T and B cell crossmatch
Haematology screen	Full blood count; coagulation studies
Biochemistry screen	Urea and electrolytes; creatinine clearance; liver function tests; blood glucose
Urinalysis	Protein; blood; sugar; culture; microscopy
Cardiovascular	Serial blood pressure measurements; electrocardiogram
Virus screen	Hepatitis B and C; human immunodeficiency virus; cytomegalovirus infection; Epstein–Barr virus; syphilis; toxoplasma
Radiology	Chest X-ray; isotope glomerular filtration rate; renal ultrasound; angiogram/spiral computed tomography/magnetic resonance angiography

FACS, flow cytometric crossmatch; HLA, human leukocyte antigen.

INITIAL INVESTIGATIONS

HLA matching

Due to advancements in immunosuppression and the excellent results for recipients of living donor transplantation, the degree of tissue matching is no longer a major issue. Histocompatibility between donor and recipient is expressed as the degree of HLA mismatch. The mismatch from donor to recipient of three HLA antigens – A, B and DR – is described in the format of three digits. If the recipient does not receive any mismatched antigens from the donor, this is described as a '000' mismatch. A haplotype (half) match will usually be a '111' mismatch, although some common antigens may be shared. Complete mismatch is described as '222'.[1]

Long-term follow-up studies have proved that the degree of matching predicts likely length of graft survival (Figure 4-1; Table 4-4).[22,23] However, in unrelated donors, such as spouses where the match is likely to be poor, graft survival is superior to cadaveric transplantation. This may be accounted for by factors such as short cold ischaemia time and a well-functioning kidney from a healthy donor.

Selection of potential donors should therefore not depend solely on matching. For example, if a recipient has the choice of a haplotype match from a parent and a complete match from a sibling, many clinicians would advise the parent donates first as the recipient may need a further transplant later in life.[7] Likewise with spousal transplantation, a dialysis-free life for the recipient is also of benefit to the donor and outweighs poor tissue matching. However, it should be remembered, as with cadaveric transplantation, that the exposure of mismatched antigens can sensitize the recipient to future transplants.

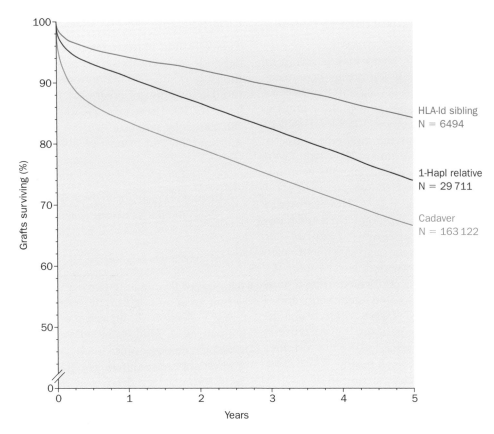

Figure 4-1 Graft survival associated with first kidney transplants (1985–2002) (courtesy of the Collaborative Transplant Study Group (CTS-K-15101-Feb2004)).[22] HLA, human leukocyte antigen.

Table 4-4 Living donor kidney transplants: unadjusted graft survival at five years (Source: OPTN/SRTR data – 1 August, 2003)[23]*

Level of HLA mismatch	N	Graft survival (%)	SE
0	1131	87.4	1.1
1	601	80.0	1.8
2	1653	77.6	1.1
3	2286	76.6	0.9
4	676	75.9	1.8
5	678	75.7	1.8
6	323	78.3	2.4
Unknown	230	75.4	3.2
Total	7578	78.6	0.5

*Cohorts are transplants performed during 1996–1997 for five-year survival.
HLA, human leukocyte antigen; SE, standard error.

Lymphocytotoxic crossmatch (T cell, B cell and FACS)

Once blood group compatibility has been established, a lymphocytotoxic crossmatch should be performed. A recipient may become sensitized to HLA types as a result of previous transplantation, pregnancy or blood transfusion. If the recipient has antibodies directed towards the potential donor HLA type, living donor transplantation has generally been precluded due to the risk of hyperacute or accelerated acute rejection.[1] However, new techniques of desensitization have made it possible to pursue successful transplantation between some donor and recipient pairs despite a positive crossmatch (see Chapter 10).

The crossmatch is performed using a sensitive assay with prolonged incubation and T and B lymphocyte target cells from the donor's blood. Furthermore, more sensitive testing may be performed using flow cytometric crossmatch (FACS). A positive FACS crossmatch is not necessarily a contraindication to transplantation, although many units would employ a regimen of stronger immunosuppression in the face of such a result.[24,25]

ASSESSMENT OF RENAL FUNCTION

Accurate measurement of kidney function during the assessment period is essential to ensure long-term adequate renal function in the donor. In addition, some studies have also suggested an impact on graft survival in the recipients of grafts from living donors who have a low glomerular filtration rate (GFR) at the time of donation.[7,9]

Measurement of renal function

Serum creatinine

Creatinine is produced from muscle at a constant rate and almost completely filtered in the glomeruli.[5] The steady-state concentration of plasma or serum creatinine depends on its excretion, which reflects GFR. However, in people with near-normal renal function, large changes in GFR correspond to only small changes in plasma creatinine.[27]

Creatinine clearance

The collection of urine over a 24-hour period depends on accuracy of sample collection by the patient and may overestimate GFR due to tubular secretion of creatinine especially at a lower GFR.[1] Creatinine clearance (CrCl) is calculated by measurement of serum creatinine and 24-hour urinary creatinine:[28]

$$\text{CrCl (mL/min)} = \frac{\text{Amount of creatinine in urine (µmol)}}{\text{Concentration in plasma (µmol/L)}} \times \frac{1000}{1440}$$

Predicted CrCl

The use of formulae to predict CrCl from the serum creatinine level removes the burden of urine collection or injection of radioisotope substances. A random blood sample and the patient's demographics such as age, height and weight are required. The most commonly used formulae are the Cockcroft–Gault equation and, more recently, the Levey formula from the Modification of Diet in Renal Disease (MDRD) trial. However, the Cockcroft–Gault formula overestimates CrCl in obese patients and those on low protein diets,[27] and the Levey formula is reported to underestimate GFR in patients with normal function.[29,30]

Isotope GFR

Due to the potential for over or underestimation of GFR by the above methods, more specific techniques are required for accurate measurement of renal function in the living donor, and such techniques are recommended. However, inulin clearance, the 'gold standard', requires continuous intravenous infusion and is not practical in most clinical settings. A radioisotope filtration marker, such as ethylenediaminetetra-acetic acid or diethylenetriaminepenta-acetic acid, can be administered by a single injection.[27] Blood samples are taken at regular intervals to estimate the GFR which can be adjusted for body surface area.

Acceptable limits

Renal function declines with age, approximately $10 \, mL/min/1.73 \, m^2$ per decade of life from the age of 40 years.[31] There is a lack of consensus about the absolute lower acceptable limit for living donors, although general recommendations suggest the lower limit for CrCl should be $80 \, mL/min/1.73 \, m^2$ and the lower limit for isotope GFR should be $70 \, mL/min/1.73 \, m^2$.[1] There is agreement that the donor's renal function should be within normal limits (and not less than two standard deviations below the mean) when adjusted for age and size (see Chapter 5).[7]

ASSESSMENT OF RENAL ANATOMY

Detailed knowledge of the renal anatomy in LDK transplantation remains important for planning the surgery. This is particularly true of laparoscopic donor nephrectomy, when the anatomy may be more difficult to appreciate at surgery than with the open technique. The primary aim of the radiological examination is to determine accurately the number, location and length of renal arteries.[32,33] Approximately 25% of potential donors have multiple arteries to one kidney and around 7% have multiple vessels to both kidneys.[34] In addition, the presence of renovascular or aortic disease, abnormalities of the renal veins and collecting systems, and parenchymal disease should be noted.[35]

Methods of assessment

Conventional angiography

The gold standard for assessment of the renal vasculature is intra-arterial angiography, either conventional or with digital subtraction (DSA).[36] DSA accurately determines the presence of multiple renal arteries but has several disadvantages: it involves administration of nephrotoxic contrast medium and radiation exposure and requires a period of several hours' inpatient recovery. Significant complications occur in 1.4% of cases and may be allergic or vascular in nature. The latter complications include haematoma, aneurysm, or distal thrombus formation.[37] An additional investigation, such as an intravenous urogram or ultrasound scan, is required to image the renal parenchyma to look for abnormalities such as cysts, tumours or calculi.

Computed tomography (CT) angiography

Due to the incidence of complications outlined above and the invasive nature of conventional intra-arterial angiography, alternative methods of assessing the renal anatomy have been sought. CT is a useful, non-invasive method of evaluating potential living donors. It is readily available at most centres and is relatively inexpensive compared with other imaging modalities. It is rapid and involves significantly lower radiation exposure than conventional angiography. CT angiography allows proper evaluation of renal arteries and veins, renal parenchyma and also the urinary tract (late phase) during a single session. The pictures may also be displayed as three-dimensional reconstruction images.[38] However, a nephrotoxic contrast medium is still required. The overall accuracy of prediction of arterial anatomy is good (>90%), but this decreases with an increasing number of renal arteries to approximately 60%.[39] Despite this, the positive predictive value of CT is high: when multiple renal arteries were seen on CT, 95.2% of patients had multiple arteries at surgery.[39] In a recent study spiral CT was used for selective determination of the GFR of each kidney. CT GFR was correlated with the standard ^{99}Tc-mercaptoacetyltriglycine (MAG3) GFR, and the results showed a good correlation between the two. It was suggested that CT may provide a single radiological diagnostic modality in living donor assessment,[40] but such an approach needs further study.

Magnetic resonance (MR) angiography

Early investigation of the role of MR angiography in evaluation of renal anatomy found that, without contrast, such techniques were unreliable in the detection of accessory renal arteries.[41] More recent studies have used gadolinium-enhanced MR angiography and have demonstrated results that are comparable with conventional and CT angiography.[42,43] Others have urged caution regarding the accuracy of MR in detecting accessory arteries,[44] and in diagnosing renal artery stenosis.[41] It should also be noted that the accuracy of MR angiography in excluding stenoses should not be judged by a study in renal donors, in whom the prevalence of renovascular disease is only 3–6%.[35] MR angiography is not validated and is probably less accurate than DSA in detecting distal stenoses and fibromuscular dysplasia (FMD). The clinical significance of FMD remains unclear: 26% of potential donors with FMD went on to develop hypertension within four to seven years, although whether this was a result of progression of FMD was not studied.[45] A more recent study has suggested that selected individuals with FMD can donate a kidney with satisfactory outcomes.[46] Other disadvantages of MR angiography are the necessity for the patient to hold their breath for several seconds and the occurrence of claustrophobia in the machine tunnel in some patients.[47] However, MR angiography has been shown to be as accurate as conventional angiography[48] and CT angiography,[47] with the advantages of avoiding exposure to ionizing radiation and the use of non-nephrotoxic contrast medium.

Summary

The use of conventional angiography in the assessment of renal anatomy in living donors can be safely replaced by contrast-enhanced CT or gadolinium-enhanced MR angiography. In many centres, conventional angiography is used only when there is some dubiety about the result from MR angiography, for example, when there is evidence of possible renal artery stenosis. Table 4-5 lists the advantages and disadvantages of each method of assessment.

RISK FACTORS AND THEIR IMPLICATIONS FOR LIVING DONATION

General risk factors

Age

It is generally accepted that children (persons under 18 years of age) should not donate, a criterion underscored at the recent Amsterdam forum.[1,6,7,10] In rare circumstances when a child might be considered as the only potential donor (such as an unaffected twin where no alternatives are available), the donor advocate, perhaps even with a legal overview, must ensure that the minor is protected.[49]

Table 4-5 Comparison of conventional, computed tomography (CT) and magnetic resonance (MR) angiography

	Advantages	*Disadvantages*
Conventional angiography	Accurate anatomical assessment	Contrast medium (nephrotoxic) Ionizing radiation Cost Bed rest required Complications: vascular, allergic Require separate investigation for parenchymal disease
CT angiography	Accurate Lower radiation exposure Rapid, cheaper Less morbidity Renal parenchymal disease identified	Intravenous contrast (nephrotoxic) Less accurate for smaller and multiple vessels
MR angiography	No ionizing radiation Non-nephrotoxic contrast medium	Breath-holding required Less ideal for identifying renal calculi

At the other end of the spectrum, setting an upper age limit for kidney donors has been difficult, related to issues of increased perioperative risk for elderly donors as well as the quality of the organ to be transplanted. Current practice varies widely. In the USA, most centres accept donors up to 70 years of age, and 3% accept even older donors.[50] Current guidelines set no upper age limit.[1,6,7] However, older donors require close attention during evaluation, in particular with regard to underlying renal function and latent cardiovascular disease or malignancy.

Obesity

Obesity is commonly defined as body mass index (BMI) over $30 \, kg/m^2$. The associated morbidity is a major health problem in the Western world, especially in the USA, and also increasingly in Europe. Obesity is a risk factor for development of diabetes, respiratory insufficiency, cardiovascular disease and also wound problems or venous embolism after surgery.[51] In a study of 107 obese donors (BMI >27), the overall complication rate (mostly wound related) was increased fivefold compared with 117 non-obese patients in whom no major complications were observed.[52] Some concern about the long-term consequences of nephrectomy was expressed by the authors due to a higher baseline blood pressure and family history of diabetes in obese donors. In a series of 871 kidney donors, a body weight over 100 kg was significantly associated with perioperative complications.[53]

Obesity is not mentioned in the US or the European guidelines. However, British guidelines regard a BMI of $30–35 \, kg/m^2$ as a relative contraindication, and recommend that those with a BMI $>35 \, kg/m^2$ should not undergo donor nephrectomy.[1]

Cigarette smoking

Smoking (current and previous) increases cardiovascular risk and is associated with perioperative cardiovascular events,[54] respiratory events,[55] and postoperative wound complications.[56] Accordingly, the British guidelines consider smoking to be a relative contraindication to kidney donation,[1] but this has not been addressed in other guidelines. There are probably few centres that would refuse kidney donation based on smoking habits alone, but consider the risk in the context of other risk factors. It appears that four to eight weeks of smoking cessation before scheduled surgery may substantially reduce the risk of complications.[56,57] In a randomized study of smoking cessation six to eight weeks before surgery, the overall complication rate (18%) was significantly lower than the rate observed in the control group (52%).[57] Therefore, any potential donor who smokes should be informed that cessation for at least four weeks before surgery reduces the risk of complications.

Medical risk factors

Hypertension

Hypertension is defined as a blood pressure higher than 140/90 mmHg.[58] The prevalence of hypertension is high and increases dramatically with age. Hypertension is a major risk factor for cardiovascular disease as well as nephrosclerosis. Consequently, blood pressure is a common reason for exclusion of donors, particularly among the elderly.[59] Although nephrectomy may not increase the incidence of hypertension, a meta-analysis of 48 studies revealed that there is probably a 2–3 mmHg increase in blood pressure after nephrectomy that would tend to increase over time.[60] According to European guidelines, well-controlled hypertension, managed with either conservative measures or antihypertensive drugs, is not considered to be an absolute contraindication for donor nephrectomy if the cardiovascular risk is otherwise low.[1,6] Although US guidelines appear somewhat more conservative, recent data have prompted consideration of potential donors with easily controlled hypertension if aged over 50, white, with normal renal function and no proteinuria.[7,61] Hypertensive and marginal donors are discussed in Chapter 5.

Diabetes

It is unknown whether unilateral nephrectomy promotes development and progression of diabetic nephropathy. Nonetheless, since diabetes mellitus is a risk factor for perioperative complications and subsequent development of chronic kidney disease, presence of either type 1 or type 2 diabetes contraindicates donor nephrectomy, as explicitly stated in all three current guidelines.[1,6,7]

Thus, exclusion of diabetes in a potential donor is critical in the medical evaluation process. Current diagnostic categories, as defined by recently published American Diabetes Association (ADA)/World Health Organization (WHO) criteria, are based on fasting blood or plasma glucose levels but may require a standard oral 75 g glucose tolerance test.[62,63] It is important to note that the values are lower for plasma than blood glucose and that the presented cut-off values are for plasma glucose measurements (Table 4-6).[62,63] The oral glucose tolerance test and measurement of glycosylated haemoglobin levels are not recommended as routine screening tests for diabetes due to cost, inconvenience and lack of sensitivity. However, a plasma glucose value below 7 mmol/L does not rule out significant glucose intolerance. A standard glucose tolerance test is required to exclude a diagnosis of diabetes and is mandatory at some centres and when other risk factors for diabetes are present. Other centres may consider a normal fasting glucose sufficient if clearly

normal.[6,7] The British guidelines define impaired fasting glucose (5.6–7.0 mmol/L) as an indication for a glucose tolerance test.[1] An oral glucose tolerance test may also reveal a condition of impaired glucose tolerance, defined as a fasting plasma glucose <7.0 mmol/L and in the range of 7.8–11.1 mmol/L after two hours. The likelihood of progression to overt diabetes after five years may be around 10%; according to the British guidelines this also contraindicates donation. The more diabetic risk factors present (including a history of gestational diabetes, older age, obesity, and a strong family history), the greater the requirement for diagnostic accuracy.

Cardiovascular disease

Clinical history or clinical signs of significant cardiovascular disease contraindicates kidney donation. More troublesome is latent or clinically silent disease, especially coronary heart disease. Older age or other risk factors such as family history of premature cardiovascular disease, smoking, male sex, hyperlipidaemia and blood pressure should be taken into consideration.[6]

High-risk patients should be screened for coronary heart disease with exercise electrocardiography (ECG) or stress nucleotide perfusion imaging (scintigraphy) or stress echocardiography. A meta-analysis of these tests performed in over 8000 patients undergoing non-cardiac vascular surgery showed that the commonly used exercise ECG had a sensitivity of about 75% as a predictor of perioperative myocardial infarction or cardiac death.[64] Stress nucleotide perfusion imaging

Table 4-6 American Diabetes Association/World Health Organization guidelines for diagnosis of diabetes and impaired fasting glucose*[62,63]

Diabetes mellitus	Fasting blood glucose (FBG) ≥126 mg/dL (7.0 mmol/L), or symptoms + casual blood glucose ≥200 mg/dL (11.1 mmol/L), or 2-hour postprandial glucose (PPG) ≥200 mg/dL after 75 g glucose load
Impaired fasting glucose	FBG >100 mg/dL (5.5 mmol/L) and <126 mg/dL (7.0 mmol/L)
Impaired glucose tolerance	2-hour PPG ≥140 mg/dL (7.8 mmol/L) and <200 mg/dL (11.1 mmol/L)

*An abnormal test should be repeated for confirmation.
To convert glucose levels from mg/dL to mmol/L, multiply by 0.05551.

(scintigraphy) and stress echocardiography were better, having a sensitivity of 85%.[64]

Anaphylaxis

Anaphylaxis and anaphylactic reactions are rare but potentially life-threatening conditions occurring during surgery. Unfortunately, such reactions frequently occur without a suspected history of allergy and the traditional risk factors (such as family history, atopy and asthma) are not valid for asssessment of such risk.[65] A review of 789 patients who experienced immune-mediated (anaphylaxis) or non-immune-mediated (anaphylactoid) reactions during surgery in 1999 revealed that two-thirds were immune mediated, 60% were due to neuromuscular blocking agents and the remainder were caused by latex or antibiotics with equal frequency.[66] Whatever the cause of such reactions during surgery, it is reasonable that a past history of such an episode should preclude future kidney donation unless the known causative agent can be avoided.

Renal risk factors

Proteinuria

Underlying renal disease must be excluded during the assessment of the potential living kidney donor. Abnormal urinary protein excretion is a marker for renal disease, increased cardiovascular disease risk, and also an independent risk factor for the progression of renal failure.[27,67–69] Thus, the accurate measurement of protein in urine is standard practice during donor assessment. The normal limit of protein excretion is <150 mg/day and albumin excretion <30 mg/day.[28] Proteinuria greater than this would indicate significant glomerular disease and usually precludes further consideration as a kidney donor, except in the case of proved orthostatic proteinuria.[1] Methods of testing for proteinuria include:

- **Dipstick urinalysis**: A simple and cost-effective method for initial screening. Most reagent strips detect only albumin. However, a recent study has suggested that qualitative testing for protein by urinalysis has high sensitivity and specificity for diagnosing or ruling out microalbuminuria. A result of trace proteinuria on dipstick analysis is usually indicative of microalbuminuria; a negative dipstick result tends to rule it out.[68]
- **24-hour urine collection**: Correctly performed 24-hour urine collection provides the most accurate assessment of protein quantity, although incomplete collection underestimates any protein leak.[1]
- **Spot analysis of the albumin**: Creatinine ratio of a single early morning urine specimen provides an accurate quantitative measurement. A ratio of <0.2 mg albumin/mg creatinine (<22 mg albumin/mmol creatinine) equates to urine albumin <0.2 g/24 hours.[27] A lower ratio may still be in the microalbuminuria range, but is, in itself, not considered as a contraindication for kidney donation.

Orthostatic proteinuria

Fixed and reproducible orthostatic proteinuria is the repeated qualitative detection of proteinuria only while the patient maintains an upright position. A 20-year follow-up evaluation study of young men with this condition showed no evidence of progressive renal disease.[70] This is a benign form of proteinuria and can be excluded by testing an early morning specimen.[27]

Pyuria and bacteriuria

If a living donor is found to have pyuria and/or bacteriuria, further investigations should be done. Urinary tract infections (UTI) and asymptomatic bacteriuria are more common in women, with about one-third having a UTI at some time. In males it is uncommon, other than in the first year of life and over the age of 60 years due to prostatic hypertrophy.[28] Pyuria is the best determinant of bacteriuria requiring therapy. Microscopy studies showing ≥8 white blood cells (WBC) per high-power field reliably predict a positive urine culture.[71]

The cause of pyuria should be established before continuing donor evaluation. If it can be confirmed pyuria is the result of an uncomplicated and reversible UTI, assessment may proceed. If the donor has a history of recurrent UTIs, or it is difficult to clear the problem, further studies such as cystocopy and intravenous pyelography should be undertaken for investigation of any underlying renal or urological abnormalities.[7]

Haematuria

Two methods are used to assess haematuria:

- **Urinary dipstick analysis**: This provides a straightforward means of detecting the presence of blood in the urine, and is routinely performed as part of the work-up for living donation. Interpretation of the results of such analyses is difficult. A few red cells can be found in some healthy people,[72] and so the concentration of detected red cells on microscopy becomes important. Studies of healthy individuals undergoing health screening suggest an incidence of asymptomatic microscopic haematuria of approximately 3% in men and 11% in women, which escalates with increasing age.[73,74] Causes of benign transient haematuria include exercise, trauma and menstruation, which can be readily excluded from a review of history and a repeated test (after one week) that is negative.
- **Urinary microscopy**: Phase-contrast microscopy of freshly voided urine is the gold standard with which results of dipstick tests should be compared. It may also reveal dysmorphic red cells and casts – signs of renal disease that cannot be assessed by dipstick testing alone. However, routine urine microscopy in the laboratory falls short of this standard. Many urinary red blood cells lyse, particularly in dilute urine, in the time between voiding and microscopy. Studies have failed to demonstrate a correlation

between results of microscopy and dipstick analysis. In one study, 49% of patients with microscopic haematuria on the basis of dipstick testing and positive microscopy were found to have an abnormal renal biopsy, in comparison with 43% of patients with haematuria on dipstick testing but not on microscopy.[75]

The diagnostic yield of investigation of microscopic haematuria depends on the age and sex of the individuals being studied. Often, no cause is found in younger individuals and the literature supports non-invasive monitoring and follow-up in this group, given the small risk of malignancy.[7] Malignancy becomes more common with increasing age, whereas young people are more likely to have renal parenchymal disease as the cause of haematuria. The diagnostic yield remains low, with one population-based study identifying only 0.5% of individuals with urological malignancy as a cause of asymptomatic microscopic haematuria.[76] However, in the context of the decision-making process of living donation, it is crucial to exclude any significant pathology. Another cause of microscopic haematuria that must be excluded is renal calculus, which has a prevalence of approximately 4% in patients with asymptomatic microscopic haematuria[77] and glomerular disease.

Having appreciated the shortcomings of the initial assessment for haematuria, it is important to note that the rate of false negative results of such tests is low. Thus a negative dipstick analysis from a potential donor requires no further investigation. In the event of a positive dipstick test, testing should be repeated. If testing is negative on three occasions, further concern is unnecessary, due to the known incidence of sporadic haematuria. Persistent microscopic haematuria requires further investigation, as outlined in the algorithm in Figure 4-2.

The methods used for investigating persistent haematuria are as follows:

- **Urinary cytology**: This allows quantification of the cellular content of the urine.

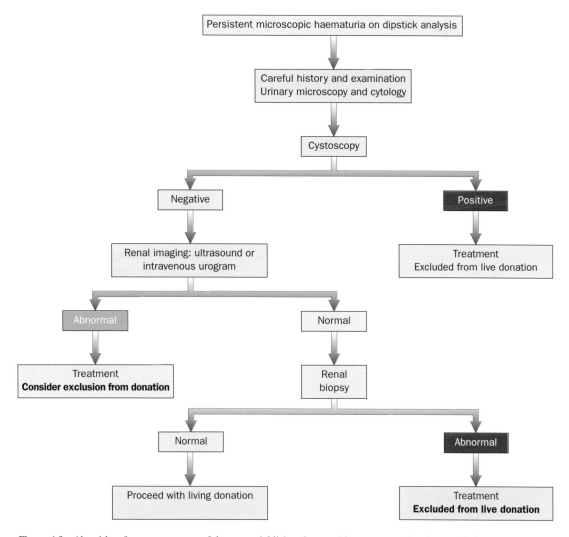

Figure 4-2   Algorithm for management of the potential living donor with asymptomatic microscopic haematuria.

- **Cystoscopy**: This is used to identify bladder mucosal abnormalities, in particular, bladder tumours that can then be treated appropriately. Such findings on cystoscopy will exclude that individual from live donation. Once significant bladder abnormalities have been excluded by negative cystoscopy, imaging of the upper urinary tract is required.
- **Upper renal tract imaging**: Renal ultrasound or intravenous urography (IVU) may be performed to visualize the kidney. IVU allows visualization of the ureters, but

is more invasive and requires an intravenous contrast medium. A CT scan may be best for overall evaluation allowing a complete anatomical assessment of the donor to be done at the same time. If these investigations are normal, a decision should be made as to whether a renal biopsy is indicated, with clear explanation to the patient of the inherent risks.
- **Renal biopsy**: Data regarding biopsy results in potential living donors are scarce. In an Egyptian study of 37 living donors with isolated microscopic haematuria, progressive

renal disease was found on biopsy in the majority: hereditary nephritis in 25, nephrolithiasis in five, bilharzial cystitis in two, isolated glomerular deposition of C3 in three and glomerular deposits of IgA and IgM in one each.[78] Whether these results apply to other populations is not clear. A survey of US transplant centres indicated that 37% are willing to accept patients with isolated microscopic haematuria if urological investigation and biopsy were negative.[50] If possible, the biopsy should be taken from the kidney that is likely to be transplanted.

If all these investigations are normal, after further discussion with the living donor–recipient pair, it would be reasonable to proceed with donation.

Nephrolithiasis

Kidney stones are common, affecting up to 5% of the population, with a lifetime risk of passing a kidney stone of about 8–10%.[79] Kidney stones are a relative contraindication to living donation because of the future risk of recurrent stones, infections and obstruction, which places the remaining kidney at an unacceptable risk.[80] In addition, the recipient may be at increased risk.[80] In one study that specifically addressed this issue, 50 patients were followed-up for longer than five years post-unilateral nephrectomy for nephrolithiasis. In total, 30% developed recurrent stones: the average number of further stones was 2.1 and the average time to recurrence was 31.1 months. Patients with metabolic stone disease had a higher recurrence rate compared with those with infection as the cause of stone formation (37% vs 13%, respectively).[81] Overall, the risk of recurrence for all types of stone is about 50% within five years.[82] This is an unacceptably high risk for living donation.

The circumstances in which an individual with a history of renal stones may be considered for living donation have been clearly defined and are as follows:

- The donor has only passed one stone.

- Stone disease has been inactive for longer than 10 years.
- No stones on current radiographic studies.
- Exclusion of metabolic abnormalities such as hyperparathyroidism and gout and other abnormalities that increase the risk of recurrent stones.[82]

Individuals should be advised of general measures that they should take to reduce the likelihood of recurrent stone formation. Such measures include increasing fluid intake to maintain a urine output of between 2 L and 3 L/day, decreasing intake of animal protein, salt and dietary oxalate (e.g. spinach, rhubarb and chocolate).[69] Such donation should go ahead only after the living donor–recipient pair have accepted the slight increased risk to the remaining kidney and possibly to the transplanted kidney. In addition, it is probably wise to transplant the kidney that had previously passed a stone.[1]

Methods used to screen living donors for renal stone disease are as follows:

- Plain X-ray often performed as part of a routine intravenous pyelogram or at the time of angiography.
- Spiral CT scan provides a sensitive method of stone detection,[83] and if this is adopted for the definition of the anatomy, the technique may also be used to detect renal stone disease.
- Ultrasound is useful for differentiating stones from a soft-tissue mass.
- 24-hour urine collection should be undertaken to screen for those at high risk of recurrent stone formation, including measurements of calcium, uric acid, and citrate excretion.

Inherited renal disease

When renal failure in the recipient is due to an inherited renal disease or there is a family history of renal disease, the focus should be on excluding the disease in the genetically related donor. Knowledge of the clinical features of the disease, age of onset and pattern of inheritance is important. Examples of such diseases are:

- Autosomal dominant adult polycystic kidney disease (ADPKD)
- Autosomal recessive juvenile PKD
- Autosomal dominant medullary cystic kidney disease
- Alport's syndrome
- Congenital nephrotic syndrome
- Vesico-ureteric reflux

In some cases, the presence of these diseases precludes transplantation from related donors.[1] The more common genetic abnormalities are considered here.

Polycystic kidney disease

Autosomal recessive juvenile PKD is not a diagnosis that is commonly made during donor evaluation, as this typically presents in infancy and is far less common than ADPKD. ADPKD occurs in 1/400 to 1/1000 live births. About one half will have the diagnosis made during their lifetime. The gene (*ADPKD1*) responsible for the majority (86–96%) of cases is located on chromosome 16; the remainder are due to an abnormal *ADPKD2* gene. The age at which the diagnosis can be made depends on the genetic defect present; the cysts are detected later in ADPKD2 than in ADPKD1.

The criteria for diagnosis of ADPKD are age dependent. In patients under 30 years of age, two cysts establish the diagnosis. The cysts may be either unilateral or bilateral. Between 30 and 59 years, at least two cysts must be present in each kidney. Over the age of 60 years, four cysts must be present in each kidney.

It is clear, therefore, that the diagnosis of PKD is based on radiological criteria and that any investigation must be highly specific and sensitive. The only alternative is genetic analysis, but this is impractical as it requires testing of two or more affected family members and from two or three generations in order to establish the linkage.[84] Ultrasound has a sensitivity of 100% in patients over the age of 30 years,[85] but carries a 10% risk of a false-negative result in younger patients.[86] Other

studies have suggested a role for CT,[87] and, more recently, magnetic resonance imaging (MRI)[84] in the assessment of younger potential donors. An alternative strategy is to exclude prospective donors who are under 30 years of age in families with PKD.[88]

In summary:

- Ultrasound is usually sufficient to diagnose ADPKD in adults over 30 years of age.
- In patients aged between 25 and 30 years, CT or MRI is indicated.
- Below the age of 25 years, genetic testing is required.

Hereditary nephritis

In families with documented evidence of hereditary nephritis, or Alport's syndrome, potential donors should be counselled with regard to the possible development of the disease. However, the genetic polymorphisms and heterogeneity of clinical presentation of Alport's syndrome make prediction of risk difficult.[89] It is most commonly inherited as an X-linked disorder of type IV collagen. Asymptomatic males do not carry the abnormality and heterozygous females are most likely to develop asymptomatic haematuria, although approximately 15% of female carriers develop end-stage renal failure.[1] In up to 15% of cases, there is no family history, suggesting a new mutation.

Screening of potential donors consists of examination for haematuria, renal function, deafness or eye abnormalities. Renal biopsy is diagnostic, but early in the course of the disease the only abnormality present may be thinning of the basement membrane, histologically similar to thin basement membrane disease, which may or may not have a more benign course.[26,90] The characteristic splitting of the basement membrane occurs in 30% of males by the age of 10 years, and in more than 90% by 30 years.[90]

In summary:

- A male relative without haematuria can be a suitable donor for a patient with hereditary nephritis.

- A female relative without haematuria may be considered a suitable donor, but if she is a carrier, it would be important to provide counselling regarding the possibility of her having a child with the disease who may require transplantation at a later stage.
- Haematuria precludes donation for both males and females.

Vesico-ureteric reflux

Vesico-ureteric reflux affects about 1% of infants and is a common reason for transplantation in young adults. A careful search for evidence of reflux or its consequences should be undertaken in any relative considering live donation. A history of enuresis or childhood urinary infections should alert the clinicians to the possibility of this condition. An isotope renal scan is a sensitive investigation for detecting renal scars, which occur as a result of reflux.[1]

FACTORS WITH RISK OF TRANSMISSION FROM DONOR

Donor malignancy

Transmission of malignancy from donor to the immunosuppressed recipient is a known risk with serious consequences in solid organ transplantation. The Council of Europe has issued guidelines on standardization of organ donor screening to prevent transmission of neoplastic diseases from multi-organ cadaveric donors. A medical history of malignancy, other than carcinoma in situ of the uterine cervix, treated low-grade, non-melanotic skin cancer or some primary brain tumours, is a contraindication to solid organ donation.[91]

It may be argued that within the living donor situation, more time is available to assess the donor with a past history of treated malignancy and screen appropriately. However, there are few data to predict the risk of disease transmission. Many types of primary malignant tumour such as breast cancer, malignant melanoma and sarcomas lead to exclusion due to risk of late recurrence.[28] If the recipient's original disease was bilateral renal cell carcinoma, there is an increased risk of transmitting familial renal cell carcinoma from a living related donor.[92] Further consideration may be given to other malignancies after a tumour-free period of 10 years,[93] however the risk/benefit balance for the recipient must be quantified and discussed with donor and recipient, though many centres would not accept such donors.

During the assessment period, the potential donor should be examined for abdominal masses, breast lumps, testicular swelling or prostate gland pathology and lymphadenopathy.[1] Information should be sought from the family practitioner concerning past medical history and may include cervical smear and mammography screening records for women. Any indication of abnormalities during the assessment process should be thoroughly investigated.

In summary, a history of malignant disease is, in most cases, a contraindication to living kidney donation, other than carcinoma in situ of the uterine cervix or treated low-grade, non-melanotic skin cancer. Careful donor examination and history taking is essential to reduce the risk of disease transmission.

Infection in the potential donor

Identification of current or previous infection in the potential donor is an important aspect of donor evaluation. The presence of active infection precludes donation. There are two areas of risk associated with donor infection: the health of the potential donor and the risk of transmission to the recipient.[1] Table 4-7 outlines the infections that are of established clinical significance.

A detailed clinical history is important and should include a psychosocial history to define 'at-risk behaviour' and information regarding residency in geographical areas where there is a high prevalence of a particular infection. Routine screening investigations will play a role in excluding infection, such as a chest X-ray for evidence of previous tuberculosis (TB), and when indicated, urine

Table 4-7 Infections of clinical significance in the donor

Viral infections	Bacterial infections	Fungal, parasitic infections
Human immunodeficiency virus	Urinary tract infections	Malaria
Human T lymphotrophic virus	*Mycobacterium tuberculosis* infection	Toxoplasmosis
Hepatitis B	Atypical *Mycobacterium* infections	Schistosomiasis
Hepatitis C	Syphilis	
Cytomegalovirus		
Varicella zoster virus		
Epstein–Barr virus		
Kaposi's sarcoma virus		
West Nile virus		

culture for TB. Specific serological tests should also be performed, as outlined in Table 4-8.[1] It is important to note that the prospective donor must be counselled prior to testing for human immunodeficiency virus (HIV), hepatitis B virus (HBV) and hepatitis C virus (HCV). Other serological tests may be undertaken, for example, for human T lymphotropic virus (HTLV), schistosomiasis and malaria, where geographically important.

Viral infections

- **HIV**: The presence of HIV or HTLV is an absolute contraindication to living donation.
- **HCV infection**: This is considered an absolute and strong contraindication to living donation by most centres, not only because of the risk of transmission of infection to the recipient, but also because the donor has a risk of developing renal complications of HCV.[94] The risk of transmission of infection from an HCV-positive

Table 4-8 Specific serological tests for living donor assessment

Donor screening	Recipient screening
HIV	HIV
CMV	CMV
EBV	VZV
HCV	EBV
HBV	HCV
Syphilis	HBV
Toxoplasmosis	

HIV, human immunodeficiency virus; CMV, cytomegalovirus; EBV, Epstein–Barr virus; HCV, hepatitis C virus; HBV, hepatitis B virus; VZV, varicella zoster virus.

donor approaches 100%.[95] An HCV polymerase chain reaction (PCR) test is recommended, as well as an HCVAb test, since HCV infection may rarely occur in seronegative individuals. A situation in which transplantation from an HCV-positive donor has been considered is in cadaveric transplantation, when the recipient is also HCV positive.[96] This cannot be recommended in the living donor situation.

- **HBV infection**: Donor infection with a positive hepatitis B antigen (HBsAg) is an absolute contraindication for transplantation. However, when HBsAg is negative, it may be considered in certain circumstances, with careful counselling of the living donor–recipient pair, although many centres would not support it. Routine serological testing of donors for HBV includes, in addition to HBsAg, anti-hepatitis B surface antibody (HBsAb) and antibody to hepatitis B core antigen (anti-HBc). HBsAb production denotes an immunological response to HBsAg and is a marker of previous infection with or effective immunization against HBV. This carries a low risk of transmission to the recipient. If such a donor is being considered, it is important to know their HBsAg status, which if positive, discloses viral replication and a high degree of infectivity,[97] thus acting as a contraindication to donation. In the event that such a donor may be considered, an HBV PCR should be performed to further exclude the risk of viral transmission. The recipient of an HBsAb-positive graft would have to

Table 4-9 Suggested use of prophylactic antimicrobial agents

HBV-positive donor (see text)	Vaccinate recipient with HBV immunoglobulin
CMV (donor positive to negative recipient)	Prophylactic antivirals
EBV (donor positive to negative recipient)	Prophylactic antivirals: aciclovir or ganciclovir
Toxoplasmosis	Sulfonamide, clindamycin or clarithromycin
Mycobacterial infection	Prophylactic isoniazid

HBV, hepatitis B virus; CMV, cytomegalovirus; EBV, Epstein–Barr virus.

have mounted an effective response to immunization against HBV, and use of HBV immunoglobulin and antiviral therapy should be considered (Table 4-9).[1] However, this has addressed the issue of likelihood of transmission of infection to the recipient without consideration of potential risks to the donor of developing extra-hepatic complications secondary to hepatitis B.[98] The living donor–recipient pair will require careful counselling.

- **Cytomegalovirus (CMV) infection**: This is one of the widely distributed herpes group of viruses, with a prevalence that increases with age, such that 40% of the population are infected by the age of 20 years and 80% by the age of 60.[99] The latent virus may be transmitted with kidney donation, causing primary CMV infection in seronegative recipients. This infection can easily be treated in the recipient with antiviral drugs (see Table 4-9), used either prophylactically or pre-emptively during viral surveillance.[100–104]

- **Primary Epstein–Barr virus (EBV) infection**: This is most likely to occur in EBV-negative paediatric recipients who receive a kidney from an EBV-positive donor. Ninety-eight percent of the adult population is EBV-positive, and because EBV is often acquired early in childhood, this is a relatively uncommon problem. Nevertheless, the consequences of transmitting EBV from donor to recipient or acquiring primary EBV post-transplantation are serious, with a significant risk of post-transplantation lymphoproliferative disorders (PTLD). Recommendations for management in this situation include: antiviral prophylaxis with aciclovir or ganciclovir (see Table 4-9) for a period of up to

six months post-transplantation, subsequent monitoring of EBV status and further treatment with antiviral therapy or reduction of immunosuppression.[105] The living donor–recipient pair must be counselled about the risks and consequences of developing PTLD.

- **Varicella zoster virus (VZV)**: The occurrence of VZV antibodies in the donor carries no risk of transfection. On the other hand, it is very important to know whether the potential recipient is VZVAb-positive, since a primary infection may be rapidly fatal in an immunocompromised host. If an individual is seronegative, they should be vaccinated prior to receiving a transplant.

Bacterial infections

The main risk of transmissible bacterial infection is from *Mycobacterium tuberculosis*, and donors should be screened for this, with a careful history and chest X-ray. If there is evidence of invasive TB adequate eradication therapy for TB is a prerequisite for future donation. If a specific bacterial infection has been diagnosed in the donor, treatment with the appropriate antibiotic regimen should be effective in preventing transmission (see Table 4-9).

CONCLUSION

In summary, evaluation of the potential living donor must be thorough and comprehensive, with the primary aim of ensuring that the risk to the donor is minimized with maximum benefit to the recipient. This chapter outlined the medical evaluation process and discussed common risk factors. In addition, a practical outline of investigation of common problems that arise during living donor evaluation was provided with supporting evidence.

REFERENCES

1. Working Party of the British Transplantation Society and the Renal Association. United Kingdom Guidelines for living donor kidney transplantation. London: British Transplantation Society, 2000: 1–82.
2. Jakobsen A, Albrechtsen D, Leivestad T. Renal transplantation – the Norwegian model. *Ann Transplant* 1996; **1**: 32–35.
3. US Renal Data System. *USRDS 2003 Annual Data Report: Atlas of End-stage Renal Disease in the United States.* Bethesda, MD: National Institutes of Health, National Institute of Diabetes and Digestive and Kidney Diseases, 2003.
4. Lumsdaine JA, Wigmore SJ, Forsythe JLR. Live kidney donor assessment in the UK and Ireland. *Br J Surg* 1999; **86**: 877–881.
5. Delmonico F. The consensus statement of the Amsterdam Forum on the Care of the Live Kidney Donor. *Transplantation* 2004; **78**: 491–492.
6. EBPG Expert Group on Renal Transplantation. European best practice guidelines for renal transplantation (Part 1). *Nephrol Dial Transplant* 2000; **15**(suppl 7): 47–58.
7. Kasiske BL, Ravenscraft M, Ramos EL et al. The evaluation of living renal transplant donors: clinical practice guidelines. Ad Hoc Clinical Practice Guidelines Subcommittee of the Patient Care and Education Committee of the American Society of Transplant Physicians. *J Am Soc Nephrol* 1996; **7**: 2288–2313.
8. Kim YS, Moon JI, Kim DK et al. Ratio of donor kidney weight to recipient bodyweight as an index of graft function. *Lancet* 2001; **357**: 1180–1181.
9. Norden G, Lennerling A, Nyberg G. Low absolute glomerular filtration rate in the living kidney donor: a risk factor for graft loss. *Transplantation* 2000; **70**: 1360–1362.
10. Najarian JS, Chavers BM, McHugh LE, Matas AJ. 20 years or more of follow-up of living kidney donors. *Lancet* 1992; **340**: 807–810.
11. Lennerling A, Forsberg A, Meyer K, Nyberg G. Motives for becoming a kidney donor. *Nephrol Dial Transplant* 2004; **10**: 1–6.
12. Prasad S, Russ G, Faull R. Live donor renal transplantation in Australia 1964–1999: an evolving practice. *Intern Med J* 2002; **32**: 569–574.
13. Humar A, Durand B, Gillingham K et al. Living unrelated donors in kidney transplants: better long-term results than with non-HLA-identical living related donors? *Transplantation* 2000; **69**: 1942–1945.
14. Park K, Kim SI, Kim YS et al. Results of kidney transplantation from 1979 to 1997 at Yonsei University. *Clin Transpl* 1997: 149–156.
15. Foss A, Leivestad T, Brekke IB et al. Unrelated living donors in 141 kidney transplantations: a one-center study. *Transplantation* 1998; **66**: 49–52.
16. Abecassis M, Adams M, Adams P et al. Consensus statement on the live organ donor. *JAMA* 2000; **284**: 2919–2926.
17. Smith MD, Kappell DF, Province MA et al. Living-related kidney donors: a multicenter study of donor education, socioeconomic adjustment, and rehabilitation. *Am J Kidney Dis* 1986; **8**: 223–233.
18. Westlie L, Leivestad T, Holdaas H et al. Report from the Norwegian National Hospitals Living Donor Registry: one-year data, January 1, 2002. *Transplant Proc* 2003; **35**: 777–778.
19. Westlie L, Fauchald P, Talseth T et al. Quality of life in Norwegian kidney donors. *Nephrol Dial Transplant* 1993; **8**:1146–1150.
20. Lennerling A, Nyberg G. Written information for potential living kidney donors. *Clin Transpl* 2004: (in press).
21. Gaston RS, Thomas C. Psychosocial and psychiatric issues in renal transplantation. In: Weir MR (ed) *Medical Management of Kidney Transplantation.* Philadelphia: Lippincott Williams & Wilkins, 2005; 231–237.
22. www.ctstransplant.org.
23. www.optn.org.
24. Sonnenday CJ, Ratner LE, Zachary AA et al. Pre-emptive therapy with plasmapheresis/intravenous immunoglobulin allows successful live donor renal transplantation in patients with a positive cross-match. *Transplant Proc* 2002; **34**: 1614–1616.
25. Jordan SC, Vo A, Bunnapradist S et al. Intravenous immune globulin treatment inhibits crossmatch positivity and allows for successful transplantation of incompatible organs in living-donor and cadaver recipients. *Transplantation* 2003; **76**: 631–636.
26. Van Paassen P, van Breda Vriesman PJ, van Rie H, Tervaert JW. Signs and symptoms of thin basement membrane nephropathy: a prospective regional study on primary glomerular disease – The Limburg Renal Registry. *Kidney Int* 2004; **66**: 909–913.
27. Johnson RJ, Feehally J. *Comprehensive Clinical Nephrology.* Harcourt Publishers, 2000.
28. Haslett C, Chilvers ER, Boon NA et al. *Davidson's Principles of Medicine.* Edinburgh: Churchill Livingstone, 2002.
29. Stoves J, Lindley EJ, Barnfield MC et al. MDRD equation estimates of glomerular filtration rate in potential living kidney donors and renal transplant recipients with impaired graft function. *Nephrol Dial Transplant* 2002; **17**: 2036–2037.
30. Bertolatus JA, Goddard L. Evaluation of renal function in potential living kidney donors. *Transplantation* 2001; **71**: 256–260.
31. Gonwa TA, Atkins C, Zhang YA et al. Glomerular filtration rates in persons evaluated as living-related donors – are our standards too high? *Transplantation* 1993; **55**: 983–985.

32. Spring D, Salvatierra O Jr, Palubinskas AJ et al. Result and significance of angiography in potential kidney donors. *Radiology* 1979; **133**: 45–47.

33. Walker T, Geller S, Delmonico F et al. Donor renal angiography: its influence on the decision to use the right or the left kidney. *Am J Roentgenol* 1988; **151**: 1149–1151.

34. Weinstein S, Navarre R, Loening S, Corry R. Experiences with live donor nephrectomy. *J Urol* 1980; **124**: 321–323.

35. Frick M, Goldberg M. Uro- and angiographic findings in a 'normal' population: screening of 151 symptom free potential transplant donors for renal disease. *Am J Roentgenol* 1980; **134**: 503–505.

36. Flechner S, Sandler C, Houston G et al. 100 living-related kidney donor evaluations using digital subtraction angiography. *Transplantation* 1985; **40**: 675–678.

37. Egglin T, O'Moore P, Feinstein A, Waltman A. Complications of peripheral arteriography, a new system to identify patients at risk. *J Vasc Surg* 1995; **22**: 787–794.

38. Watarai Y, Kubo K, Hirano T et al. Intravenous digital subtraction angiography and helical computed tomography in evaluation of living renal donors. *Int J Urol* 2001; **8**: 417–422.

39. Janoff D, Davol P, Hazzard J et al. Computerized tomography with 3-dimensional reconstruction for the evaluation of renal size and arterial anatomy in the living kidney donor. *J Urol* 2004; **171**: 27–30.

40. El-Diasty T, Shokeir A, El-Ghar M et al. Contrast enhanced spiral computerized tomography in live kidney donors: a single session for anatomical and functional assessment. *J Urol* 2004; **171**: 31–34.

41. Gourlay W, Yucel E, Hakaim A et al. Magnetic resonance angiography in the evaluation of living-related renal donors. *Transplantation* 1995; **60**: 1363–1366.

42. Buzzas G, Shield III C, Pay N et al. Use of gadolinium-enhanced, ultrafast, three-dimensional, spoiled gradient-echo magnetic resonance angiography in the preoperative evaluation of living renal allograft donors. *Transplantation* 1997 **64**: 1734–1737.

43. Bakker J, Ligtenberg G, Beek F et al. Preoperative evaluation of living renal donors with gadolinium-enhanced magnetic resonance angiography. *Transplantation* 1999; **67**: 1167–1172.

44. Vallet C, Bettschart V, Meuli R et al. Preoperative assessment of laparoscopic live kidney donors by gadolinium-enhanced magnetic resonance angiography. *Transplant Proc* 2002; **34**: 795–796.

45. Cragg A, Smith T, Thompson B et al. Incidental fibromuscular dysplasia in potential renal donors: long-term clinical follow-up. *Radiology* 1989; **172**: 145–147.

46. Kolettis P, Bugg C, Lochkhart M et al. Outcomes for live donor renal transplantation using kidneys with medial fibroplasia. *Urology* 2004; **63**: 656–659.

47. Halpern E, Mitchell D, Wechsler R et al. Preoperative evaluation of living renal donors: comparison of CT angiography and MR angiography. *Radiology* 2000; **216**: 434–439.

48. Giessing M, Krencke T, Taupitz M et al. Gadolinium-enhanced three-dimensional magnetic resonance angiography versus conventional digital subtraction angiography: which modality is superior in evaluating living kidney donors? *Transplantation* 2003; **76**: 1000–1002.

49. Delmonico FL, Harmon WE. The use of a minor as a live kidney donor. *Am J Transplant* 2002; **2**: 333–336.

50. Bia MJ, Ramos EL, Danovitch GM et al. Evaluation of living renal donors. The current practice of US transplant centers. *Transplantation* 1995; **60**: 322–327.

51. Flancbaum L, Choban PS. Surgical implications of obesity. *Annu Rev Med* 1998; **49**: 215–234.

52. Pesavento TE, Henry ML, Falkenhain ME et al. Obese living kidney donors: short-term results and possible implications. *Transplantation* 1999; **68**: 1491–1496.

53. Johnson EM, Remucal MJ, Gillingham KJ et al. Complications and risks of living donor nephrectomy. *Transplantation* 1997; **64**: 1124–1128.

54. Gedebou TM, Barr ST, Hunter G et al. Risk factors in patients undergoing major nonvascular abdominal operations that predict perioperative myocardial infarction. *Am J Surg* 1997; **174**: 755–758.

55. Schwilk B, Bothner U, Schraag S, Georgieff M. Perioperative respiratory events in smokers and non-smokers undergoing general anaesthesia. *Acta Anaesthesiol Scand* 1997; **41**: 348–355.

56. Chang DW, Reece GP, Wang B et al. Effect of smoking on complications in patients undergoing free TRAM flap breast reconstruction. *Plast Reconstr Surg* 2000; **105**: 2374–2380.

57. Moller AM, Villebro N, Pedersen T, Tonnesen H. Effect of preoperative smoking intervention on postoperative complications: a randomised clinical trial. *Lancet* 2002; **359**: 114–117.

58. World Health Organization, International Society of Hypertension Writing Group. 2003 World Health Organization (WHO)/International Society of Hypertension (ISH) statement on management of hypertension. *J Hypertens* 2003; **21**: 1983–1992.

59. Riehle RA Jr, Steckler R, Naslund EB et al. Selection criteria for the evaluation of living related renal donors. *J Urol* 1990; **144**: 845–848.

60. Kasiske BL, Ma JZ, Louis TA, Swan SK. Long-term effects of reduced renal mass in humans. *Kidney Int* 1995; **48**: 814–819.

61. Textor SC, AbuAttieh M, Mahale A et al. Predictive differences and misclassification between clinic, ambulatory, and hypertension nurse blood pressure measurements in kidney recipients one year after transplantation [abstract]. *Am J Transplant* 2004; **4**(suppl 8): 546.

62. Expert Committee on the Diagnosis and Classifica-

tion of Diabetes Mellitus. Report of the expert committee on the diagnosis and classification of diabetes mellitus. *Diabetes Care* 2003; **26**(suppl 1): S5–S20.

63. Expert Committee on the Diagnosis and Classification of Diabetes Mellitus. Follow-up report on the diagnosis of diabetes mellitus. *Diabetes Care* 2003; **26**: 3160–3167.

64. Kertai MD, Boersma E, Bax JJ et al. A meta-analysis comparing the prognostic accuracy of six diagnostic tests for predicting perioperative cardiac risk in patients undergoing major vascular surgery. *Heart* 2003; **89**: 1327–1334.

65. Fisher MM, Doig GS. Prevention of anaphylactic reactions to anaesthetic drugs. *Drug Saf* 2004; **27**: 393–410.

66. Mertes PM, Laxenaire MC, Alla F, Groupe d'Etudes des Reactions Anaphylactoides Peranesthesiques. Anaphylactic and anaphylactoid reactions occurring during anesthesia in France in 1999–2000. *Anesthesiology* 2003; **99**: 536–545.

67. Tryggvason K, Pettersson E. Causes and consequences of proteinuria: the kidney filtration barrier and progressive renal failure. *J Intern Med* 2003; **254**: 216–224.

68. Atkins RC, Briganti EM, Zimmet PZ, Chadban SJ. Association between albuminuria and proteinuria in the general population: the AusDiab Study. *Nephrol Dial Transplant* 2003; **18**: 2170–2174.

69. Sam R, Shayka MS, Pegoraro AA et al. The significance of trace proteinuria. *Am J Nephrol* 2003; **23**: 483–484.

70. Springberg PD, Garrett LE, Thompson AL et al. Fixed and reproducible orthostatic proteinuria: results of a 20-year follow-up study. *Ann Intern Med* 1982; **97**: 516–519.

71. Young JL, Soper DE. Urinalysis and urinary tract infection: update for clinicians. *Infect Dis Obstet Gynecol* 2001; **9**: 249–255.

72. Addis T. The number of formed elements in the urinary sediment of normal individuals. *J Clin Invest* 1926; **2**: 409–415.

73. Carel R, Silverberg D, Kaminsky R, Aviram A. Routine urinalysis (dipstick) findings in mass screening of healthy adults. *Clin Chem* 1987; **33**: 2106–2108.

74. Iseki K, Iseki C, Ikemiya Y, Fukiyama K. Risk of developing end-stage renal disease in a cohort of mass screening. *Kidney Int* 1996; **49**: 800–805.

75. Topham P, Harper S, Furness P et al. Glomerular disease as a cause of isolated microscopic haematuria. *Q J Med* 1994; **87**: 329–335.

76. Mohr D, Offord K, Owen R, Melton L. Asymptomatic microhaematuria and urological disease. *JAMA* 1986; **256**: 224–229.

77. Khadra M, Pickard R, Charlton M et al. A prospective analysis of 1930 patients with haematuria to evaluate current diagnostic practice. *J Urol* 2000; **163**: 524–527.

78. Sobh M, Moustafa F, el-Din Saleh M et al. Study of asymptomatic haematuria in potential living related kidney donors. *Nephron* 1993; **65**: 190–195.

79. Asplin J, Favus M, Coe F. Nephrolithiasis. In: Brenner B. (ed) *Brenner and Rector's The Kidney*. Philadelphia: Saunders, 1996: 1893–1895.

80. Kar P, Popili S, Hatch D. Renal transplantation: donor with renal stone disease. *Clin Nephrol* 1994; **42**: 347–348.

81. Lee Y, Huang W, Chang L et al. The long-term recurrence rate and renal function change in unilateral nephrectomy urolithiasis patients. *J Urol* 1994; **152**: 1386–1388.

82. Parmar M. Kidney stones. *BMJ* 2004; **328**: 1420–1424.

83. Smith R. Acute flank pain: comparison of non-contrast enhanced CT and intravenous urography. *Radiology* 1995; **194**: 789–794.

84. Zand M, Strang J, Dumlao M et al. Screening a living kidney donor for polycystic disease using heavily T2-weighted MRI. *Am J Kidney Dis* 2001; **37**: 612–619.

85. Ravine D, Gibson R, Walker R et al. Evaluation of ultrasonographic diagnostic criteria for autosomal dominant polycystic kidney disease. *Lancet* 1994; **343**: 824–827.

86. Nicolau C, Torra R, Badenas C et al. Autosomal dominant polycystic kidney disease types 1 and 2: assessment of US sensitivity for diagnosis. *Radiology* 1999; **213**: 273–276.

87. Levine E, Grantham J. The role of computed tomography in the evaluation of adult polycystic kidney disease. *Am J Kidney Dis* 1981; **1**: 99–105.

88. Bay W, Hebert L. The living donor in kidney transplantation. *Ann Intern Med* 1987; **106**: 719–727.

89. Lemmink HH, Schroder CH, Monnens LA, Smeets HJ. The clinical spectrum of type IV collagen mutations. *Hum Mutat* 1997; **9**: 477–499.

90. Rumpelt H. Correlation of clinical data with glomerular basement membrane alterations. *Clin Nephrol* 1980; **13**: 203–207.

91. Council of Europe Guidelines. Standardisation of organ donor screening to prevent transmission of neoplastic diseases. Council of Europe, 1997.

92. Cohen F.L. Familial bilateral renal cell carcinoma in a prospective living related donor. *Mt Sinai J Med* 1994; **61**: 70–71.

93. Penn I. Donor transmitted disease: cancer. *Transplant Proc* 1991; **23**: 2629–2631.

94. Johnson RJ, Gretch D, Yamabe H et al. Membranoproliferative glomerulonephritis associated with hepatitis C virus infection. *N Engl J Med* 1993; **328**: 465–470.

95. Pereira BJ, Milford EL, Kirkman RL et al. Prevalence of hepatitis C virus RNA in organ donors positive for hepatitis C antibody and in the recipients of their organs. *N Engl J Med* 1992; **327**: 910–915.

96. Natov S, Pereira B. Transmission of viral hepatitis by

kidney transplantation: donor evaluation and transplant policies (Part 2: hepatitis C virus). *Transplant Infect Dis* 2002; **4**: 124–131.

97. Natov S, Pereira B. Transmission of viral hepatitis by kidney transplantation: donor evaluation and transplant policies (Part 1: hepatitis B virus). *Transplant Infect Dis* 2002; **4**: 117–123.

98. Davis CL. Evaluation of the living kidney donor: current perspectives. *Am J Kidney Dis* 2004; **43**: 508–530.

99. British Transplantation Guidelines for the prevention and management of cytomegalovirus disease after solid organ transplantation. 2004: London: British Society for Histocompatibility and Immunogenetics, Leeds and London: British Transplantation Society.

100. Lowance D, Neumayer H, Legendre C et al. Valaciclovir for the prevention of cytomegalovirus disease after renal transplantation. International Valaciclovir Cytomegalovirus Prophylaxis Transplantation Study Group. *New Engl J Med* 1999; **340**: 1462–1470.

101. Newstead C. Cytomegalovirus and Epstein-Barr virus following solid organ transplantation. In: Forsythe JLR (ed) *Transplantation Surgery: Current Dilemmas* Philadelphia: WB Saunders, 2001.

102. Hart G, Paya C. Prophylaxis for CMV should now replace pre-emptive therapy in solid organ transplantation. *Rev Med Virol* 2001; **11**: 73–81.

103. Emery V. Prophylaxis for CMV should not now replace pre-emptive therapy in solid organ transplantation. *Rev Med Virol* 2001; **11**: 838–836.

104. Sagedal S, Nordal KP, Hartmann A et al. Pre-emptive therapy of CMVpp65 antigen positive renal transplant recipients with oral ganciclovir: a randomized, comparative study. *Nephrol Dial Transplant* 2003; **18**: 1899–1908.

105. Ellis D, Jaffe R, Green M et al. Epstein-Barr virus-related disorders in children undergoing renal transplantation with tacrolimus-based immunosuppression. *Transplantation* 1999; **68**: 997–1003.

Living kidney donors with isolated medical abnormalities: the SOL-DHR experience 5

Gilbert T Thiel, Christa Nolte, Dimitrios Tsinalis

INTRODUCTION

Transplant professionals traditionally define optimal living kidney donors as those who are younger than 65 years of age, with a creatinine clearance (CrCl) $\geq 80\,\text{mL/min}$ (standardized for a body surface area of $1.73\,\text{m}^2$) and normal body habitus (body mass index (BMI) $<30\,\text{kg/m}^2$), glucose tolerance, blood pressure and urinalysis.[1] In reality, however, highly motivated potential donor candidates do not always fulfil all of these requirements.

Extending donor selection criteria beyond the generally defined rules may be hazardous and requires that donors be fully informed about additional risks. The problem is made more difficult by a paucity of data that can be used to quantify the added extra risk. It is true that a plethora of long-term follow-up data exist, but they are retrospective, incomplete and, most importantly, are not related to specific risk factors before donation (e.g. obesity, hypertension or age).[2–23] As such, potential donor candidates with one or more added risks are usually informed on the basis of data inappropriate to address the issue(s) at hand.

In this chapter we will attempt to quantify the risks for donor candidates who present with one or more pre-existing risk factors. The analysis is based on data collected by the Swiss Organ Donor Health Registry (SOL-DHR) over a 10-year period (1993–2003). Reference will also be made to published data that help define long-term risks associated with nephrectomy. Approaches for evaluation and acceptance of donors under more standard circumstances are discussed in Chapter 4.

DONORS, METHODS AND DEFINITIONS

The SOL-DHR contains prospective and sequential data for all living kidney donors managed at all six Swiss transplant centres. In November 2003, the database contained pre- and post-nephrectomy information (1, 3, 5, 7 and 10 years) on 631 donors. We analysed these data in an attempt to understand better the factors that influence donor outcomes, particularly in subjects with renal and cardiovascular risk factors (age >65 years, BMI $>30\,\text{kg/m}^2$, CrCl $<80\,\text{mL/min}$, hypertension or albuminuria) prior to nephrectomy. We also sought to determine whether the use of strict selection criteria results in better outcomes for donors, and which preoperative variables predicted an uncomplicated course at five years after nephrectomy.

The analysis of donors with known renal and cardiovascular risk factors was confined to those with complete 5-year follow-up data for each variable. This group included 171 donors (115 females and 56 males) with a mean follow-up of 6.2 ± 1.5 years (range 5–10 years). Seventy-two donors (42%) had at least one risk factor, 29 of whom had more than one risk factor; the remaining 99 donors (58%) did not have any of the mentioned risks. Data from 583 prospective kidney donors of all ages were used to calculate the projected decline in CrCl due to aging; for calculation of the mean loss of CrCl after nephrectomy, data from 353 actual donors were included.

All chemical analyses were performed in the same laboratory (Viollier AG, Basel), using the same methodology for measurement of creatinine and albumin in serum and urine. Creatinine was measured by Jaffé's technique (Roche Diagnostica). Urine albumin was measured using a polyclonal antibody technique (Roche Diagnostica) in spot urine. CrCl was calculated as a transformation of the measured serum value, using Dettli's modified formula adapted by him later to serum creatinine levels determined by enzymatic technique:[24]

$$CrCl = (150 - age) \times body\ weight \times$$

$$\left(\frac{gender\ factor\ (0.9\ for\ females\ and\ 1.1\ for\ males)}{serum\ creatinine\ [\mu mol/l]} \right)$$

Albuminuria was defined as urine albumin >5 mg/mmol creatinine, which corresponds to approximately 50 mg urine albumin/24 h. Expressed per gram of creatinine instead of mmol, this corresponds to >44 mg albumin/g creatinine and is slightly higher than >30 mg/g creatinine as proposed by the National Kidney Foundation Practice Guidelines.[25]

Blood pressure was determined as the mean value of three forearm measurements at an ambulatory examination. Hypertension was defined as a mean diastolic blood pressure >90 mmHg or maintenance therapy with antihypertensive agents, a definition enabling comparison of Swiss data with Swedish data classified by the same criteria (see Chapter 7). Elevated systolic pressure alone was also recorded and used in the multivariate analysis.

WHAT IS THE MINIMAL CLEARANCE REQUIRED FOR KIDNEY DONATION?

The 171 donors with complete 5-year follow-up were divided into three groups according to their CrCl before nephrectomy (Table 5-1):

- Group I (n=124) – good function (>80 mL/min/1.73 m^2)
- Group II (n=27) – borderline function (70–80 mL/min/1.73 m^2)
- Group III (n=20) – low function (<70 mL/min/1.73 m^2).

Table 5-1 Living donor characteristics before and five years after nephrectomy

	Group I (n=124)	Group II (n=27)	Group III (n=20)
Demographics			
Age (years)	46 ± 11 (25–68)	58 ± 7 (47–72)	61± 8 (44–80)
>60 years	15 (12%)	7 (26%)	11 (55%)
Female	74 (60%)	24 (89%)	17 (85%)
Before nephrectomy			
Serum creatinine (μmol/L)	82 ± 13 (54–120)	84 ± 8 (71–100)	96 ± 15 (72–129)
CrCL (mL/min/1.73 m^2)	101 ± 16 (81–143)	76 ± 3 (70–79)	65 ± 5 (52–69)
Hypertensive	15 (12%)	9 (33%)	7 (35%)
Albuminuria (>5 mg/mmol)	5 (4%)	4 (15%)	1 (5%)
ACEI or ARA therapy	4 (3%)	4 (15%)	3 (15%)
5 years post-nephrectomy			
Serum creatinine (μmol/L)	105 ± 16 (74–172)	106 ± 19 (66–155)	115 ± 17 (91–158)
CrCl (mL/min/1.73 m^2)	76 ± 15 (43–116)	58 ± 11(40–88)	52 ± 11(31–79)
Hypertensive (%)	31 (25%)	8 (30%)	10 (50%)
Albuminuria (>5 mg/mmol)	7 (6%)	6 (22%)	1 (5%)
ACEI or ARA therapy	17 (14%)	5 (18%)	4 (20%)

All values are mean ± standard deviation (range).
Group I, good renal function (>80 mL/min/1.73 m^2); group II, borderline function (70–80 mL/min/1.73 m^2); group III, low function (<70 mL/min/1.73 m^2).
CrCl, creatinine clearance; ACEI, angiotensin-converting enzyme inhibitor; ARA, angiotensin-receptor antagonist.

Groups II and III comprised mostly female subjects (~87%); about one-third were hypertensive, 15% had microalbuminuria before nephrectomy and 34% were females over 60 years of age. The change in renal function in all three groups over a 7-year period is shown in Figure 5-1. The initial decline in CrCl was smaller in group III (23%) than in group II (26%) or group I (28%). This suggests that the capacity for early functional adaptation (i.e. hyperfiltration accomplished by changes in glomerular haemodynamics) is well maintained even in donors with lower renal function (group III) and higher age. Thereafter, the improvement in CrCl was best in group I followed by group II. In group III, almost no further improvement was apparent.

The mechanism for further functional recuperation after initial adaptation to nephrectomy (given a finite number of nephrons) is believed to be achieved by hypertrophy of single nephrons, producing an increase in the glomerular filtration surface area (via stretching of podocytes which cannot divide and multiply) and hyperplasia of tubular cells (tubular epithelium can divide and multiply). The driving force for these changes is thought to be ongoing hyperfiltration, but the factors involved are not yet fully recognized.

In group III, antihypertensive drug use (i.e. angiotensin-converting enzyme inhibitors (ACEI) and angiotensin-receptor antagonists (ARAs)) before nephrectomy was five times higher than in group I and remained higher afterwards. The lack of CrCl improvement in group III donors might, therefore, be interpreted as successful protection against hyperfiltration as a result of appropriate pharmacological treatment. A more negative interpretation would be that only minimal functional reserve remains

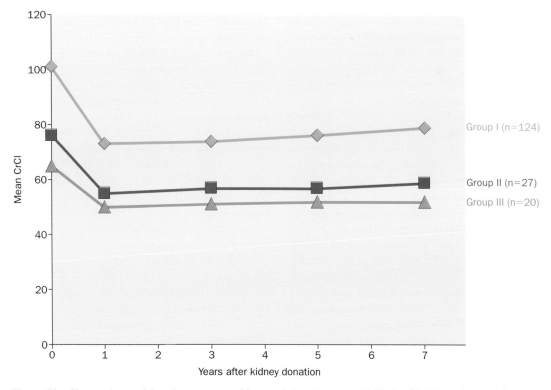

Figure 5-1   Changes in renal function, as assessed by creatinine clearance (CrCl), in 171 kidney donors followed-up for seven years after nephrectomy (stratified by baseline values). Group I, good renal function (>80 mL/min/1.73 m²); group II, borderline function (70–80 mL/min/1.73 m²); group III, low function (<70 mL/min/1.73 m²).

following nephrectomy due to pre-existing hypertrophy of the remnant nephrons. Thus, following the initial haemodynamic adaptation in these donors, there may be inadequate functional reserve to compensate for age-related nephron loss over the next 30–40 years of life. Since the youngest person in group III was 44 years old at the time of donation, and some former kidney donors in the USA are now in need of transplantation themselves,[26] this interpretation raises concern particularly for younger donors with borderline low renal function.

Life expectancy is, therefore, an important consideration if the criterion regarding CrCl for donor acceptance is to be lowered to $<80 \, mL/min/1.73 \, m^2$. Clearly, the lowest acceptable CrCl cannot be the same for both a 20- and a 70-year-old person. With a life expectancy of at least 60 years, the younger donor needs more renal reserve.

The estimation of adequacy of renal reserve begins with defining the expected physiological decline in CrCl associated with aging. Using SOL–DHR-derived data from 583 living donors (390 females and 193 males) prior to nephrectomy (i.e. based on two functioning kidneys), the average loss in CrCl is $1.00 \, mL/min/year$ in males and $0.85 \, mL/min/year$ in females (Figure 5-2A and B). Data on the expected decline in renal function after unilateral nephrectomy are more difficult to obtain. A Scandinavian study in 348 donors followed for 12 ± 8 years after donation,[8] and data from Germany in 87 donors followed for 11 ± 1 years after nephrectomy,[19] indicate that the annual loss of CrCl following nephrectomy is also approximately $1 \, mL/min$. Accelerated loss of renal function was not reported in the Swedish analysis,[8] however, both studies were cross-sectional (single point examinations) and neither used standardized laboratory techniques. Our analysis of the SOL-DHR data showed no decline in CrCl with aging in the first five to seven years after nephrectomy, either in the group with initial low clearance (group III, see Figure 5-1) or in donors older than 65 years at the time of donation (see below and also Figure 5-9 later in this chapter).

The apparent lack of age-dependent decline of CrCl in the first years after nephrectomy is incomprehensible. Indeed, one might expect the opposite (i.e. a more rapid deterioration as a consequence of hyperfiltration). It may be that functional hyperfiltration is obscuring the normal ongoing process of 'morphological' aging in the kidney. It remains uncertain as to whether these trends will continue indefinitely, or whether, especially in older adults, adverse effects will become evident in the future. To address this issue, we assumed that CrCl declines over time at a usual rate of $1 \, mL/min/year$ and that most donors will survive to the age of 80 years. Although Swedish data indicate donors may survive longer than the general population, the former is a realistic assumption. In Switzerland, two-thirds of current donors are healthy females (mean age 50.1 ± 11.0 years) and mean life expectancy for such persons is currently 34.5 additional years. The mean age of male donors is 49.1 ± 12.0 years, with an average life expectancy of 32.5 additional years.

Rather than a fixed limit on adequacy of renal function for donor acceptance, we calculated a 'minimal creatinine clearance required' (MCCR) before donation in order to ensure that CrCl at age 80 was at least $40 \, mL/min/1.73 \, m^2$. After broad discussions with nephrologists and a gerontologist in Switzerland, we considered a CrCl of $40 \, mL/min$ to be adequate to maintain fluid and electrolyte homeostasis and for the donor to remain independent of a need for calcitriol and erythropoietin supplementation at the age of 80 a second calculation was made targeting a CrCl of at least $30 \, mL/min/1.73 \, m^2$ at the age of 80, which we thought to be the absolute minimum acceptable voluntarily for an elderly person (but which may necessitate some intervention to maintain normal, age-related quality of life).

In order to determine the MCCR, we used the SOL-DHR data to obtain the average loss of renal function during the first year after nephrectomy. The mean decline in CrCl after nephrectomy was relatively stable over all age groups, being 27% in males and 25% in

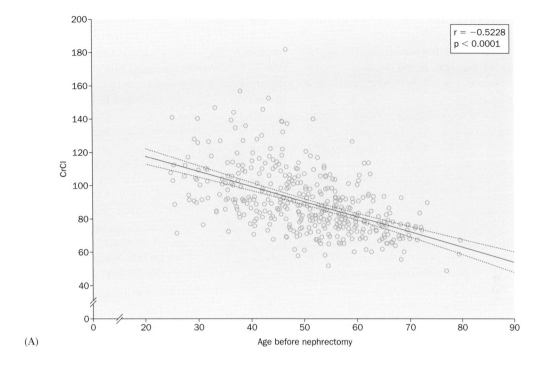

(A)

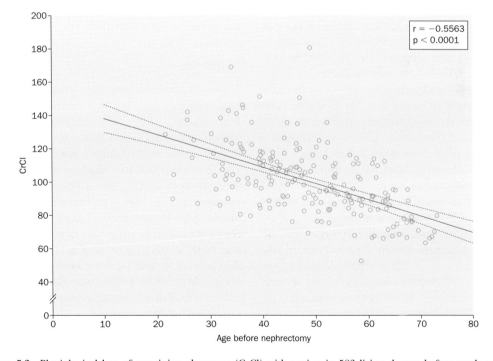

(B)

Figure 5-2 Physiological loss of creatinine clearance (CrCl) with ageing in 583 living donors before nephrectomy (390 females and 193 males). Mean loss in CrCl by age: (A) 0.85 mL/min/year in females; (B) 1.00 mL/min/year in males (p<0.0001 for both). CrCl corrected for 1.73 m² body surface area.

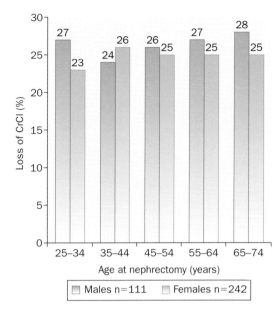

Figure 5-3 Percentage loss of creatinine clearance (CrCl) due to nephrectomy, stratified by age. Mean decline in CrCl in males = 27% and in females = 25%.

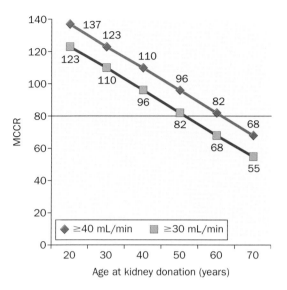

Figure 5-4 Minimal creatinine clearance required (MCCR) before nephrectomy to obtain a creatinine clearance of 30 or 40 mL/min/1.73 m^2 at age 80, estimated from living donors in the SOL-DHR from 1993 to 2003.

females (Figure 5-3). There was a trend towards an increased loss in CrCl in males older than 65, but for ease of calculation 27% was used for both sexes and all ages. The formula used to calculate MCCR is shown in Table 5-2 and a nomogram for determining MCCR at different ages is given in Figure 5-4. For example, a 30-year-old potential donor would require a CrCl of at least 123 mL/min/1.73 m^2 to maintain a clearance of at least 40 mL/min/1.73 m^2 at 80 years old. However, for a 70-year-old donor, the MCCR would be as low as 68 mL/min/1.73 m^2. The formula failed in two of the oldest donors because the loss of renal function due to nephrectomy was exceptionally high and was not compensated for by hyperfiltration (see below).

These arguments and calculations do not incorporate the impact of projected outcomes in the kidney recipients. Indeed, poor renal function and small mass of the donated kidney may each exert a negative impact on long-term graft survival, especially in younger recipients.[27] Alternatively, a kidney from a small and slim 70-year-old female may be sufficient when donated to her uraemic husband of similar age and size to provide a decade of good-quality life for both.

Summary

It is evident from the data presented above that it makes little sense to use a fixed limit for MCCR. The conventional limit of >80 mL/min/1.73 m^2 fails to adequately define donor acceptability, being too low for young donors and too high for older ones. In determining MCCR, two aspects need to be considered: (i) the life expectancy of the donor (ensuring adequate renal function in older age); and (ii) the kidney recipient's age and body weight (good donor renal function is required for young recipients with a large body surface area). The formula used to calculate MCCR has been based on hypothetical, but reasonable, assumptions. It utilizes the observed age-related decline in CrCl in patients with two kidneys and assumes that the decline in CrCl after nephrectomy will continue unchanged (1 mL/min/year). Although at present this assumption is not well documented, the increasing number of

Table 5-2   Example calculations of minimal creatinine clearance (CrCl) required (MCCR)

Definitions	
CC_{y0}	CrCl immediately before nephrectomy
CC_{nx1}	CrCl 1 year post-nephrectomy (nephrectomy = nx)
CC_{nx80}	CrCl at 80 years of age
AD	Age difference between 80 and age at nephrectomy
NF	Nephrectomy factor (27% loss = 0.73)
$MCCR_{40}$	Minimal CrCl required before nx to maintain donor CrCl at age of 80 of $\geq 40\,mL/min/1.73\,m^2$

Derivation	
Step 1	Calculation of $CC_{nx1} = CC_{y0} \times NF$
	$CC_{nx1} = CCy0 \times 0.73$
Step 2	Calculation of $CC_{nx80} = CC_{nx1} - (AD \times 1mL/min$ predicted loss per year)
	$CC_{nx80} = (CCy0 \times 0.73) - (AD \times 1\,ml/min) = (CCy0 \times 0.73) - AD$
Step 3	Calculation of $MCCR_{40} = (CCy0 \times 0.73) - AD = 40\,mL/min/1.73\,m^2$
	Transformation: $CCy0 = (40\,mL/min/1.73\,m^2 + AD)/0.73$

Final formula	
	$MCCR_{40} = (40\,mL/min/1.73m^2 + AD)/0.73$

Example	
	Calculation of $MCCR_{40}$ for a 60-year-old donor:
	$MCCR_{40} = (40\,mL/min/1.73\,m^2 + 20)/0.73 = \mathbf{82\,mL/min/1.73\,m^2}$

donors and duration of follow-up in the SOL-DHR should enable us to refine the calculations in years to come.

DONORS WITH PRE-EXISTING HYPERTENSION

Prior to 1990, potential donors with hypertension were usually rejected in Switzerland. Based on the absence of evidence that unilateral nephrectomy impedes treatment of hypertension, an expert panel from the Swiss League Against High Blood Pressure ultimately supported using donors with well-controlled hypertension, provided there was no evidence of target organ damage (microalbuminuria, left ventricular hypertrophy, retinopathy).[28] More recently, a single study of 24 donors who were hypertensive prior to kidney donation found no adverse effects at one year post-nephrectomy and concluded that selected hypertensive candidates can be accepted for renal donation.[29]

Among the 171 donors in our analysis, 29 (17%) were hypertensive before nephrectomy. Despite the recommendation of the expert panel, three of the hypertensive donors also had slight microalbuminuria. Eight of the 26 without microalbuminuria were receiving antihypertensive therapy with either ACEI or ARAs, which may have masked proteinuria. This group of hypertensive donors was, on average, 10 years older than their normotensive counterparts (58±9 vs 48±11 years). During the 5-year follow-up, 8/29 (28%) hypertensive donors became normotensive without any treatment, suggesting that the diagnosis of hypertension may have been erroneous. These findings support those of Textor et al, i.e. candidates should not be excluded as donors on the basis of hypertension diagnosed from office-based readings, particularly those based on automated devices in donors older than 50 years.[30] Textor et al's recommendation that 24-hour blood pressure monitoring or a similar approach is needed for accurate decision making appears reasonable.

In the SOL-DHR, hypertension was well controlled at five years post-nephrectomy in 41% (12/29) of these donors. The reason for persistent hypertension despite treatment in six other donors (21%) may have been suboptimal use of antihypertensive agents (too low dosage). Mean CrCl at five years was 61 ± 14 mL/min among the 29 hypertensive donors and 72 ± 17 mL/min in the normotensive donors, findings that are within the expected range given the 10-year age difference between the groups. Furthermore, the decline in CrCl during the first year after nephrectomy was similar among normotensive (24%) and hypertensive (26%) donors. Three of the 29 hypertensive donors (10%) did not take any antihypertensive medication; one of these donors developed albuminuria at three years post-nephrectomy. This progressed in parallel with a steadily deteriorating CrCl (45 mL/min) after 10 years of follow-up.

An interesting observation from the 5-year data is that antihypertensive drug use was up to three times higher among donors who were hypertensive before donation than among those who developed hypertension after nephrectomy (Figure 5-5). Thus, potential donors with hypertension should be advised of the potential need for more intensive antihypertensive therapy after nephrectomy. While exacerbation of hypertension is not causally related to nephrectomy, the risk of developing progressive glomerular damage due to untreated hypertension may be (see Chapter 7). For this reason, hypertensive individuals known to be non-compliant with medical treatment should not be accepted as kidney donors.

The percentage of donors with albuminuria at five years was three times higher among hypertensive (6/29; 21%) than normotensive (8/142; 6%) donors, but the magnitude of albumin excretion in those with hypertension was low (mean 7.7 mg/mmol); this was less than half the amount seen at five years among normotensive donors who later acquired hypertension (21.2 mg/mmol). This difference may be due to the fact that 48% (14/29) of initially hypertensive donors were receiving ACEI or ARAs at five years post-nephrectomy compared with 11% (15/142) of initially normotensive donors.

Summary

Our results, with limited follow-up, indicate that moderate hypertension alone may not

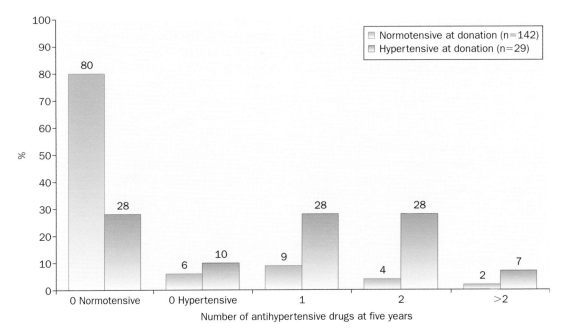

Figure 5-5 Number of drugs used to control hypertension at five years post-nephrectomy. Of those not receiving antihypertensive drugs at 5 years, most were normotensive, but some hypertensive.

pose a significant hazard to the kidney. Donor candidates with hypertension can be accepted if blood pressure is well controlled, microalbuminuria is absent compliance with treatment is good and the candidate is aware of/accepts the fact that he or she may need ongoing antihypertensive treatment is rising quantity. Regular medical follow-up and access to antihypertensive drugs are required. If these prerequisites cannot be met, hypertensive candidates should not be considered for kidney donation. Potential donors with newly diagnosed hypertension should undergo 24-hour blood pressure monitoring or similar procedures to confirm or reject the diagnosis. Any potential donor with end-organ damage attributable to hypertension must be excluded.

DONORS WITH PRE-EXISTING MICROALBUMINURIA

As noted in Chapter 7, albuminuria is a more reliable outcome measure than proteinuria. Data from the Heart Outcomes Prevention Evaluation (HOPE) study indicate that even low levels of microalbuminuria (>2 mg/mmol) are a risk factor for cardiovascular events in individuals with or without diabetes.[31–33]

Based on our definition of microalbumin-uria (urine albumin >5 mg/mmol creatinine), 5% (8/171) of donors had microalbuminuria prior to donation (mean 8.1±3.2 mg/mmol); none of these donors had microhaematuria. Comparison of these donors with the 163 without initial microalbuminuria showed the only difference between the two groups was the frequency of hypertension before donation, which was more than twice as common among donors with initial microalbuminuria (38% vs 16%; Table 5-3). After five years, albuminuria persisted in only one of these donors: despite treatment with an ACEI, albumin excretion was 5.8 mg/mmol. Even in the presence of pre-existing proteinuria (>15 mg/mmol), both albuminuria and proteinuria normalized in all others. Three donors were accepted despite pre-existing hypertension and microalbumin-uria. Albumin excretion normalized or improved in two with ACEI/ARA therapy. However, in the oldest of the three donors (a 68-year-old male), CrCl decreased from 79 to 44 mL/min at one year post-nephrectomy and remained low at five years. His hypertension was not normalized until the third year, and elevated blood pressures proved difficult to control in the other two despite administration of as many as four antihypertensive agents. Warning against the acceptance of hypertensive donors with microalbuminuria seems well justified.

Table 5-3   Five-year follow up of living donors with microalbuminuria prior to nephrectomy

	Normal (Urinary albumin ≤5 mg/mmol; n = 163)	Microalbuminuria (Urinary albumin >5 mg/mmol; n = 8)
Age at donation (years)	50 ± 11	51 ± 11
Female	109 (67%)	6 (75%)
CrCl (mL/min/1.73 m²)		
Year 0	93 ± 20	91 ± 19
Year 5	70 ± 17	68 ± 17
Albuminuria		
Year 0	0	100
Year 5	13 (8%)	1 (12%)
Hypertension		
Year 0	26 (16%)	3 (38%)
Year 5	45 (28%)	3 (38%)
ACEI or ARA therapy		
Year 0	10 (6%)	1 (12%)
Year 5	26 (16%)	3 (38%)

CrCl, creatinine clearance; ACEI, angiotensin-converting enzyme inhibitor; ARA, angiotensin-receptor antagonist.

Among the seven donors who later developed clinically relevant microalbuminuria (>20 mg/mmol), only one had had microalbuminuria before nephrectomy. Thus, pre-existing mild microalbuminuria was of limited value in predicting the future development of relevant albuminuria. There was no sex imbalance among donors with pre-donation microalbuminuria, but among those who later developed relevant microalbuminuria (>20 mg/mmol) and proteinuria (>30 mg/mmol), there was a predominance of male subjects (71% vs 33% males in the population as a whole).

Summary

Our findings indicate that mild microalbuminuria (5–15 mg/mmol) (documented in at least two consecutive urine samples) in the absence of microhaematuria, hypertension or obvious renal or systemic disease is not a strict exclusion criterion for renal donation. However, in potential donors who are relatives of the proposed recipient, microalbuminuria should be considered an initial sign of underlying kidney disease. In these circumstances, evaluation should be undertaken by an experienced nephrologist and extensive diagnostic evaluation, including renal biopsy, may be indicated. If no apparent reason for microalbuminuria is found, an observation period of at least 12 months is recommended before accepting the donor. In the presence of albuminuria and co-existing hypertension, donor nephrectomy is discouraged. Overall, the experience to date in the SOL-DHR with pre-existing microalbuminuria is too limited to support any other recommendation.

PRE-EXISTING OBESITY (BMI >30 kg/m^2) OR DIABETES

One in 20 donors in the SOL-DHR was obese prior to nephrectomy; at five years post-nephrectomy, the incidence of obesity had almost tripled to 14%. Donors were stratified into three groups based on pre-donation BMI (kg/m^2): <25 (n=96); 25–30 (n=66); and >30

(n=9). The analysis indicated that BMI decreased over the 5-year period in half the donors with a pre-donation BMI of >30 kg/m^2. However, at year 5, the number of donors with a BMI >30 kg/m^2 had increased to 24, of whom 19 had a BMI of 25–30 kg/m^2 prior to donation. The age (50±8.5 years) and sex distribution (71% female) of these obese donors were similar to the entire donor population.

Donors with a body weight >100 kg have been reported to have a significantly increased operative complication rate.[12] Only one of the nine obese Swiss donors in our analysis weighed more than 100 kg at the time of nephrectomy, and no particular postoperative complications were observed.

We attempted to investigate whether nephrectomy in obese donors is accompanied by an accelerated loss of renal function and occurrence of proteinuria, as suggested recently by Praga et al.[34] Our analysis of SOL-DHR data found no differences in 5-year prospective CrCl values between any of the three BMI groups, nor in the 24 donors who became obese after five years (Figure 5-6). A similar scenario was observed with regard to the incidence of albuminuria. Of note, however, was the finding that more than half with a BMI >30 kg/m^2 at donation or at five years were also hypertensive (Figure 5-7).

The reason why hypertension was not accompanied by a higher rate of albuminuria is probably explained by antihypertensive treatment (ACEI or ARA) use in a third of the donors with a BMI >30 kg/m^2 at five years. The high incidence of hypertension among obese subjects is well recognised. Since unilateral nephrectomy in obese subjects may also increase the risk of hypertensive renal damage, especially if hypertension is not appropriately treated, access to long-term medical care is of utmost importance in obese donors.[35]

Another potential risk in obese donors is the development of diabetes. Obesity alone increases the risk of type 2 diabetes. If an obese donor continues to gain weight after nephrectomy, the risks of developing hypertension, diabetes and hyperlipidaemia increase still further, with all three variables

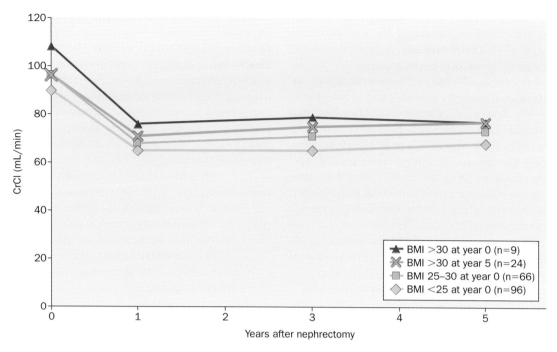

Figure 5-6   Effect of body mass index (BMI in kg/m²) on creatinine clearance (CrCl) in 171 living kidney donors followed for five years.

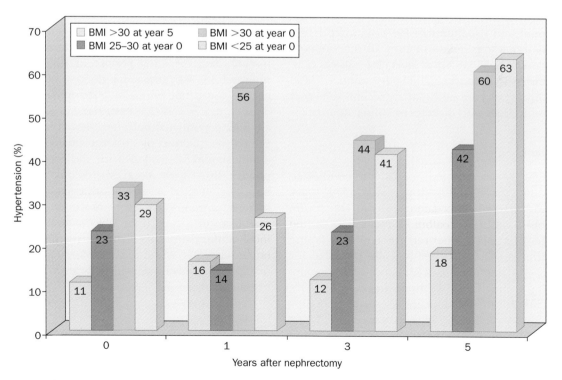

Figure 5-7   Relation between body mass index (BMI in kg/m²) and hypertension in 171 living kidney donors followed for five years.

exerting a potentially synergistic negative impact on the remaining kidney. Only two donors in the SOL-DHR registry developed diabetes so far. One was a 33-year-old female with a BMI of $36.5\,kg/m^2$ before donation; she developed diabetes mellitus during pregnancy in the third year, at which point her BMI had increased to $45.4\,kg/m^2$. The other was a 59-year-old male with a BMI of $27\,kg/m^2$ at donation who developed diabetes after his BMI had increased to $29\,kg/m^2$ in the fifth year. The overall follow-up in the SOL-DHR is too limited to evaluate at present the long-term incidence of new-onset diabetes in obese donors.

It is a mistake to accept any donor candidate with insulin-dependent diabetes. There was one such case in the SOL-DHR: a 66-year-old insulin-dependent male, who donated a kidney to his female partner. The argument in favour of accepting him has been the lack of hypertension, micro-albuminuria and retinopathy before nephrectomy despite more than a decade of insulin treatment. After three years however, the donor developed hypertension (172/92 mmHg), profound albuminuria (110 mg/mmol) and deteriorating renal function. In our opinion, good renal function and the absence of microalbuminuria, hypertension and retinopathy are not valid arguments to accept individuals with diabetes as kidney donors.

Summary

Obesity per se is not an absolute contraindication for renal donation. Nevertheless, transplant teams should be reluctant to accept obese people as donors. Obese donors should be informed regarding risks of developing hypertension, diabetes and the potential for accelerated decline of function in the remaining kidney. Those without access to ongoing clinical care and appropriate medical therapy should not donate. Without exception, donor candidates with diabetes should be rejected.

MICROHAEMATURIA

The decision of whether to accept a donor candidate with microhaematuria very much depends on its cause, which can range from residual vaginal blood related to menstruation to renal stones to kidney or urinary tract tumour, glomerulonephritis, hereditary renal disease, thin basement membrane syndrome etc. Consistent dysmorphic erythrocyturia is usually regarded as a sign of glomerulopathy and therefore a reason to exclude the candidate from donating.

The SOL-DHR data concerning microhaematuria before renal donation do not unfortunately distinguish between dysmorphic and non-dysmorphic erythrocyturia. Isolated microscopic haematuria (>10 cells per high power field, without evidence of microalbuminuria) was present in four of the 171 donors. In all but one case erythrocyturia disappeared post-nephrectomy.

A '1+' positive dipstick test for haemoglobinuria was reported in 11 of the 171 donors prior to nephrectomy. Post-nephrectomy tests were negative for five of these donors, and alternated between positive and negative for the other six. None of the 11 donors had initial microalbuminuria, but two developed microalbuminuria, one during the first year and one during the seventh year. A '2+' positive dipstick was reported in two additional donors prior to nephrectomy, but normalized afterwards. The dipstick test is very sensitive, but not specific enough. A positive dipstick test should be confirmed by microscopic urinary analysis. No donor should be excluded on the base of a positive dipstick test alone. Microscopic hematuria documented in several urine samples is, however, a good reason to exclude the candidate from donating. Even if a usually benign renal abnormality like thin basement membrane syndrome is the cause for hematuria, it may be rarely associated with progressive renal dysfunction later on.[36]

Summary

Microhaematuria found in kidney donor candidates may indicate significant pathology within the urinary tract, and adequate diagnostic work-up is required to determine the reason for bleeding. Potential donors with kidney or urinary tract tumours or stone disease with high recurrence rate should be rejected.[37] A biopsy may be necessary to eliminate important intrarenal pathology, especially if there is any suggestion of hereditary renal disease. In all cases, extreme caution is in order.

DONORS OLDER THAN 65 YEARS

There are three reasons why one should be reluctant to accept kidneys from elderly donors:

- the higher morbidity rate in the perioperative phase
- the potential for coexistence of a small malignancy in the donated kidney, which

may be difficult to detect and then emerge to the detriment of an immunosuppressed recipient
- inadequate renal function to provide long-lasting benefit in the recipient.

It is likely, especially in a younger recipient, that progressive nephron loss associated with aging will continue in grafts from old donors regardless of how young the recipient is, and complications will ensue. However, kidney donation from an older person to another older person, is often an excellent option, prolonging quality of life and expressing 'togetherness' in couples of advanced age or between older siblings with strong emotional ties. Furthermore, evidence from a Collaborative Transplant Study analysis has

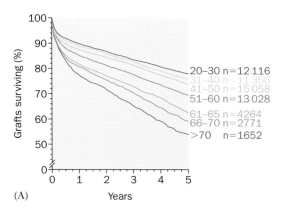
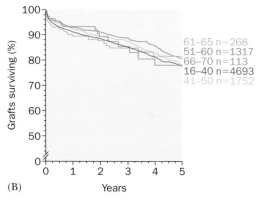

Figure 5-8 Effect of donor age on kidney graft survival in (A) deceased donors (1995–2003) and (B) living-unrelated donors: a Collaborative Transplant Study analysis (data kindly provided by G Opelz).

Table 5-4 Comparison of living donors >65 and <45 years of age at nephrectomy with regard to creatinine clearance, hypertension and albuminuria

	<45 years (n=55)		>65 years (n=14)	
	Pre-nx	5 years post-nx	Pre-nx	5 years post-nx
CrCl (mL/min/1.73 m²)				
Mean ± SD	108 ± 18	82 ± 16	72 ± 10	49 ± 10
Range	67–143	53–116	55–95	31–65
Decrease at 5 years		24 ± 13%		32 ± 17%
Hypertension	2 (4%)	3 (5%)	6 (43%)	11 (79%)
Albuminuria				
>5 mg/mmol (%)	2 (4%)	2 (4%)	1 (7%)	4 (29%)
Range (mg/mmol)	0.2–10.0	0.2–67.4	1.2–7.4	0.2–71.5

CrCl, creatinine clearance; nx, nephrectomy.

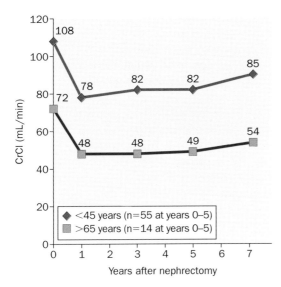

Figure 5-9 Seven-year follow-up of creatinine clearance (CrCl; mL/min/1.73 m²) in young (<45 years; n=55) and elderly (>65 years; n=14) living kidney donors.

shown that, in contrast with deceased donors, transplant survival rates with kidney grafts from living donors are not negatively affected by increasing age (Figure 5-8A and B; G Opelz, personal communication in December 2004).

In the SOL-DHR, 8% (14/171) of donors were older than 65 years of age (mean 69±4 years) at the time of donation. The major differences (Table 5-4) between this group and those <45 years of age were:

• a larger decline in CrCl
• a substantially greater frequency of hypertension before and five years after nephrectomy
• a seven times greater prevalence of microalbuminuria at five years.

Comparison of the mean CrCl demonstrated that clearance is much lower in the older age group, but the slope after nephrectomy is parallel (Figure 5-9). In general, no accelerated decline in CrCl due to advanced aging or hypertension was seen in the elderly donors up to seven years post-nephrectomy.

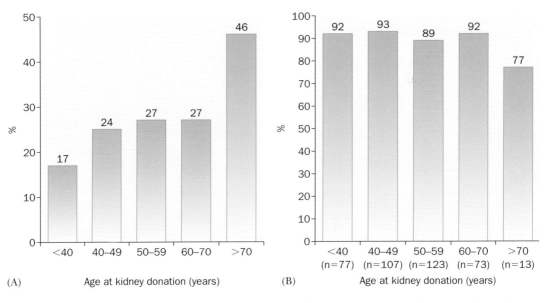

Figure 5-10 Early complications in 393 kidney donors followed for five years after nephrectomy: effect of age at nephrectomy: (A) incidence of all early complications across the age groups; (B) proportion of donors free from important early complications.

The worst cases were two elderly female donors, aged 71 and 80 years at nephrectomy, in whom CrCl almost halved following kidney removal. Thereafter, clearance decreased at a rate of 1.25–2.75 mL/min/year until year 5. If this rate of decline were to remain unchanged, end-stage renal failure (CrCl ≤5 mL/min/1.73 m^2) would be reached after another 9 years in the 80-year-old donor (who would then be 94 years of age) and in 20 years in the 71-year-old donor (who would then be 96 years of age).

Perioperative complications appear to be commoner in elderly donors. We analysed a cohort of 393 kidney donors in the SOL-DHR in whom early postoperative complications were recorded. In the 13 donors over 70 years of age, the risk of developing any complication was between 19 and 29% higher than in younger donors (Figure 5-10A). Considering only important complications (e.g. severe bleeding necessitating blood transfusions, chyloperitoneum, myocardial infarction, relevant depression), the risks were 7–11% in younger donors but 23% in donors older than 70 years (Figure 5-10B).

SUMMARY

Age above 65 years is not a strict contraindication for renal donation, but caution is indicated. The "old for old" concept achieves strikingly better results in living than in cadaveric donation and is an attractive solution for life partners in advanced age. The medical work-up before accepting an older donor should be more extensive, including adequate tests for coronary disease and malignancy. The elderly incur a higher risk of acute complications during or early after surgery. Treatment of hypertension is mandatory and older donors known not to tolerate antihypertensive drugs should not be accepted.

POTENTIAL BENEFITS OF APPLYING CONSERVATIVE DONOR SELECTION CRITERIA

The conservative selection criteria defined for the analysis were as follows:

- CrCl ≥80 mL/min/1.73 m^2
- Age ≤65 years
- BMI ≤30 kg/m^2
- No albuminuria (≤5 mg urine albumin/mmol urine creatinine)
- No hypertension (diastolic blood pressure ≤90 mmHg and no antihypertensive treatment)
- No diabetes (normal blood glucose).

Three categories describing the clinical course during the first five years post-nephrectomy ('perfect', 'moderate' and 'worrisome') are defined in Table 5-5. A perfect

Table 5-5 Three categories of clinical course after kidney donation (restricted to blood pressure, renal function and albuminuria)

Category	Definition
Perfect	• Good function of the remaining kidney: CrCl ≥56 mL/min/1.73 m^2* • No albuminuria (urine albumin/urine creatinine ≤5 mg/mmol)[†] • No hypertension (diastolic blood pressure ≤90 mmHg and no antihypertensive treatment)[‡]
Moderate	• Deteriorating renal function: CrCl 45–55 mL/min/1.73 m^2; or • Slight albuminuria (5–15 mg/mmol)[§] • Easily controllable hypertension: diastolic blood pressure ≤100 mmHg
Worrisome	• Deteriorating renal function: CrCl <45 mL/min/1.73 m^2 or serum creatinine >160 µmol/L; or • Albuminuria >15 mg/mmol[¶]; or • Hypertension with diastolic blood pressure >100 mmHg with or without antihypertensive treatment

*56 is derived from a pre-donation CrCl of 80 mL/min/1.73 m^2 less 30%; [†]equivalent to <50 mg albumin/24 h urine; [‡]excluding hypertension during the first 4 weeks after nephrectomy; [§]corresponding to 50–150 mg albumin/24 h urine; [¶]corresponding to >150 mg albumin/24 h urine.

Table 5-6   Characteristics of donors with a perfect or worrisome 5-year course after nephrectomy, as presented before donation

Characteristics before nephrectomy	Perfect course (n = 74)	Worrisome course (n = 33)	p value
Age at donation (years)	42 ± 10 (25–63)	57 ± 10 (31–80)	<0.0001
Donors >65 years	0	8 (24%)	<0.0001
Female	49 (66%)	20 (61%)	
BMI (kg/m²)	24 ± 3 (17–36)	25 ± 3 (20–32)	
BMI >30kg/m²	2 (3%)	3 (9%)	
Serum creatinine (μmol/L)	82 ± 12 (54–120)	87 ± 13 (69–119)	
Serum creatinine >120 μmol/L	0	0	
CrCl (mL/min/1.73 m²)	102 ± 18 (69–143)	86 ± 19 (55–124)	<0.0005
CrCl <80mL/min/1.73 m²	6 (8%)	15 (45%)	<0.0001
History of hypertension			
SBP (mmHg)	118 ± 11 (90–148)	133 ± 18 (100–185)	<0.0001
DBP (mmHg)	74 ± 9 (46–93)	82 ± 14 (57–113)	<0.001
SBP >140 mmHg	1 (1%)	10 (30%)	0.0001
DBP >90 mmHg	2 (3%)	7 (21%)	<0.005
Hypertensive	2 (3%)	11 (33%)	<0.0001
Treated for hypertension	0	6 (18%)	<0.001
Two antihypertensive agents	0	3 (9%)	<0.05
Criteria fulfilled			
All fullfilled	62 (84%)	9 (27%)	<0.0001
One missed	12 (16%)	10 (33%)	
Two missed	0	10 (33%)	<0.0001
Three missed	0	3 (9%)	<0.05
Four missed	0	1 (3%)	

All values are mean ± SD (range).
BMI, body mass index; CrCl, creatinine clearance; SBP, systolic blood pressure; DBP, diastolic blood pressure.
*Conservative selection criteria before donation fulfilled.

course after nephrectomy was documented for 74/171 (43%) donors; 57% experienced either a moderate (n=64, 38%) or worrisome (n=33, 19%) course. The pre-nephrectomy characteristics of the donors in the perfect and worrisome groups are compared in Table 5-6.

When trying to identify those destined to have a perfect course using the six selection criteria stated above (Table 5-7), 73 donors (43%) would have been rejected for donation and 98 (57%) would have been selected. The sensitivity of this approach would have been 84% (identifying 62 of 74 donors with a perfect course) but the specificity only 63% (62 of 98 included donors showed a perfect clinical course). The high rate of 37% false inclusions (36 of 97 donors showing a non-perfect clinical course would have been included) indicates that even applying all six conservative selection criteria does not ensure safety. Indeed, over one-third of

donors selected using these criteria may require medical intervention within 5–10 years of donation. At the other extreme is the rate of 16% false exclusions (12 of 74 donors having a perfect clinical course would have been excluded) or one out of 6.

The next step in the analysis was to examine whether applying fewer than six criteria offered greater predictability. Applying criteria for CrCl (≥80 mL/min) and no hypertension only, 109 donor candidates would have been accepted and 62 rejected (Table 5-8). The sensitivity for identifying donors with perfect outcomes was 89% (66/74), so eight (11%) of the 74 candidates who achieved a perfect follow-up would not have been accepted. More importantly, the rate of false inclusions increased to 44% inclusions (43 of 97 donors with a non-perfect course would be included), rendering this approach of little value.

Multivariate analysis of variance and classi-

Table 5-7 Attempt to identify donors with a perfect clinical course using all six conservative selection criteria

	Perfect clinical course	Non-perfect clinical course	Total
Donors matching all six criteria	62	36	98
Donors not matching all six criteria	12	61	73
Total	74	97	171

Table 5-8 Attempt to identify donors with a perfect clinical course using 'CrCl ($\geqslant$80 mL/min)' and 'no hypertension' criteria only

	Perfect clinical course	Non-perfect clinical course	Total
Donors matching both criteria	66	43	109
Donors not matching both criteria	8	54	62
Total	74	97	171

Table 5-9 Attempt to identify donors with a perfect clinical course using the three criteria derived from multivariate analysis (CrCl 82 mL/min; diastolic blood pressure 83 mmHg; age 56 years)

	Perfect clinical course	Non-perfect clinical course	Total
Donors matching all three criteria	59	14	73
Donors not matching all three criteria	15	83	98
Total	74	97	171

fication-tree techniques were applied to the complete set of pre-nephrectomy data (including systolic blood pressure) to define criteria and cut-off points with highest significance in identifying those donors destined to experience perfect and non-perfect outcomes. Three significant ($p<0.0001$) criteria emerged from this analysis:

- CrCl $\geqslant$ 82 mL/min
- Diastolic blood pressure $\leqslant$ 83 mmHg
- Age $\leqslant$ 56 years

The use of these three cut-off points (Table 5-9) would decrease the sensitivity for identifying perfect donors only slightly to 80% (59 of all 74 with a perfect course), but the rate of falsely-included donors would roughly be cut to one third or 14% (14 of 97). However, adopting these criteria would still result in every seventh donor needing a careful medical follow-up and in falsely excluding 20% (15 of 74) of donors who achieved a perfect course after nephrectomy.

Summary

From the data collected prior to donation, it was not possible to predict a perfect 5-year outcome with sufficient sensitivity and specificity and, more importantly, with an acceptable rate of false inclusions or exclusions of potential donors. There is no simple and guaranteed algorithm for donor selection. The use of fixed cut-off points for donor acceptance, such as age, CrCl and blood pressure, cannot replace clinical judgement and does not allow us to neglect the medical follow-up of kidney donors. No criteria can accurately predict pre-operatively which donors will need medical care and treatment after nephrectomy. Thus, medical follow-up has to be given to all donors.

CONCLUSION

Extending criteria for donor acceptance beyond the generally defined rules, without paying attention to all the prerequisites as discussed in this chapter, may be hazardous and negligent. If one is contemplating accepting donors with one or more isolated medical abnormalities, adequate follow-up and assurance of lifelong access to medications are mandatory. Such a recommendation was recently adopted in the consensus statement of the Amsterdam Forum, and its implementation is essential to ensure that preservation of donor health remains the primary focus in living donor transplantation.[35,36]

ACKNOWLEDGEMENTS

The main sponsors of the SOL-DHR are Novartis Switzerland and Viollier AG, Basel. All laboratory data used by the SOL-DHR were obtained from Viollier AG, without charge. SOL-DHR is also sponsored by Roche, Fresenius, Fujisawa, Wyeth and the Swiss League Against Renal Disease.

REFERENCES

1. Davis C. Evaluation of the living kidney donor: current perspectives. *Am J Kidney Dis* 2004; **43**: 508–530.
2. Bay WH, Heber LA. The living donor in kidney transplantation. *Ann Int Med* 1987; **106**: 719–727.
3. Bia MJ, Ramos EL, Danovitch GM et al. Evaluation of living renal donors. *Transplantation* 1995; **60**: 322–327.
4. Dunn JF, Richie RE, MacDonell RC Jr et al. Living related kidney donors: a 14-year experience. *Ann Surg* 1986; **203**: 637–643.
5. Eberhard OK, Kliem V, Offner G et al. Assesment of long-term risks for living related kidney donors: 24-h blood pressure monitoring and testing for microalbuminuria. *Clin Transplant* 1997; **11**: 415–419.
6. Fehrmann-Ekholm I, Elinder C-G, Stenbeck M et al. Kidney donors live longer. *Transplantation* 1997; **64**: 976–978.
7. Fehrman-Ekholm I, Brink B, Ericsson C et al. Kidney donors don't regret. Follow-up of 370 donors in Stockholm since 1964. *Transplantation* 2000; **69**: 2067–2071.
8. Fehrman-Ekholm I, Duner F, Brink B et al. No evidence of accelerated loss of kidney function in living

9. kidney donors: results from a cross-sectional follow-up. *Transplantation* 2001; **72**: 444–449.
9. Hakim RM, Goldszer RC, Brenner BM. Hypertension and proteinuria: long-term sequelae of uninephrectomy in humans. *Kidney Int* 1984; **25**: 930–936.
10. Hartmann A, Fauchald P, Westlie L et al. The risk of living kidney donation. *Nephrol Dial Transplant* 2003; **18**: 871–873.
11. Higashihara E, Horie S, Takeuchi T et al. Long-term consequences of nephrectomy. *J Urol* 1990; **143**: 239–243.
12. Johnson EM, Remucal MJ, Gillingham KJ et al. Complications and risks of living donor nephrectomy. *Transplantation* 1997; **64**: 1124–1128.
13. Johnson EM, Anderson JK, Jacobs CJ et al. Long-term follow-up of living kidney donors: quality of life after donation. *Transplantation* 1999; **67**: 717–721.
14. Matas AJ, Bartlett ST, Leichtman AB, Delmonico FL. Morbidity and mortality after living kidney donation, 1999–2001: survey of United States transplant centers. *Am J Transplant* 2003; **3**: 830–834.
15. Miller IJ, Suthanthiran M, Riggio RR et al. Impact on renal donation. Long-term clinical and biochemical follow-up of living donors in a single centre. *Am J Med* 1985; **79**: 201–208.
16. Najarian JS, Chavers BM, McHugh LE, Matas AJ. 20 years or more of follow-up of living kidney donors. *Lancet* 1992; **340**: 807–810.
17. Narkun-Burgess DM, Nolan CR, Norman J et al. Forty-five year follow-up after uninephrectomy. *Kidney Int* 1993; **43**: 1110–1115.
18. Ramcharan T, Matas AJ. Long-term (20–37 years) follow-up of living kidney donors. *Am J Transplant* 2002; **2**: 959–946.
19. Schumann V, Fritschka E, Goepel M et al. Langzeitnierenfunktion nach unilateraler nephrectomie. *Nieren und Hochdruck-Krankheiten* 1994; **23**: 125–131.
20. Talseth T, Fauchald P, Skrede S et al. Long-term blood pressure and renal function in kidney donors. *Kidney Int* 1986; **29**: 1072–1078.
21. Torres VE, Offord KP, Andertson CF et al. Blood pressure determinants in living-related allograft donors and their recipients. *Kidney Int* 1987; **31**: 1383–1390.
22. Weidland D, Sutherland DER, Chavers B et al. Information on 628 living-related kidney donors at a single institution, with long-term follow-up in 472 cases. *Transplant Proc* 1984; **16**: 5–7.
23. Zucchelli P, Cagnoli L, Casanova S, Donini U, Pasquali S. Focal glomerulosclerosis in patients with unilateral nephrectomy. *Kidney Int* 1983; **24**: 649–655.
24. Hallynck T, Soep HH, Thomis J et al. Prediction of creatinine clearance from serum creatinine concentration based on lean body mass. *Clin Pharmacol Ther* 1981; **30**: 414–421.
25. Levey AS, Coresh J, Balk E et al. National Kidney

Foundation Practice Guidelines for chronic renal disease: evaluation, classification and stratification. *Ann Int Med* 2003; **139**: 137–147.

26. Ellison MD, McBride MA, Taranto SE, Delmonico FL, Kauffman HM. Living kidney donors in need of kidney transplants: a report from the organ procurement and transplant network. *Transplantation* 2002; **74**: 1349–1351.

27. Kim YS, Kim MS, Han DS et al. Evidence that the ratio of donor kidney weight to recipient body weight, donor age, and episodes of acute rejection correlate independently with live-donor graft function. *Transplantation* 2002; **74**: 280–283.

28. Official response letter addressed to G Thiel after written demand to the expert board of the Swiss League Against High Blood Pressure (1989).

29. Textor SC, Taler SJ, Driscoll N et al. Blood pressure and renal function after kidney donation from hypertensive living donors. *Transplantation* 2004; **78**: 276–282.

30. Textor SC, Taler SJ, Larson TS et al. Blood pressure evaluation among older living kidney donors. *J Am Soc Nephrol* 2003; **14**: 2159–2167.

31. Gerstein HC, Mann JFE, Yi Q et al. Albuminuria and risk of cardiovascular events, death and heart failure in diabetic and nondiabetic individuals. *JAMA* 2001; **286**: 421–426.

32. Mann JFE, Gerstein HC, Pogue J, Bosch J, Salim Y. Renal insufficiency as a predictor of cardiovascular outcome and the impact of ramipril: the HOPE randomized trial. *Ann Int Med* 2001; **134**: 629–636.

33. Mann JF, Gerstein HC. Albuminuria as a predictor of cardiovascular and renal outcome of people with known atherosclerotic cardiovascular disease. *Kidney Int* 2004; **66**: S59–S62.

34. Praga M, Hernandez E, Herrero JC et al. Influence of obesity on the appearance of proteinuria and renal insufficiency after unilateral nephrectomy. *Kidney Int* 2000; **58**: 2111–2118.

35. Delmonico F. The consensus statement of the Amsterdam Forum on the Care of the Live Kidney Donor. *Transplantation* 2004; **78**: 491–492.

36. Van Paassen P, van Breda Vriesman PJ, van Rie H, Tervaert JW. Signs and symptoms of thin basement membrane nephropathy: a prospective regional study on primary glomerular disease – The Limburg Renal Registry. *Kidney Int* 2004; **66**: 909–913.

37. A Report of the Amsterdam Forum on the Care of the Live Kidney Donor Data and Medical Guidelines. *Transplantation* 2005; **79** (2S): S53–S66.

Living donor nephrectomy

6

Jonas Wadström

INTRODUCTION

Live donor nephrectomy, with major surgery performed on a healthy person who receives no direct therapeutic benefit, exposes the surgeon to unusual and specific challenges: the benefit accrues to the recipient and the principle of '*primum non nocere*' remains of utmost importance. It is the duty of the operating surgeon to scrutinize the donor evaluation, making sure that all potential issues have been addressed so that mortality and morbidity can be minimized. It is also incumbent upon the surgeon to inform the donor and to document informed consent, especially if there are any circumstances that might increase the risk for either donor or recipient. The main emphasis of this chapter is on the surgical procedure. However, the issues the surgeon has to consider to minimize risks in the pre-, peri- and the postoperative period will also be addressed.

PREOPERATIVE EVALUATION

The donor evaluation serves to assess not only perioperative anaesthetic and surgical risks, but also long-term prognosis. The ideal is that the donor is completely healthy. However, medical abnormalities that might be associated with an increased perioperative risk can often be attenuated with prophylaxis or treatment before the operation. If this is not possible, the potential donor should be advised not to undergo nephrectomy.

Assessing risk is often difficult, and it is seldom possible to specify the degree of risk involved in an individual case. It is, therefore, of value that the donor evaluation is reviewed by a nephrologist, surgeon, anaesthesiologist and a psychiatrist and/or social worker in order to obtain information from each perspective. In addition, it is important that both donor and recipient are informed and are involved in the final decision.

Anaesthesiological aspects

Anaesthesiological assessment is generally based on anamnesis (history), physical examination and laboratory findings. The personal and family history can reveal if the donor or any other member of the family has had any adverse reactions in connection with previous surgery or dental treatment. These include unexpected bleeding, thrombosis, allergic reactions, difficulties during intubation and hyperthermic reactions.

Donors should generally be ASA (American Association of Anesthesiologists Physical Status Classification) class I. In this group of patients, perioperative complications are rare.[1] Although extensive preoperative screening laboratory tests, chest radiographs and electrocardiograms are often performed during the donor evaluation, for an ASA class I patient, there is only a very small chance of detecting any abnormality that signifies increased risk or that might lead to changes in anaesthetic management.[2,3] However, given the special circumstances that surround live donor nephrectomy, most centres follow a meticulous preoperative assessment. Some centres include a stress electrocardiogram in all patients over 50 years of age,[4] since it is known that potential donors sometimes deny symptoms of coronary ischaemia in the interest of donating, despite themselves having cardiac risk factors (A Hartmann, personal communication). Indeed, donor mortality due to coronary ischaemia has been reported even during recent times.[5]

It is important that the anaesthesiologist is prepared for possible problems and complications related to the donor operation. A specific issue is the positioning of the patient. Both flank and laparoscopic nephrectomy often require the patient to be placed in a full flank position with a broken operating table for a fairly long time (especially laparoscopic procedures). This position may have an impact on the haemodynamics and gas exchange, as well as promote atelectasis.[6,7] The anaesthesiologist should also be familiar with the perioperative surveillance needed for lengthy laparoscopic procedures that can result in carbon dioxide (CO_2) retention and significant adverse cardiopulmonary effects. It is important to recognize that increased intra-abdominal pressure decreases renal blood flow and glomerular filtration rate (GFR), and can even cause oliguria.[8–10] However, the adverse effects on kidney function can be ameliorated by providing adequate intraoperative volume.[11,12]

The renin–angiotensin–aldosterone system (RAAS) can be activated by both open and endoscopic nephrectomy.[13] Volume loading is, therefore, also important in open procedures and many anaesthesiologists add mannitol and/or furosemide to maintain good diuresis. Unfortunately, during the donor operation vascular clamps or clips can slip, or endovascular staplers can malfunction, sometimes resulting in injuries to the major vessels as well as sudden major bleeding.[14,15] If this happens, the anaesthesiologist must be prepared for rapid infusion of fluids and blood products.

Surgical aspects

Some of the investigations during the donor evaluation specifically address surgical issues and risk factors. In addition to those already discussed in this and other chapters, coagulation disorders and obesity are probably the most important surgical risk factors.

Pulmonary embolism is the single most common cause of perioperative death in live donors.[16] It does not necessarily lead to donor death but it is still a severe, life-threatening complication that is seen in most larger series of donor follow-up.[14,17,18] Risk factors for thromboembolic events must, therefore, be investigated thoroughly as part of the preoperative assessment. A summary of the prevalence of common risk factors and their associated relative risk for venous thromboembolism is presented in Table 6-1.[19–21] Some risk factors are rare but associated with a high risk of venous thromboembolism, whereas others are frequent but carry a low risk. The total risk is thus a product of relative risk and prevalence. It should further be noted that the presence of two risk factors can significantly increase the hazard of thromboembolic events. For instance, the combination of oral contraceptive use and a prothrombin gene mutation dramatically increases risk for cerebral venous thrombosis 149-fold even though the relative risk of each individual factor is much smaller.[19] With a marginally increased risk, such as heterozygous carrier of activated protein C resistance, the operation might still be justified, but with a more potent prophylactic regimen. In this case, at our institution, the procedure would be to give the donor a higher dose of low molecular weight heparin, and to prolong prophylaxis for six weeks after surgery.

Obesity is often said to be associated with increased morbidity and mortality, although there is no strong evidence to support this. The increased risk in obese patients seems to be more or less limited to wound infections and haematoma.[22,23] This seems also true for laparoscopic surgery, although such a contention is controversial.[23–25] Obesity can also increase the risk of respiratory complications.[22]

From a purely surgical point of view, moderate obesity is probably not a contraindication for live donor nephrectomy. However, over the long term, obese patients are at

Table 6-1 Prevalence of risk factors and their associated relative risk for venous thromboembolism (VTE)[19-21]

Risk factor	Prevalence (%)	Relative risk for VTE
Antithrombin deficiency	0.02	10–20
Protein C deficiency	0.2–0.4	5–10
Protein S deficiency	0.03–0.3	5–10
Factor V Leiden, heterozygous	5–15	3–6
Factor V Leiden, homozygous	0.1–1	30–50
Prothrombin mutation, heterozygous	1–4	2–5
Prothrombin mutation, homozygous	0.01	?
Homocysteinaemia	5	5–10
Lupus anticoagulant	1	10
Cardiolipin antibodies	2	10
History of earlier VTE	2	5–10
Hormone contraceptives	Culture dependent	2–4

dramatically increased risk of developing hypertension, hyperlipidaemia and type 2 diabetes.[26] There is also a report that obese patients have a significantly increased risk of developing renal insufficiency after unilateral nephrectomy.[27] While these issues are discussed in greater detail elsewhere in this book, it is important for the operating surgeon to be aware of these risks before contemplating donor nephrectomy in an obese person.

BEFORE THE OPERATION

The surgeon has the overall responsibility of ensuring maximal safety of both the nephrectomy and the perioperative course. The commonest reason for perioperative complications is human error.[28,29] The surgeon in charge must, therefore, confirm that all personnel (including the surgeon) involved in the operation are appropriately qualified, that surgical equipment is functioning (and that the personnel know how to handle the equipment), and that relevant information about the donor and proposed operation has been shared with all involved.

Often, the operation is stressful for the donor, who many times has never previously undergone a surgical procedure. Additionally, there is also concern about the recipient. The surgeon, anaesthesiologist and the rest of the staff should be aware of these issues and take time to inform the donor about the procedure and what is to be expected during the hospital stay. We also let the donor meet a physiotherapist prior to the operation, who gives instructions about early postoperative mobilization, measures peak expiratory flow and provides adjusted compression stockings. To be effective, thrombosis and antibiotic prophylaxis should also be started prior to surgery.

THE DONOR OPERATION

Choice of kidney

It is generally accepted that the best kidney should stay with the donor. Factors influencing which kidney to harvest include split function, arterial, venous and ureteral anatomy, and any other renal abnormalities (e.g. cysts). Extrarenal findings such as previous operations and scars or perceived difficulty in positioning on one side may also play a role. When all factors, including function and quality, are equivalent, the kidney with the lowest risk for surgical complications in the recipient is selected. It is then generally preferable to remove the left kidney since it has a longer renal vein that makes the recipient operation easier. There also seems to be a lower risk for venous thrombosis with the left kidney, from both deceased and live donors.[30]

Arterial anatomy

The presence of multiple renal arteries to one or both of the kidneys is a common finding, present in as many as 20–30% of potential donors.[31–33] Harvesting a kidney with two or more arteries is more complex. The operating time, and the warm and cold ischaemia times, are longer due to the greater effort required to establish perfusion in two arteries and the back table reconstruction of the arteries. One can also expect more vascular complications in the recipient, such as bleeding, thrombosis, stenosis or hypertension. Although earlier reports indicate that complications are more common with multiple vessels,[34,35] more recent publications refute this contention.[33,36–38] However, the studies are small and general experience continues to lead most surgeons to harvest the kidney with the least number of arteries.

There are some additional caveats regarding vascular anatomy. A small upper polar artery can, in most cases, be ligated or thrombosed without dramatic consequences. However, lower polar arteries supply the ureteral vasculature and an occlusion can lead to necrosis that may involve not only the ureter but also the renal pelvis. Sometimes a localized plaque, renal artery aneurysm or fibromuscular dysplasia is seen on the preoperative angiogram. The presence of these lesions should, in general, disqualify the donor, which is in the interest of both donor and recipient. However, successful reports of transplantation of kidneys with these lesions do exist.[39,40] If such donors are used, it is essential that the diseased kidney is removed for transplantation, with the affected vessel modified on the back table.

Venous anatomy

As previously mentioned, the left renal vein is longer than the right. This is especially important in endoscopic surgery since the vascular stapler shortens the length of the vessels by 1–1.5 cm. Nonetheless, some surgeons prefer the right side since there are no gonadal, suprarenal or lumbar branches into the right renal vein.[41–43] Utilizing the right kidney, however, may make the recipient operation more difficult, at times necessitating use of a venous graft to lengthen the vein.

This adds to risk for the recipient, and because the back wall of the right renal vein can be thin, a venous graft can result in bleeding, kinking or avulsion.[44,45]

Although less common than in the arterial circulation, venous anomalies can also influence the choice of kidney.[46,47] In the case of multiple veins, one or more can normally be ligated. More complicated anomalies such as retroaortic left renal vein types I and II, circumaortic venous collar, duplication of the inferior vena cava (IVC), transposition or left-sided IVC, and preaortic iliac confluence can be an indication to remove the contralateral kidney.[44] However, in most cases this is not necessary.[48,49]

Ureteral anatomy

Anomalies of the ureter such as duplication and cysts are not uncommon,[50,51] and can be associated with obstruction, vesicoureteral reflux and infections.[52] In most cases the finding is asymptomatic.[51] There is little information in the literature on how to handle ureteral anomalies in a donor but it is probably wise to harvest the affected side even if it is asymptomatic. It has been suggested that the right kidney should be used in women of childbearing age since it is postulated that the right kidney is more susceptible to hydronephrosis and obstruction during pregnancy.[19,53] However, this view is not widely shared.[54]

Kidney anatomy and function

To evaluate the function of each individual kidney, many centres rely on the size of the kidney in the radiogram.[44,55] Others use radionuclide scanning.[42,56] Neither of these techniques is uniformly accurate, since the kidney does not always demonstrate its maximal length in the vertical plane and the distance to the gamma camera is not always symmetrical. Recently, a new technique has been proposed to calculate split function with spiral computerized tomography. With this method the arterial, venous and ureteral anatomy can be displayed together with split function in one examination.[57,58] Regardless, it is generally accepted that the best functioning kidney should remain in the donor. If the discrepancy is so large that either donor or recipient may be left with inadequate renal mass, it may be advisable to abandon the proposed transplantation. Occasionally, other anatomical variants such as simple cysts may also influence which kidney to harvest.[55,56]

Choice of method

When choosing the surgical technique for donor nephrectomy, a number of sometimes conflicting variables and interests must be considered. The donor's interests must always be primary, with emphasis on reducing risks for morbidity and mortality as much as possible. Of secondary importance, but still essential, is the optimization of factors influencing graft outcome. The choice between open and laparoscopic (endoscopic) operations impacts on the risks for both donor and recipient. Open procedures include either flank or anterior incisions and laparoscopic approaches can be divided into

hand-assisted and traditional laparoscopic procedures. Furthermore, both open and laparoscopic operations can be performed intra- or extraperitoneally. The operation can also be performed as a mixture of open and laparoscopic procedures. Each of these surgical techniques and approaches is associated with different risks for mortality, morbidity and postoperative kidney function. A summary of the possible combinations is depicted in Figure 6-1.

Irrespective of the surgical approach, positioning of the patient on the operating table may influence morbidity. For flank incisions and most laparoscopic procedures the donor is generally placed in a full flank position with a broken table. This position is awkward and can cause longlasting discomfort and even lead to severe complications such as neuromuscular injuries and rhabdomyolysis.[59–63] To reduce the risk of such complications it is essential that all pressure points are padded meticulously, that the table is not broken more than necessary and that the operating time is as short as possible.[63]

In the following sections, risks of mortality, morbidity and the quality of the procured

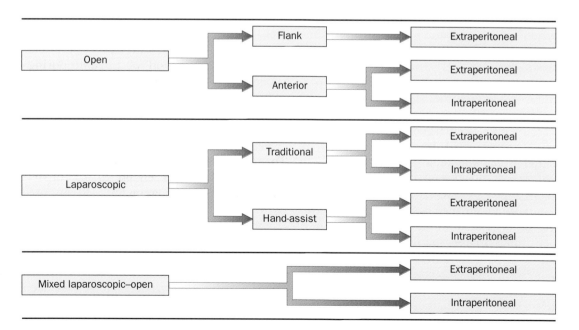

Figure 6-1   The different operative procedures used for live donor nephrectomy.

kidney will be discussed by surgical technique. Risks and complications that are common for all types of surgery will not be addressed here, nor a detailed description of each operative procedure. For description of the technical details of the operations, the reader should refer to references cited in each section. A short summary of each type of operation is given in the corresponding tables (see Tables 6-2 and 6-4–6-7 below).

Intraperitoneal versus extraperitoneal

Gustav Simon performed the first described nephrectomy in 1869.[63] The operation was retroperitoneal with a vertical paravertebral incision. By the mid-1880s, reviews of more than 100 nephrectomies were published with both the extraperitoneal and intraperitoneal approach. Mortality was high, both for the lumbar extraperitoneal approach (37%) and for the transperitoneal approach (51%). The higher mortality rate for the transperitoneal approach was due to septic complications.[65]

The extraperitoneal flank incision has since been the gold standard for many years,[19,66] but with the introduction of laparoscopic nephrectomy the intraperitoneal route has now found widespread use.[67] In addition, a minority of operations (6.2% in the USA) are performed intraperitoneally but with an open approach.[68]

There is no indication that the choice of intra- or extraperitoneal route per se influences renal allograft integrity or function. It has, however, been argued that the intraperitoneal route gives better access, allowing minimal manipulation of the kidney and its vessels, which in turn minimizes vasospasm.[69,70] However, gas insufflated into the peritoneum may have an adverse effect on kidney function when the operation is performed laparoscopically.[8–11,71–73]

Intraperitoneal

Nowadays, infectious complications are uncommon, but morbidity with the intraperitoneal route still remains higher than the

extraperitoneal approach. Some complications (bleeding, wound infection, seroma, etc.) are not affected by the operative approach. Other complications (visceral injuries, bowel obstruction and adhesions), however, are almost exclusively seen with the intraperitoneal approach. In laparoscopic urological procedures, bowel injuries occur at a frequency of 0.4–2.5%,[74–78] and almost 70% of cases are not detected intraoperatively.[75] The delay in diagnosis of complications may worsen the prognosis, with substantial risk of mortality.[75,76] Intraperitoneal adhesions can cause chronic abdominal pain, female infertility, small bowel obstruction or ileus, often resulting in additional operations that are often more difficult and more risky than the original procedure. The incidence of postoperative intra-abdominal adhesion is 70–90% and is responsible for 60–70% of all small bowel obstructions. The lifetime risk of developing adhesive obstruction is about 5%.[79] However, it appears that adhesions are less frequent after laparoscopy compared with open transperitoneal operations.[79,80]

Intraperitoneal operations also cause early perioperative complications more frequently, such as nausea, vomiting, constipation, diarrhoea and small bowel obstruction, as recently confirmed in a large survey of living donor programmes in the USA.[14]

There are few published data on risks with open transperitoneal nephrectomy in donors. Most of our knowledge about complications associated with the procedure is derived from nephrectomy for urological indications (mainly tumours). Splenic injuries are common in this population, occurring in 2–13% of patients.[70,81–83] Intestinal complications are seen less frequently, in approximately 2% of cases.[82] Dunn et al[18] have reported a fairly large series (314 cases) of open intraperitoneal nephrectomies in live donors. In this series, major perioperative complications occurred in 7% of cases, whereas major late complications were seen in 20%. Complications specifically associated with the intraperitoneal approach were pancreatitis (1%) and injuries to the spleen (1%)

or adrenal gland (0.3%). Late complications related to the intraperitoneal route included bowel obstruction (2%) and chronic pancreatitis (0.4%). Other smaller studies have reported similar complications and frequency rates.[69,70,84]

Extraperitoneal

Although rare, visceral injuries can also occur in extraperitoneal operations, involving the bladder, colon, pancreas, small bowel, spleen or liver. The type of lesion is somewhat dependent on the type of procedure performed. These lesions are generally caused when the peritoneum is inadvertently perforated.[74,85]

There also seems to be an advantage in avoiding the intraperitoneal route for endoscopic procedures. With the extraperitoneal procedure, the retroperitoneal space is created by balloon or manual finger dissection before inserting the trocars, which potentially reduces the rate of visceral injuries caused by the trocars.[86] Morbidity with the endoscopic retroperitoneal operation is related to the location of the incision, anterior or flank, and this is discussed later.

Open versus endoscopic

Endoscopic

After Ratner introduced laparoscopic live donor nephrectomy in 1995 rapid developments have been made.[67] Modifications have included both better instruments and new operative techniques such as introduction of hand-assist,[87] retroperitoneal approaches,[86] and finally hand-assisted retroperitoneal techniques.[88] These developments have reduced the risks associated with the operation. In addition, availability of endoscopic procedures has also stimulated greater emphasis on reduction of morbidity with open operations.[89–92]

In general, endoscopic procedures are associated with a lower morbidity. As yet, however, it remains unclear whether there is a greater risk of severe, life-threatening complications and mortality associated with current endoscopic techniques. A recent United Network for Organ Sharing (UNOS) survey, with incomplete response rates that may indicate underreporting, indicates low risk with endoscopic approaches, but that the risk may be greater than that associated with open donor nephrectomy.[14] Nonetheless, it is important to address all possible complications associated with endoscopic nephrectomy and to try to reduce those risks.

Risks associated with all types of endoscopic surgery
Some surgical complications can be associated with endoscopic surgery regardless of the organ involved in the operation. Such complications may reasonably be expected to complicate donor nephrectomy as well, and include:

- emphysema, pneumomediastinum, pneumothorax and pneumopericardium
- gas embolism
- trocar injuries
- malfunctioning of endoscopic instruments
- impaired handling of major complications (bleeding)
- hidden late complications – bleeding, cautery.

Emphysema: Subcutaneous emphysema is fairly common, but usually not severe. In 2–5% of cases, insufflated gas leaks into the thoracic space and may cause any combination of pneumomediastinum, pneumothorax and pneumopericardium.[93,94] These complications are associated with high insufflation pressure, large number of ports, long operative time, age of the patient and type of surgical procedure.[93] The complication seems to be slightly less common in urological surgery, and in most cases is asymptomatic.[94] The incidence is higher when the procedure is retroperitoneal since gas is thought to follow the psoas muscle into the thorax. However, one should bear in mind that pneumothorax remains more frequent when the open flank incision is used compared with endoscopic procedures.[94]

Gas embolism: Insufflated gas can embolize in the circulation. Subclinical air embolism is relatively common, being observed in up to 69% of the cases in connection with cholecystectomy,[95] and in 6% of cases with nephrectomy.[96] A gas embolus has also been reported as a complication of live donor nephrectomy.[97]

This potentially lethal complication is more common when large amounts of gas rapidly enter a vessel.[98–101] The risk of fatality is, therefore, larger early during the operation when pneumoperitoneum is created with the Verres needle and a large vessel is inadvertently punctured. The risk is also potentially greater when the operation is performed close to large vessels as in live donor nephrectomy. To prevent gas embolism, CO_2 insufflation should begin with a slow flow rate and low pressure. Clinical signs of gas embolism are cardiac murmur, arrhythmia, sudden increase in end-tidal CO_2 and cyanosis. Detection of gas embolism is best done by transesophageal echocardiography.[95,96] If air embolism is suspected or diagnosed, gas insufflation should be stopped immediately. Treatment includes high-fraction inspired oxygen ventilation, left lateral decubitus positioning, gas aspiration through a central venous catheter and cardiac massage.[99]

Trocar injuries: Insertion of trocars or a Verres needle is always associated with some risk. These instruments are known to have injured vessels in the abdominal wall and almost all intra-abdominal organs or vessels. The incidence is probably below 1% for general surgical as well as for urological procedures, including live donor nephrectomy.[76,102,103] It is, however, a severe and life-threatening complication often necessitating conversion to the open procedure.

This risk as well as the risk of gas embolism can be reduced by using the open Hassan technique or a hand-assisted technique from the start of the operation, which enables the first trocar to be inserted under direct vision without organ injury and the gas to be insufflated in the right spacium. Subsequent ports can then be inserted under direct vision. The use of trocars with safety shields or optical access devices has, so far, not convincingly reduced the incidence of injuries.[102] However, by using radially expandable needles instead of cutting trocars the risk of injuring vessels or nerves of the abdominal wall can be reduced.[104]

Malfunctioning of endoscopic instruments: Endoscopic instruments are sophisticated and complex, subject to both malfunction and, not infrequently, human error. Handling a malfunctioning instrument is more difficult in an endoscopic operation than in open surgery. Malfunction during dissection and division of major vessels, such as the renal vein or artery, during live donor nephrectomy is especially dangerous. Malfunctioning linear cutters have been known to cause death: numerous cases of malfunction have been reported in connection with live donor nephrectomy, some causing donor mortality.[105] Malfunction can occur with any type of stapler or clip[15,106–108] (O Oyen, ML Nicholson, H Gjertsen, personal communication). It is, therefore, important that the surgeon and assisting nurse are familiar with the instruments, that the instruments are thoroughly checked before use, and that they are used properly. In addition, a stapler or clip should not be placed across a previously placed clip. The artery should be ligated with a transfixational technique and not with clips, since clips have been shown to slip more frequently, both intra- and postoperatively, causing life-threatening bleeding.[108]

Impaired handling of major complications (bleeding): Bleeding is the commonest major intraoperative complication in urological endoscopic surgery as well as in endoscopic live donor nephrectomy.[76,109,110] It is also the commonest reason for conversion to open surgery and the most important surgical risk factor for donor mortality.[103,111] At least two patients are known to have died as a result of massive bleeding during general laparoscopic surgery.[105] Donors have died and one patient is in a permanent vegetative state after massive bleeding and hypotension during laparoscopic live donor nephrectomy.[14,108] However, it should be pointed out that incidence of bleeding is low (1–4%) and comparable with that seen in open surgery.[15] In addition, there was no mortality due to bleeding in the large US study that included several thousand endoscopic live donor nephrectomies, although one donor was in a permanent vegetative state.[14,110]

Hidden late complications: In contrast to open approaches, where visceral injury is likely to be detected intraoperatively, in endoscopic surgery, it is possible for lesions (mainly representing visceral injury) to go undetected during the operation. Such injuries can be caused by retractors or cautery inflicting damage outside the optical field. Thus, a specific drawback with endoscopic surgery is the risk of delayed diagnosis, which can worsen the condition and lead to fatal complications.[75,76]

Venous and capillary bleeding is another complication that might not become evident until after surgery since the increased intra- or retroperitoneal pressure from insufflated gas exerts a counterpressure until it is removed. By this time, the instruments have been removed and the bleeding remains undetected. Reoperation for bleeding is also commoner after laparoscopic surgery than after open nephrectomy. But once again, the overall frequency is very low, 0.18–0.45%.[14]

Traditional laparoscopic nephrectomy
Despite the potential dangers associated with endoscopic surgery, the technique has rapidly gained widespread acceptance. A large number of reports now provide substantial evidence that the endoscopic technique offers equivalent graft survival with less donor morbidity than open techniques.[68,110,112] Laparoscopic nephrectomy (in retrospective, case–control and even prospective, randomized studies) is associated with less pain, shorter hospital stays and an earlier return to work[90,113–120] (O Oyen, personal communication). Other benefits include early mobilization (which could have an impact on thromboembolic and pulmonary complica-

tions) and better cosmetic results. Some maintain that it has also contributed to increased willingness of some reluctant potential donors to undergo nephrectomy. A summary of the operative procedure is given in Table 6-2.[120–122]

However, at times the operation is difficult, with a steep learning curve that impedes implementation of the technique without a high frequency of complications. Almost all studies have demonstrated longer operating times and warm ischaemia time.[110,116,118,119,123–125] Initial reports indicated a higher frequency of ureteral complications.[126,127] However, if care is taken to leave as much tissue as possible around the ureter (with or without the gonadal vein), and perform the periureteral dissection with an ultrasonic device instead of cautery, the frequency of ureteral complications can be minimized.[118,126,128]

Pneumoperitoneum results in a transient decrease in renal blood flow and GFR, and can lead to oliguria.[8–11,72,73] These effects have raised concerns about early and late graft function. Indeed, there is fairly strong evidence in the literature, especially the UNOS survey, of higher serum creatinine levels in the early postoperative period and a slower decline in serum creatinine after transplantation.[14] Later on, however, this difference is no longer evident and the rate of delayed graft function seems equal to that encountered with open nephrectomy.[68,116,125,127] To improve early graft function it is important to keep the insufflation pressure as low as possible ($\leq 12\,mmHg$), avoid long operating times and keep the donor well hydrated.[11,129,130]

Another disadvantage that can be associated with laparoscopic nephrectomy is rhabdomyolysis.[59–62] Orchialgia is a rare complication of unknown aetiology that can occur in up to 9% of the male population.[131] The condition seems difficult to treat, but in many cases microsurgical testicular denervation is successful.[132,133] Thigh paraesthesia can also occur, and is best avoided by careful and precise dissection and division of the ureter.[103,134–136]

Table 6-2   Nephrectomy with traditional laparoscopic nephrectomy

Positioning	• Lateral decubitus ± broken operating table
	• Pressure points carefully padded
	• Table ± tilted
Incision	• Generally one paraumbilical port and two to four ports along the costal margin from midline to the flank
	• Incision for kidney removal: Pfannenstiel, lower midline, paraumbilical or transverse abdominal
Pneumoperitoneum	• Verres needle or Hassan trocar
	• CO_2 insufflation, pressure below 12 mmHg
Dissection	• Dissection with ultrasonic dissector. Colon (and spleen on left side) reflected medially
	• On right side, retraction of liver with retractor or grasper
	• Open Gerotta's facia
	• Kidney freed from its attachments
	• Dissecting vessels without traction
	• Local spasmolytic agents optional as well as intravenous heparin prior to dividing vessels
Vessels	*Right side:*
	• Division of artery behind IVC with endovascular stapler (clips dangerous)
	• Division of vein with rim of IVC if open division, otherwise with endovascular stapler
	Left side:
	• Ligation and division of gonadal, lumbar and suprarenal vein
	• Division of artery close to aorta with endovascular stapler (clips dangerous)
	• Division of renal vein proximal to the suprarenal vein with endovascular stapler
Ureter	• Preservation of tissue around the ureter (± gonadal vein)
	• Division + ligation of ureter as it enters the true pelvis
Kidney extraction	• Extraction bag
Wound closure	• Closure of trocar sites ≥10 mm.
	• Closure of kidney extraction site
	• Skin closure, preferably intracutaneous
	• No drainage

IVC, inferior vena cava.

Laparoscopic procedures are associated with increased costs due to longer operating times and the use of disposable instruments. This can be offset by shorter hospitalization, but the overall cost-equation is dependent on the local economic healthcare environment.[112,137]

Endovascular stapling devices consume 1–1.5 cm of vessel length. This is a disadvantage of laparoscopic nephrectomy, especially on the right side, since the right renal vein is much shorter than the left. A short vein makes the recipient operation more difficult, and it was speculated to be the reason for a high rate of venous thrombosis in the initial experience from the Johns Hopkins centre.[55] Higher rates of venous thrombosis have also been reported in cadaveric transplants, indicating that this concern could be relevant.[30] Several subsequent publications have, however, reported successful outcomes after harvesting the right kidney. The final division of the right renal vein is sometimes made through a minilaparotomy, which makes the

procedure more of a mixed operation.[41,42,44,45,56] Nonetheless, the two centres with the longest and largest experience still use the left kidney in 95–96% of donors.[103,107] This predilection for the left kidney poses a potential problem, since it implies that the best kidney does not always remain in the donor. When both kidneys are equally good but there are more arteries on the left side, by employing a policy to almost always harvest the left kidney, it is also possible that the kidney with the lowest risk for vascular complications does not always go to the recipient.

Endoscopic techniques have been used in donors with multiple vessels without significant impact on operation time, warm ischaemia time or graft outcome, although operation and warm ischaemia times tend to be somewhat longer.[33,37,38,138] Laparoscopic nephrectomy has also been used in obese or elderly donors, as well as in an adult donor when the recipient is a small child. The operating times are longer in obese donors, who are also more likely to require conversion to open surgery. However, donor morbidity and recipient outcomes do not appear compromised.[26,139] Elderly donors also seem to tolerate the procedure well.[140]

Some have been reluctant to use laparoscopic nephrectomy when the recipient is a child due to the risk of delayed graft function, a complication that makes the postoperative course more complicated in this patient population. However, in the literature there is no real indication of increased risk of delayed graft function.[125,141,142] For paediatric recipients, it is important that the donor, often one of the parents, has a quick recovery, which makes laparoscopic nephrectomy particularly attractive.

Hand-assisted laparoscopic nephrectomy

As noted earlier, the inherent risks and a steep learning curve associated with laparoscopic nephrectomy have dissuaded some from the procedure.[143–145] Hand-assisted techniques have been introduced to increase safety and to facilitate the operation. They offer the same benefits as laparoscopic nephrectomy,[124,146–151] as well as a number of additional advantages that increase patient safety (Table 6-3). In the hand-assisted technique, the incision for extracting the kidney is used to insert a hand in the operative field while still maintaining intact pneumoperitoneum or retroperitoneum. The operation preferably begins with placing the hand port so that the trocars can thereafter be introduced in a safe manner under direct vision. A summary of the operative procedure is given in Table 6-4.

Massive bleeding is probably the single most important risk factor for intraoperative mortality and is the primary reason for emergency conversion.[76,103,108–111] With a hand in the operating field the surgeon can immediately achieve haemostasis. The hand also gives a tactile feedback, which gives better control and can prevent torsion of the kidney, something that can occur when all the attachments of the kidney have been dissected free. The tactile feedback dimension makes it easier to learn the procedure and reduces the operating time (and costs) compared with traditional laparoscopic nephrectomy.[148,152–155]

A critical part of the operation is ligation and division of the major vessels, as well as retrieval of the kidney. Problems such as stapler malfunction are much more readily addressed with the hand-assisted approach. In traditional laparoscopy it can be difficult to extract the kidney and this can lead to excessively long warm ischaemia times of 10–30 minutes.[41,42,118,156] Warm ischaemia times above 10 minutes are associated with a high frequency of delayed graft function.[156] In this respect, it is important to note that secure and rapid placement of vascular staplers and retrieval of the kidney both reduce warm ischaemia time.[148,152–155]

Retroperitoneoscopic nephrectomy

Retroperitoneoscopic techniques reduce the risks associated with intraperitoneal operations (see the 'Intraperitoneal' section above). The advantages are summarized in Table 6-3. The technique has found fairly wide acceptance in the urological community, but there are very few publications on retroperitoneoscopic live donor nephrectomy. The results so far are encouraging,

Table 6-3   Advantages of combined hand-assisted and retroperitoneoscopic nephrectomy

Compared with traditional laparoscopic nephrectomy	Compared with transperitoneal laparoscopic nephrectomy
Safer trocar placement	Reduced risk of visceral injuries
Better control of potential bleeds	Reduced risk of bowel obstruction
Prevention of torsion of the kidney	Reduced risk of postoperative adhesions
Reduces operating time (cost reduction)	No risk of internal herniation
Secure and rapid placement of vascular staplers	
Secure and rapid retrieval of the kidney	
Reduces warm ischaemia time	

Table 6-4 Nephrectomy with hand-assisted laparoscopic nephrectomy

Positioning	• Lateral decubitus ± broken operating table • Pressure points carefully padded • Table ± tilted
Incision	• Incision for kidney removal: Pfannenstiel, lower midline, paraumbilical or transverse abdominal • Also used for entering hand. Pneumoperitoneum kept intact with hand-assist device • One port lateral to the hand port, generally two to four additional ports along the costal margin from midline to the flank, introduced after introduction of hand
Pneumoperitoneum	• Preferably generated after introduction of hand, pressure below 12 mmHg
Dissection	• Dissection with ultrasonic dissector. Colon (and spleen on left side) reflected medially • On right side, retraction of liver with retractor or grasper • Open Gerotta's facia • Kidney freed from its attachments • Dissection of vessels without traction • Local spasmolytic agents optional as well as intravenous heparin prior to vessel division
Vessels	*Right side:* • Division of artery behind IVC with endovascular stapler (clips dangerous) • Division of vein with rim of IVC if open division, otherwise with endovascular stapler *Left side:* • Ligation and division of gonadal, lumar and suprarenal vein • Division of artery close to aorta with endovascular stapler (clips dangerous) • Division of renal vein proximal to the suprarenal vein with endovascular stapler
Ureter	• Preservation of tissue around the ureter (± gonadal vein) • Division + ligation of ureter as it enters the true pelvis
Kidney extraction	• Manual extraction
Wound closure	• Closure of trocar sites ≥10 mm • Closure of kidney extraction site • Skin closure, preferably intracutaneous • No drainage

IVC, inferior vena cava.

though the smaller operative field is a potential disadvantage.[157–161]

Retroperitoneal hand-assisted nephrectomy
Retroperitoneoscopic hand-assisted nephrectomy combines the benefits of hand-assistance and the retroperitoneal approach. There is no need for mobilizing the colon or the spleen, and the splenocolic ligament is left intact, with no risk of internal herniation.[162] A summary of the operative procedure is given in Table 6-5. Experience with the technique, although limited, is promising, indicating even shorter operating times and less pain.[13]

The technique involves the hand port being placed in a lower midline or Pfannenstiel incision. Thus there is no division of muscles or nerves, which eliminates the risk of paraesthesia or bulging.[13,48,88,163–165] According to the US survey, gastrointestinal complications are the commonest cause for reoperation or readmission after traditional and hand-assisted laparoscopic neph-

rectomy,[14] and the largest single-centre report notes that 'the major postoperative problem in laparoscopic donors is bowel function'.[103] These complications are apparently minimized with the hand-assisted retroperitoneoscopic approach.

Open

The open procedure can be performed with a retroperitoneal flank incision or an intra- or extraperitoneal anterior incision. Aspects of intra- and extraperitoneal procedures have already been discussed; in this section, advantages and disadvantages of the location (flank or anterior) will be discussed.

Flank
The flank incision has been the gold standard for many years. A summary of the operative procedure is given in Table 6-6. The procedure is fairly safe, with a calculated mortality of 0.03%.[18,166] Morbidity and perioperative complications are, however, fairly high, reported in

Table 6-5   Nephrectomy with hand-assisted retroperitoneal endoscopic nephrectomy

Positioning	• Lateral decubitus
	• Operating table not broken
	• Pressure points carefully padded
Incision	• Incision for kidney removal: Pfannenstiel or lower midline
	• Also used for entering hand. Pneumoretroperitoneum kept intact with hand-assist device
	• Generally three additional ports: paraumbilical, subcostal, flank, introduced after introduction of hand
Pneumoretroperitoneum	• Generated after manual dissection of peritoneum from abdominal wall
	• Retroperitoneal CO_2 insufflation with pressure below 12 mmHg
Dissection	• Introduction of hand and further loosening of peritoneum from anterior and posterior abdominal wall
	• Dissection with ultrasonic dissector
	• Open Gerotta's facia
	• Kidney freed from its attachments
	• Dissection of vessels without traction
	• Local spasmolytic agents optional as well as intravenous heparin prior to vessel division
Vessels	*Right side:*
	• Division of artery behind IVC with endovascular stapler (clips dangerous)
	• Division of vein with rim of IVC if open division, otherwise with endovascular stapler
	Left side:
	• Ligation and division of gonadal, lumbar and suprarenal vein
	• Division of artery close to aorta with endovascular stapler (clips dangerous)
	• Division of renal vein proximal to the suprarenal vein with endovascular stapler
Ureter	• Preservation of tissue around the ureter (± gonadal vein)
	• Division + ligation of ureter as it enters the true pelvis
Kidney extraction	• Manual extraction
Wound closure	• Closure of trocar sites ≥ 10 mm
	• Closure of kidney extraction site
	• Skin closure, preferably intracutaneous
	• No drainage

IVC, inferior vena cava.

Table 6-6   Nephrectomy with flank incision

Positioning	• Lateral decubitus with broken operating table
	• Pressure points carefully padded
Incision	• Dorsolateral over the 11th, 12th or just below the ribs
Dissection	• Division of abdominal and part of latissimus muscle
	• Resection of one rib (optional)
	• Avoid injuring intercostal nerves and entering the pleura
	• Open Gerotta's facia
	• Removal of perinephric fat
	• Dissection of vessels without traction
	• Local spasmolytic agents optional as well as intravenous heparin prior to dividing vessels
Vessels	*Right side:*
	• Division of artery behind IVC
	• Division of vein with rim of IVC
	• Closure of IVC with sutures
	• Double ligature (suture) of arterial stump
	Left side:
	• Ligation and division of gonadal, lumbar and suprarenal vein
	• Division of artery close to aorta
	• Division of renal vein proximal to the suprarenal vein
	• Suturing of venous stump
	• Double ligature (suture) of artery
Ureter	• Preservation of tissue around the ureter
	• Division + ligation of ureter as it enters the true pelvis
Kidney extraction	• Manual extraction
Wound closure	• Local nerve blockade of intercostal nerves (optional)
	• Closure of muscular layer without injuring nerves
	• Skin closure, preferably intracutaneous
	• Drainage optional

IVC, inferior vena cava.

up to 48% of patients.[19,89,115,123,167–178] The majority of the complications are either wound- or pulmonary-related. Intraoperative iatrogenic pneumothorax is not uncommon, being seen in up to 39% of donors.[171] This is an independent risk factor for other complications such as postoperative atelectasis or pneumonia.[172] Pneumothorax-associated morbidity, however, tends to be short lived. Wound complications affect as many as 25% of donors.[89] Infections or seroma are easily dealt with, but postoperative pain can cause considerable morbidity.[90,107,114–119] Rib resection may be responsible for some of the pain. However, the flank incision, with or without rib resection, is made close to the intercostal nerves and may also be responsible for some of the pain, due to the risk of nerve damage and chronic neuralgia.[89,179] The nerve lesion causes paresis of the muscle and leads to disturbing bulging of the flank in as many as 50% of patients undergoing flank incision.[176,179–181] A patient with bulging after live donor nephrectomy is shown in Figure 6-2.

In studies evaluating quality of life after nephrectomy with flank incision, 33–53% of donors claimed to have long-term wound-site pain, which is significantly greater than that after laparoscopic nephrectomy.[90,168,179,182–184] Bulging rarely heals and is difficult to treat.[185] Thus, the major disadvantages of flank incision are short- and long-term scar discomfort and pain.

Anterior

Anterior intraperitoneal: An anterior intraperitoneal incision is not commonly used for living donor nephrectomy and only a limited number of publications report short- and long-term morbidity. These studies indicate that most complications are related to the intraperitoneal approach and not to the anterior location of the incision as such.[69,70,84] Complications and other aspects of intra- or extraperitoneal procedures have already been discussed above.

Anterior retroperitoneal: There are more publications on the experience with an anterior retroperitoneal than with the anterior intraperitoneal approach incision. With this procedure, the incision is more or less horizontal or vertical. This approach seems to have a low frequency of short- and long-term complications. Wound infections, seromas

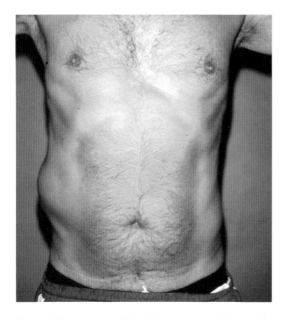
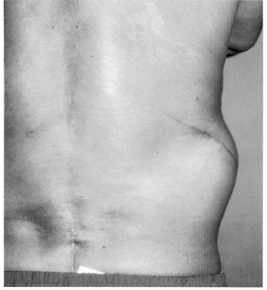

Figure 6-2 A patient with bulging and neuralgia after live donor nephrectomy with flank incision.

Table 6-7   Nephrectomy with anterior retroperitoneal incision

Positioning	• Roll or pillow behind the back and/or table tilted 30°
	• Table extended
Incision	• Horizontal or curvilinear incision from mid-rectus muscle cranial to umbilicus
	• Extended to mid-axillary line
	• Avoid too lateral incision that can injure intercostal nerves
Dissection	• Division of abdominal muscles, leaving (most of) the rectus intact
	• Loosening of peritoneum from abdominal wall without entering the abdomen
	• Medial reflection of the peritoneum
	• Open Gerotta's facia
	• Removal of perinephric fat
	• Dissection of vessels without traction
	• Local spasmolytic agents optional as well as intravenous heparin prior to dividing vessels
Vessels	*Right side:*
	• Division of artery behind IVC
	• Division of vein with rim of IVC
	• Closure of IVC with sutures
	• Double ligature (suture) of arterial stump
	Left side:
	• Ligation and division of gonadal, lumbar and suprarenal vein
	• Division of artery close to aorta
	• Division of renal vein proximal to the suprarenal vein
	• Suturing of venous stump
	• Double ligature (suture) of artery
Ureter	• Preservation of tissue around the ureter
	• Division + ligation of ureter as it enters the true pelvis
Kidney extraction	• Manual extraction
Wound closure	• Local nerve blockade of intercostal nerves (optional)
	• Closure of muscular layer without injuring nerves
	• Skin closure, preferably intracutaneous
	• Drainage optional

IVC, inferior vena cava.

and hernias may develop, but bulging and long-term neuralgia are uncommon. Perioperative pain is mild and long-term scar discomfort is rare.[13,43,186–189] When the incision is extended dorsally to get better access to the upper pole of the kidney (sometimes including rib resection), there is a risk of nerve damage.[190,191] Normally, however, one can achieve good access without extending the incision dorsally. The intraoperative site of an anterior retroperitoneal approach is depicted in Figure 6-3. The transverse incision allows better conservation of the intercostal nerves.[192] A summary of the operative procedure is given in Table 6-7.

Mixed

A number of centres in Asia have described a hybrid open–endoscopic technique, where the operation starts with a small pararectal anterior incision. Special retractors or lift devices are then used to create working space without insufflating gas. Additional port(s) are then introduced for a videotelescope and for endoscopic instruments that allow a minimal incision. The operation is performed mainly with normal surgical instruments, and the majority are performed retroperitoneally. The number of patients reported is fairly small, but the authors claim good results and minimal morbidity.[193–200] Another approach is to start with a laparoscopic operation and at the end perform a minilaparotomy for division of the vessels. This approach has been used predominantly

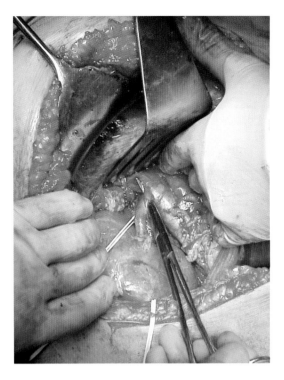

Figure 6-3 Intraoperative view of an anterior retroperitoneal approach shows good exposure of the kidney and its vessels.

on the right side, mainly to achieve maximal vessel length.[44,55,130,201]

The mixed procedure has both the advantages and the disadvantages of the open and endoscopic techniques. Thus, the primarily laparoscopic operation has the risks of laparoscopy with increased intraperitoneal pressure and gastrointestinal complications. The only remaining benefit is avoidance of the flank incision. However, the gasless intraperitoneal technique reduces the risk of pneumoperitoneum. The retroperitoneal gasless technique removes all these disadvantages but still has a cosmetic deficit compared with the lower midline or Pfannenstiel incision used in pure endoscopic techniques. The major advantages are good vessel length, better control of potential bleeding and the three-dimensional view of the operative field.

Thus, the gasless retroperitoneal technique may be the best mixed alternative despite some unresolved problems. Suzuki

and colleagues, who have one of the largest experiences with the technique, have, for instance, started to use an additional hand port (with an additional incision) to reduce operating times.[202] They have further reported that some patients have pain, especially if the retractors are lifted too strongly, and that the upper abdominal incision poses a cosmetic problem. The surgical field is also slightly smaller than that achieved using a pneumoperitoneum.

POSTOPERATIVE CARE

The postoperative care of the living donor is not fundamentally different from any other surgery. Reduction of postoperative pain has been an issue in lowering donor morbidity and a stimulus for the introduction of laparoscopic techniques. Postoperative analgesia should preferably be discussed with the patient before the operation. Pain is subjective with wide interpatient variability in severity and duration as well as analgesic requirements. Donors may benefit from perioperative regional or local analgesia used alone and/or in combination with patient-controlled analgesia and oral analgesics.[116,170,190,203,204] Even for patients undergoing laparoscopic donor nephrectomy, where pain should be less intense, local infiltration with bupivacaine has been shown to reduce the postoperative use of narcotics and reduce the length of hospital stay.[204] Good pain control is essential for early mobilization, which in turn promotes rapid recovery. Early mobilization is important in preventing pulmonary complications and thromboembolism. Pulmonary complications may also be reduced by active breathing exercises, such as physiotherapy and incentive spirometry.[172,205] Pulse oximetry can be used to monitor the pulmonary status. Adequate thrombosis prophylaxis helps to reduce the risk of perioperative death and should be given even when the hospital stay is less than 24 hours.[203]

Monitoring urinary production and kidney function is important, but a moderate rise in creatinine is to be expected and needs no special attention. However, in rare cases rhabdomyolysis may occur, being characterized by significant impairment of kidney function necessitating treatment and even dialysis.[14,61,63]

Short-term follow-up is within the domain of the surgeon; surgical reports of follow-up generally focus on time to recovery and time lost from work. The duration is often claimed to be short, especially after endoscopic procedures. It should, however, be recognized that in quality-of-life studies the duration to full recovery is often longer, and depression is not uncommon. This might be related to the psychological and emotional stress that accompanies the operation and concerns about the recipient outcome. Negative reactions are more frequent in cases of unfavourable recipient outcome and for more distant relatives.[182,183,186,206] Keeping in contact with the donor after discharge is, therefore, important in recognizing and attending to any such problem.

FUTURE DEVELOPMENTS

Future developments will focus on reducing perioperative mortality, short- and long-term morbidity, as well as optimizing kidney function and integrity in both the donor and recipient. This will require attention to issues throughout the process, including donor evaluation, perioperative management and long-term follow-up. Registry data regarding donor outcomes will be beneficial in focusing attention on specific issues and potential interventions.

From a surgical standpoint, the most crucial issues appear to be better screening of thromboembolic risk factors and prevention of thrombosis. Increased safety and quality of surgical techniques and instruments, especially endoscopic instruments, are also important. Robotic surgery may be of value, but the ability to intervene immediately to achieve control of major bleeding remains of utmost importance. Thus, robotics will probably be combined with either hand-assisted or open techniques.

In terms of improving kidney function,

new gasless technology and pharmacological treatments to reduce vasospasm and reduce ischaemia/reperfusion damage both need to be developed.

SUMMARY

The ideal live donor operation should have no mortality or morbidity, and procure a kidney with optimal function. This will not be possible in 100% of cases, but with this goal in mind the surgical team must take meticulous care of all details in the pre-, peri- and postoperative periods. Donor mortality is very low, and it will not be possible to perform prospective randomized trials to evaluate which operative methods are the safest. On theoretical grounds, applying empirical data, two techniques now seem the best options: for the open procedure, the anterior retroperitoneal approach and for the endoscopic, the hand-assisted retroperitoneal approach. Both methods have the best potential to reduce the most significant complications associated with mortality and morbidity, namely sudden massive bleeding, visceral injuries, adhesions and wound-related problems. The endoscopic technique has the advantage of retrieving the kidney from a lower midline or Pfannenstiel incision, and the open technique is probably safer in cases of massive bleeding. Ultimately, the choice of method depends on which kidney is to be removed, together with the experience of the surgical team with each technique.

REFERENCES

1. Wolters U, Wolf T, Stutzer H, Schroder T. ASA classification and perioperative variables as predictors of postoperative outcome. *Br J Anaesth* 1996; **77**: 217–222.
2. Archer C, Levy AR, McGregor M. Mayo. Value of routine preoperative chest x-rays: a meta-analysis. *Can J Anaesth* 1993; **40**: 1022–1027.
3. Narr BJ, Hansen TR, Warner MA. Preoperative laboratory screening in healthy Mayo patients: cost-effective elimination of tests and unchanged outcomes. *Clin Proc* 1991; **66**: 155–159.
4. www.acc.org/clinical/guidelines/perio/update/pdf/perio_update.pdf (Accessed 16 March 2004).

5. Hazebroek EJ, Gommers D, Schreve MA et al. Impact of intraoperative donor management on short-term renal function after laparoscopic donor nephrectomy. *Ann Surg* 2002; **236**: 127–132.

6. Kwik RS. Complications associated with surgery in the flank position for urological procedures. *Middle East J Anaesthesiol* 1980; **5**: 485–494.

7. Fujise K, Shingu K, Matsumoto S et al. The effects of the lateral position on cardiopulmonary function during laparoscopic urological surgery. *Anesth Analg* 1998; **87**: 925–930.

8. Lindstrom P, Kallskog O, Wadstrom J, Persson AE. Blood flow distribution during elevated intraperitoneal pressure in the rat. *Acta Physiol Scand* 2003; **177**: 149–156.

9. Razvi HA, Fields D, Vargas JC et al. Oliguria during laparoscopic surgery: evidence for direct renal parenchymal compression as an etiologic factor. *J Endourol* 1996; **10**: 1–4.

10. Chang DT, Kirsch AJ, Sawczuk IS. Oliguria during laparoscopic surgery. *J Endourol* 1994; **8**: 349–352.

11. Lindstrom P, Wadstrom J, Ollerstam A, Johnsson C, Persson AE. Effects of increased intra-abdominal pressure and volume expansion on renal function in the rat. *Nephrol Dial Transplant* 2003; **18**: 2269–2277.

12. Harman PK, Kron IL, McLachlan HD, Freedlender AE, Nolan SP. Elevated intra-abdominal pressure and renal function. *Ann Surg* 1982; **196**: 594–597.

13. Sundqvist P, Feuk U, Haggman M et al. Hand-assisted retroperitoneoscopic live donor nephrectomy in comparison to open and laparoscopic procedures: a prospective study on donor morbidity and kidney function. *Transplantation* 2004; **78**: 147–153.

14. Matas AJ, Bartlett ST, Leichtman AB, Delmonico FL. Morbidity and mortality after living kidney donation, 1999–2001: survey of United States transplant centers. *Am J Transplant* 2003; **3**: 830–834.

15. Hsu TH, Su LM, Ratner LE, Kavoussi LR. Renovascular complications of laparoscopic donor nephrectomy. *Urology* 2002; **60**: 811–815.

16. Najarian JS, Chavers BM, McHugh LE, Matas AJ. 20 years or more of follow-up of living kidney donors. *Lancet* 1992; **340**: 807–810.

17. Waples MJ, Belzer FO, Uehling DT. Living donor nephrectomy: a 20-year experience. *Urology* 1995; **45**: 207–210.

18. Dunn JF, Nylander WA Jr, Richie RE et al. Living related kidney donors. A 14-year experience. *Ann Surg* 1986; **203**: 637–643.

19. McGlennen RC, Key NS. Clinical and laboratory management of the prothrombin G20210A mutation. *Arch Pathol Lab Med* 2002; **126**: 1319–1325.

20. Seligsohn U, Lubetsky A. Genetic susceptibility to venous thrombosis. *N Engl J Med* 2001; **344**: 1222–1231.

21. Siegbahn A. Koagulation och fibrinolys. In: Nordgren L (ed) *Vensjukdommar* Studentlitteratur: Lund, 2002: 79–86.

22. Flancbaum L, Choban PS. Surgical implications of obesity. *Annu Rev Med* 1998; **49**: 215–234.

23. Dindo D, Muller MK, Weber M, Clavien PA. Obesity in general elective surgery. *Lancet* 2003; **361**: 2032–2035.

24. Jacobs SC, Cho E, Dunkin BJ et al. Laparoscopic nephrectomy in the markedly obese living renal donor. *Urology* 2000; **56**: 926–929.

25. Pesavento TE, Henry ML, Falkenhain ME et al. Obese living kidney donors: short-term results and possible implications. *Transplantation* 1999; **68**: 1491–1496.

26. Haffner SM, Valdez RA, Hazuda HP et al. Prospective analysis of the insulin-resistance syndrome (syndrome X). *Diabetes* 1992; **41**: 715–722.

27. Praga M, Hernandez E, Herrero JC et al. Influence of obesity on the appearance of proteinuria and renal insufficiency after unilateral nephrectomy. *Kidney Int* 2000; **58**: 2111–2118.

28. Sigurdsson GH, McAteer E. Morbidity and mortality associated with anaesthesia. *Acta Anaesthesiol Scand* 1996; **40**: 1057–1063.

29. Spencer FC. Human error in hospitals and industrial accidents: current concepts. *J Am Coll Surg* 2000; **191**: 410–418.

30. Bakir N, Sluiter WJ, Ploeg RJ, van Son WJ, Tegzess AM. Primary renal graft thrombosis. *Nephrol Dial Transplant* 1996; **11**: 140–147.

31. Patil UD, Ragavan A, Nadaraj et al. Helical CT angiography in evaluation of live kidney donors. *Nephrol Dial Transplant* 2001; **16**: 1900–1904.

32. Kawamoto S, Montgomery RA, Lawler LP, Horton KM, Fishman EK. Multidetector CT angiography for preoperative evaluation of living laparoscopic kidney donors. *Am J Roentgenol* 2003; **180**: 1633–1638.

33. Johnston T, Reddy K, Mastrangelo M, Lucas B, Ranjan D. Multiple renal arteries do not pose an impediment to the routine use of laparoscopic donor nephrectomy. *Clin Transplant* 2001; **15**(suppl 6): 62–65.

34. Roza AM, Perloff LJ, Naji A, Grossman RA, Barker CF. Living-related donors with bilateral multiple renal arteries: a twenty-year experience. *Transplantation* 1988; **47**: 397–399.

35. Loughlin KR, Tilney NL, Richie JP. Urologic complications in 718 renal transplant patients. *Surgery* 1984; **95**: 297–302.

36. Oesterwitz H, Strobelt V, Scholz D, Mebel M. Extracorporeal microsurgical repair of injured multiple donor kidney arteries prior to cadaveric allotransplantation. *Eur Urol* 1985; **11**: 100–105.

37. Hsu TH, Su LM, Ratner LE, Trock BJ, Kavoussi LR. Impact of renal artery multiplicity on outcomes of renal donors and recipients in laparoscopic donor nephrectomy. *Urology* 2003; **61**: 323–327.

38. Troppmann C, Wiesmann K, McVicar JP, Wolfe BM, Perez RV. Increased transplantation of kidneys with multiple renal arteries in the laparoscopic live

donor nephrectomy era: surgical technique and surgical and nonsurgical donor and recipient outcomes. *Arch Surg* 2001; **136**: 897–907.

39. Indudhara R, Kenney, Bueschen AJ, Burns JR. Live donor nephrectomy in patients with fibromuscular dysplasia of the renal arteries. *J Urol* 1999; **162**: 678–681.

40. Nahas WC, Lucon AM, Mazzucchi E et al. Kidney transplantation: the use of living donors with renal artery lesions. *J Urol* 1998; **160**: 1244–1247.

41. Lind MY, Hazebroek EJ, Hop WC et al. Right-sided laparoscopic live-donor nephrectomy: is reluctance still justified? *Transplantation* 2002; **74**: 1045–1048.

42. Bettschart V, Boubaker A, Martinet O et al. Laparoscopic right nephrectomy for live kidney donation: functional results. *Transpl Int* 2003; **16**: 419–424.

43. Blohme I, Fehrman I, Norden G. Living donor nephrectomy. Complication rates in 490 consecutive cases. *Scand J Urol Nephrol* 1992; **26**: 149–153.

44. Buell JF, Edye M, Johnson M et al. Are concerns over right laparoscopic donor nephrectomy unwarranted? *Ann Surg* 2001; **233**: 645–651.

45. Swartz DE, Cho E, Flowers JL et al. Laparoscopic right donor nephrectomy: technique and comparison with left nephrectomy. *Surg Endosc* 2001; **15**: 1390–1394.

46. Karkos CD, Bruce IA, Thomson GJ, Lambert ME. Retroaortic left renal vein and its implications in abdominal aortic surgery. *Ann Vasc Surg* 2001; **15**: 703–708.

47. Satyapal KS, Kalideen JM, Haffejee AA, Singh B, Robbs JV. Left renal vein variations. *Surg Radiol Anat* 1999; **21**: 77–81.

48. Wadstrom J, Lindstrom P. Retroaortic renal vein not a contraindication for hand-assisted retroperitoneoscopic living donor nephrectomy. *Transplant Proc* 2003; **35**: 784.

49. Lin CH, Steinberg AP, Ramani AP et al. Laparoscopic live donor nephrectomy in the presence of circumaortic or retroaortic left renal vein. *J Urol* 2004; **171**: 44–46.

50. Hartman GW, Hodson CJ. The duplex kidney and related abnormalities. *Clin Radiol* 1969; **20**: 387–400.

51. Privett JT, Jeans WD, Roylance J. The incidence and importance of renal duplication. *Clin Radiol* 1976; **27**: 521–530.

52. Fernbach SK, Feinstein KA, Spencer K, Lindstrom CA. Ureteral duplication and its complications. *Radiographics* 1997; **17**: 109–127.

53. Lowell JA, Taylor RJ. The evaluation of the living renal donor, surgical techniques and results. *Semin Urol* 1994; **12**: 102–107.

54. Ratner LE. Preferential laparoscopic live donor left nephrectomy in women of childbearing age. *Arch Surg* 2002; **137**: 225.

55. Mandal AK, Cohen C, Montgomery RA, Kavoussi LR, Ratner LE. Should the indications for laparoscopic live donor nephrectomy of the right kidney be the same as for the open procedure? Anomalous left renal vasculature is not a contraindication to laparoscopic left donor nephrectomy. *Transplantation* 2001; **71**: 660–664.

56. Boorjian S, Munver R, Sosa RE, Del Pizzo JJ. Right laparoscopic live donor nephrectomy: a single institution experience. *Transplantation* 2004; **77**: 437–440.

57. el-Diasty TA, Shokeir AA, el-Ghar ME et al. Contrast enhanced spiral computerized tomography in live kidney donors: a single session for anatomical and functional assessment. *J Urol* 2004; **171**: 31–34.

58. Nilsson H, Wadström D, Andersson LG et al. Measuring split renal function in renal donors: can computed tomography replace renography? *Acta Radiol* 2004; **45**: 474–480.

59. Wolf JS Jr, Marcovich R, Gill IS et al. Survey of neuromuscular injuries to the patient and surgeon during urologic laparoscopic surgery. *Urology* 2000; **55**: 831–836.

60. Mathes DD, Assimos DG, Donofrio PD. Rhabdomyolysis and myonecrosis in a patient in the lateral decubitus position. *Anesthesiology* 1996; **84**: 727–729.

61. Kuang W, Ng CS, Matin S et al. Rhabdomyolysis after laparoscopic donor nephrectomy. *Urology* 2002; **60**: 911.

62. Kozak KR, Shah S, Ishihara KK, Schulman G. Hand-assisted laparoscopic radical nephrectomy-associated rhabdomyolysis with ARF. *Am J Kidney Dis* 2003; **41**: E5.

63. Troppmann C, Perez RV. Rhabdomyolysis associated with laparoscopic live donor nephrectomy and concomitant surgery: a note of caution. *Am J Transplant* 2003; **3**: 1457–1458.

64. Moll F, Karenberg A. Gustav Simon (1824–1877) and the development of nephrectomy: the surgeon and his intention. *J Med Biogr* 2000; **8**: 140–145.

65. Lauridsen L. Gustav Simon and the beginning of kidney surgery. *Acta Chir Scand Suppl* 1973; **433**: 31–41.

66. Cosimi AB. The donor and donor nephrectomy. In: Morris PJ (ed) *Kidney Transplantation*, 4th edn Philadelphia: WB Saunders, 1994: 56–70.

67. Ratner LE, Ciseck LJ, Moore RG et al. Laparoscopic live donor nephrectomy. *Transplantation* 1995; **60**: 1047–1049.

68. Troppmann C, Ormond DB, Perez RV. Laparoscopic (vs open) live donor nephrectomy: a UNOS database analysis of early graft function and survival. *Am J Transplant* 2003; **3**: 1295–1301.

69. Mehraban D, Nowroozi A, Naderi GH. Flank versus transabdominal living donor nephrectomy: a randomized clinical trial. *Transplant Proc* 1995; **27**: 2716–2717.

70. Ruiz R, Novick AC, Braun WE, Montague DK, Stewart BH. Transperitoneal live donor nephrectomy. *J Urol* 1980; **123**: 819–821.

71. Hamilton BD, Chow GK, Inman SR, Stowe NT, Winfield HN. Increased intra-abdominal pressure during pneumoperitoneum stimulates endothelin

release in a canine model. *J Endourol* 1998; **12**: 193–197.

72. Dolgor B, Kitano S, Yoshida T et al. Vasopressin antagonist improves renal function in a rat model of pneumoperitoneum. *J Surg Res* 1998; **79**: 109–114.

73. Chiu AW, Chang LS, Birkett DH, Babayan RK. The impact of pneumoperitoneum, pneumoretroperitoneum, and gasless laparoscopy on the systemic and renal hemodynamics. *J Am Coll Surg* 1995; **181**: 397–406.

74. Gill IS, Clayman RV, Albala DM et al. Retroperitoneal and pelvic extraperitoneal laparoscopy: an international perspective. *Urology* 1998; **52**: 566–571.

75. Bishoff JT, Allaf ME, Kirkels W et al. Laparoscopic bowel injury: incidence and clinical presentation. *J Urol* 1999; **161**: 887–890.

76. Fahlenkamp D, Rassweiler J, Fornara P, Frede T, Loening SA. Complications of laparoscopic procedures in urology: experience with 2,407 procedures at 4 German centers. *J Urol* 1999; **162**: 765–770.

77. Soulie M, Seguin P, Richeux L et al. Urological complications of laparoscopic surgery: experience with 350 procedures at a single center. *J Urol* 2001; **165**: 1960–1963.

78. Soulie M, Salomon L, Seguin P et al. Multi-institutional study of complications in 1085 laparoscopic urologic procedures. *Urology* 2001; **58**: 899–903.

79. Liakakos T, Thomakos N, Fine PM, Dervenis C, Young RL. Peritoneal adhesions: etiology, pathophysiology, and clinical significance. Recent advances in prevention and management. *Dig Surg* 2001; **18**: 260–273.

80. Kavic SM. Adhesions and adhesiolysis: the role of laparoscopy. *JSLS* 2002; **6**: 99–109.

81. Carmignani G, Traverso P, Corbu C. Incidental splenectomy during left radical nephrectomy: reasons and ways to avoid it. *Urol Int* 2001; **67**: 195–198.

82. Mejean A, Vogt B, Quazza JE, Chretien Y, Dufour B. Mortality and morbidity after nephrectomy for renal cell carcinoma using a transperitoneal anterior subcostal incision. *Eur Urol* 1999; **36**: 298–302.

83. Swanson DA, Borges PM. Complications of transabdominal radical nephrectomy for renal cell carcinoma. *J Urol* 1983; **129**: 704–707.

84. Siebels M, Theodorakis J, Schmeller N et al. Risks and complications in 160 living kidney donors who underwent nephroureterectomy. *Nephrol Dial Transplant* 2003; **18**: 2648–2654.

85. Rassweiler JJ, Seemann O, Frede T, Henkel TO, Alken P. Retroperitoneoscopy: experience with 200 cases. *J Urol* 1998; **160**: 1265–1269.

86. Wolf JS Jr, Tchetgen MB, Merion RM. Hand-assisted laparoscopic live donor nephrectomy. *Urology* 1998; **52**: 885–887.

87. Gill IS, Rassweiler JJ. Retroperitoneoscopic renal surgery: our approach. *Urology* 1999; **54**: 734–738.

88. Wadstrom J, Lindstrom P. Hand-assisted retroperi-toneoscopic living-donor nephrectomy: initial 10 cases. *Transplantation* 2002; **73**: 1839–1840.

89. Srivastava A, Tripathi DM, Zaman W, Kumar A. Subcostal versus transcostal mini donor nephrectomy: is rib resection responsible for pain related donor morbidity. *J Urol* 2003; **170**: 738–740.

90. Perry KT, Freedland SJ, Hu JC et al. Quality of life, pain and return to normal activities following laparoscopic donor nephrectomy versus open mini-incision donor nephrectomy. *J Urol* 2003; **169**: 2018–2021.

91. Shenoy S, Lowell JA, Ramachandran V, Jendrisak M. The ideal living donor nephrectomy 'mini-nephrectomy' through a posterior transcostal approach. *J Am Coll Surg* 2002; **194**: 240–246.

92. Greenstein MA, Harkaway R, Badosa F, Ginsberg P, Yang SL. Minimal incision living donor nephrectomy compared to the hand-assisted laparoscopic living donor nephrectomy. *World J Urol* 2003; **20**: 356–359.

93. Murdock CM, Wolff AJ, Van Geem T. Risk factors for hypercarbia, subcutaneous emphysema, pneumothorax, and pneumomediastinum during laparoscopy. *Obstet Gynecol* 2000; **95**: 704–709.

94. Abreu SC, Sharp DS, Ramani AP et al. Thoracic complications during urological laparoscopy. *J Urol* 2004; **171**: 1451–1455.

95. Derouin M, Couture P, Boudreault D, Girard D, Gravel D. Detection of gas embolism by transesophageal echocardiography during laparoscopic cholecystectomy. *Anesth Analg* 1996; **82**: 119–124.

96. Fahy BG, Hasnain JU, Flowers JL et al. Transesophageal echocardiographic detection of gas embolism and cardiac valvular dysfunction during laparoscopic nephrectomy. *Anesth Analg* 1999; **88**: 500–504.

97. Martay K, Dembo G, Vater Y et al. Unexpected surgical difficulties leading to hemorrhage and gas embolus during laparoscopic donor nephrectomy: a case report. *Can J Anaesth* 2003; **50**: 891–894.

98. Lantz PE, Smith JD. Fatal carbon dioxide embolism complicating attempted laparoscopic cholecystectomy – case report and literature review. *J Forensic Sci* 1994; **39**: 1468–1480.

99. Blaser A, Rosset P. Fatal carbon dioxide embolism as an unreported complication of retroperitoneoscopy. *Surg Endosc* 1999; **13**: 713–714.

100. Cottin V, Delafosse B, Viale JP. Gas embolism during laparoscopy: a report of seven cases in patients with previous abdominal surgical history. *Surg Endosc* 1996; **10**: 166–169.

101. Beck DH, McQuillan PJ. Fatal carbon dioxide embolism and severe haemorrhage during laparoscopic salpingectomy. *Br J Anaesth* 1994; **72**: 243–245.

102. Munro MG. Laparoscopic access: complications, technologies, and techniques. *Curr Opin Obstet Gynecol* 2002; **14**: 365–374.

103. Jacobs SC, Cho E, Foster C, Liao P, Bartlett ST. Laparoscopic donor nephrectomy: the University of Maryland 6-year experience. *J Urol* 2004; **171**: 47–51.

104. Feste JR, Bojahr B, Turner DJ. Randomized trial comparing a radially expandable needle system with cutting trocars. *JSLS* 2000; **4**: 11–15.

105. Deng DY, Meng MV, Nguyen HT, Bellman GC, Stoller ML. Laparoscopic linear cutting stapler failure. *Urology* 2002; **60**: 415–419.

106. Chan D, Bishoff JT, Ratner L, Kavoussi LR, Jarrett TW. Endovascular gastrointestinal stapler device malfunction during laparoscopic nephrectomy: early recognition and management. *J Urol* 2000; **164**: 319–321.

107. Montgomery RA, Kavoussi LR, Su L et al. Improved recipient results after 5 years of performing laparoscopic donor nephrectomy. *Transplant Proc* 2001; **33**: 1108–1110.

108. Friedman AL, Ratner LE, Peters TG. Fatal and nonfatal hemorrhagic complications of living kidney donation. *Am J Transplant* 2004; **8**(suppl 8): 370.

109. Parsons JK, Varkarakis I, Rha KH et al. Complications of abdominal urologic laparoscopy: longitudinal five-year analysis. *Urology* 2004; **63**: 27–32.

110. Merlin TL, Scott DF, Rao MM et al. The safety and efficacy of laparoscopic live donor nephrectomy: a systematic review. *Transplantation* 2000; **70**: 1659–1666.

111. Simon SD, Castle EP, Ferrigni RG et al. Complications of laparoscopic nephrectomy: the Mayo clinic experience. *J Urol* 2004; **171**: 1447–1450.

112. Ratner LE, Montgomery RA, Maley WR et al. Laparoscopic live donor nephrectomy: the recipient. *Transplantation* 2000; **69**: 2319–2323.

113. Ratner LE, Montgomery RA, Kavoussi LR. Laparoscopic live donor nephrectomy. A review of the first 5 years. *Urol Clin North Am* 2001; **28**: 709–719.

114. Ratner LE, Kavoussi LR, Sroka M et al. Laparoscopic assisted live donor nephrectomy – a comparison with the open approach. *Transplantation* 1997; **63**: 229–233.

115. Flowers JL, Jacobs S, Cho E et al. Comparison of open and laparoscopic live donor nephrectomy. *Ann Surg* 1997; **226**: 483–489.

116. Waller JR, Hiley AL, Mullin EJ, Veitch PS, Nicholson ML. Living kidney donation: a comparison of laparoscopic and conventional open operations. *Postgrad Med J* 2002; **78**: 153–157.

117. Hawasli A, Boutt A, Cousins G, Schervish E, Oh H. Laparoscopic versus conventional live donor nephrectomy: experience in a community transplant program. *Am Surg* 2001; **67**: 342–345.

118. Berends FJ, den Hoed PT, Bonjer HJ et al. Technical considerations and pitfalls in laparoscopic live donor nephrectomy. *Surg Endosc* 2002; **16**: 893–898.

119. Leventhal JR, Deeik RK, Joehl RJ et al. Laparoscopic live donor nephrectomy – is it safe? *Transplantation* 2000; **70**: 602–606.

120. Schweitzer EJ, Wilson J, Jacobs S et al. Increased rates of donation with laparoscopic donor nephrectomy. *Ann Surg* 2000; **232**: 392–400.

121. Ratner LE, Hiller J, Sroka M et al. Laparoscopic live donor nephrectomy removes disincentives to live donation. *Transplant Proc* 1997; **29**: 3402–3403.

122. Kuo PC, Johnson LB. Laparoscopic donor nephrectomy increases the supply of living donor kidneys: a center-specific microeconomic analysis. *Transplantation* 2000; **69**: 2211–2213.

123. Simforoosh N, Bassiri A, Ziaee SA et al. Laparoscopic versus open live donor nephrectomy: the first randomized clinical trial. *Transplant Proc* 2003; **35**: 2553–2554.

124. Velidedeoglu E, Williams N, Brayman KL et al. Comparison of open, laparoscopic, and hand-assisted approaches to live-donor nephrectomy. *Transplantation* 2002; **74**: 169–172.

125. Troppmann C, Pierce JL, Wiesmann KM et al. Early and late recipient graft function and donor outcome after laparoscopic vs open adult live donor nephrectomy for pediatric renal transplantation. *Arch Surg* 2002; **137**: 908–915.

126. Philosophe B, Kuo PC, Schweitzer EJ et al. Laparoscopic versus open donor nephrectomy: comparing ureteral complications in the recipients and improving the laparoscopic technique. *Transplantation* 1999; **68**: 497–502.

127. Nogueira JM, Cangro CB, Fink JC et al. A comparison of recipient renal outcomes with laparoscopic versus open live donor nephrectomy. *Transplantation* 1999; **67**: 722–728.

128. Lind MY, Hazebroek EJ, Kirkels WJ et al. Laparoscopic versus open donor nephrectomy: ureteral complications in recipients. *Urology* 2004; **63**: 36–39.

129. London ET, Ho HS, Neuhaus AM et al. Effect of intravascular volume expansion on renal function during prolonged CO_2 pneumoperitoneum. *Ann Surg* 2000; **231**: 195–201.

130. Kavoussi LR. Laparoscopic donor nephrectomy. *Kidney Int* 2000; **57**: 2175–2186.

131. Kim FJ, Pinto P, Su LM et al. Ipsilateral orchialgia after laparoscopic donor nephrectomy. *J Endourol* 2003; **17**: 405–409.

132. Levine LA, Matkov TG. Microsurgical denervation of the spermatic cord as primary surgical treatment of chronic orchialgia. *J Urol* 2001; **165**: 1927–1929.

133. Heidenreich A. Re: Microsurgical testicular denervation of the spermatic cord as primary surgical treatment of chronic orchialgia. *J Urol* 2001; **166**: 2322–2323.

134. Chan DY, Fabrizio MD, Ratner LE, Kavoussi LR. Complications of laparoscopic live donor nephrectomy: the first 175 cases. *Transplant Proc* 2000; **32**: 778.

135. Lee BR, Chow GK, Ratner LE, Kavoussi LR. Laparoscopic live donor nephrectomy: outcomes equivalent to open surgery. *J Endourol* 2000; **14**: 811–819.

136. Sandford R, Nicholson ML. Genito-femoral nerve entrapment: a complication of stapling the ureter during laparoscopic live donor nephrectomy. *Nephrol Dial Transplant* 2001; **16**: 2090–2091.

137. Berney T, Malaise J, Mourad M, Morel P, Squifflet JP. Laparoscopic and open live donor nephrectomy: a cost/benefit study. *Transpl Int* 2000; **13**: 35–40.

138. Giessing M, Deger S, Ebeling V et al. Laparoscopic living donor nephrectomy of kidneys with multiple renal vessels. *Urologe A* 2003; **42**: 225–232.

139. Kuo PC, Plotkin JS, Stevens S, Cribbs A, Johnson LB. Outcomes of laparoscopic donor nephrectomy in obese patients. *Transplantation* 2000; **69**: 180–182.

140. Hsu TH, Su LM, Ratner LE, Kavoussi LR. Laparoscopic donor nephrectomy in the elderly patient. *Urology* 2002; **60**: 398–401.

141. Abrahams HM, Meng MV, Freise CE, Stoller ML. Laparoscopic donor nephrectomy for pediatric recipients: outcomes analysis. *Urology* 2004; **63**: 163–166.

142. Hsu TH, Su LM, Trock BJ et al. Laparoscopic adult donor nephrectomy for pediatric renal transplantation. *Urology* 2003; **61**: 320–322.

143. Morrissey PE, Madras PN, Gohh RY, Monaco AP. Laparoscopic versus open donor nephrectomy. *Kidney Int* 2000; **58**: 2596–2597.

144. Novick AC. Laparoscopic live donor nephrectomy: con. *Urology* 1999; **53**: 668–670.

145. Serota AI. Laparoscopic live donor nephrectomy: debating the benefits. Con: persistent complications do not justify replacing 'the gold standard'. *Nephrol News Issues* 1999; **13**: 90–94.

146. Wolf JS Jr, Merion RM, Leichtman AB et al. Randomized controlled trial of hand-assisted laparoscopic versus open surgical live donor nephrectomy. *Transplantation* 2001; **72**: 284–290.

147. Wolf JS Jr, Marcovich R, Merion RM, Konnak JW. Prospective, case matched comparison of hand assisted laparoscopic and open surgical live donor nephrectomy. *J Urol* 2000; **163**: 1650–1653.

148. Gershbein AB, Fuchs GJ. Hand-assisted and conventional laparoscopic live donor nephrectomy: a comparison of two contemporary techniques. *J Endourol* 2002; **16**: 509–513.

149. El-Galley R, Hood N, Young CJ, Deierhoi M, Urban DA. Donor nephrectomy: A comparison of techniques and results of open, hand assisted and full laparoscopic nephrectomy. *J Urol* 2004; **171**: 40–3.

150. Rudich SM, Marcovich R, Magee JC et al. Hand-assisted laparoscopic donor nephrectomy: comparable donor/recipient outcomes, costs, and decreased convalescence as compared to open donor nephrectomy. *Transplant Proc* 2001; **33**: 1106–1107.

151. Stifelman MD, Hull D, Sosa RE et al. Hand assisted laparoscopic donor nephrectomy: a comparison with the open approach. *J Urol* 2001; **166**: 444–448.

152. Slakey DP, Wood JC, Hender D, Thomas R, Cheng S. Laparoscopic living donor nephrectomy: advantages of the hand-assisted method. *Transplantation* 1999; **68**: 581–583.

153. Lindstrom P, Haggman M, Wadstrom J. Hand-assisted laparoscopic surgery (HALS) for live donor nephrectomy is more time- and cost-effective than standard laparoscopic nephrectomy. *Surg Endosc* 2002; **16**: 422–425.

154. Slakey DP, Hahn JC, Rogers E et al. Single-center analysis of living donor nephrectomy: hand-assisted laparoscopic, pure laparoscopic, and traditional open. *Prog Transplant* 2002; **12**: 206–211.

155. Ruiz-Deya G, Cheng S, Palmer E, Thomas R, Slakey D. Open donor, laparoscopic donor and hand assisted laparoscopic donor nephrectomy: a comparison of outcomes. *J Urol* 2001; **166**: 1270–1273.

156. Sasaki TM, Finelli F, Bugarin E et al. Is laparoscopic donor nephrectomy the new criterion standard? *Arch Surg* 2000; **135**: 943–947.

157. Hoznek A, Olsson LE, Salomon L et al. Retroperitoneal laparoscopic living-donor nephrectomy. Preliminary results. *Eur Urol* 2001; **40**: 614–618.

158. Rassweiler JJ, Wiesel M, Carl S et al. Laparoscopic liver donor nephrectomy. Personal experiences and review of the literature. *Urologe A* 2001; **40**: 485–492.

159. Buell JF, Abreu SC, Hanaway MJ et al. Right donor nephrectomy: a comparison of hand-assisted transperitoneal and retroperitoneal laparoscopic approaches. *Transplantation* 2004; **77**: 521–525.

160. Gill IS, Uzzo RG, Hobart MG et al. Laparoscopic retroperitoneal live donor right nephrectomy for purposes of allotransplantation and autotransplantation. *J Urol* 2000; **164**: 1500–1504.

161. Abbou CC, Rabii R, Hoznek A et al. Nephrectomy in a living donor by retroperitoneal laparoscopy or lomboscopy. *Ann Urol* 2000; **34**: 312–318.

162. Knoepp L, Smith M, Huey J, Mancino A, Barber H. Complication after laparoscopic donor nephrectomy: a case report and review. *Transplantation* 1999; **68**: 449–451.

163. Wadstrom J, Lindstrom P, Engstrom BM. Hand-assisted retroperitoneoscopic living donor nephrectomy superior to laparoscopic nephrectomy. *Transplant Proc* 2003; **35**: 782–783.

164. Iinuma M, Satoh S, Tsuchiya N et al. Retroperitoneoscopic hand-assisted nephrectomy for live donor: Akita University experience. *Nippon Hinyokika Gakkai Zasshi* 2002; **93**: 721–726.

165. Wadström J. Hand-assisted retroperitoneoscopic nephrectomy. Experience with the first 50 consecutive cases [abstract]. *Am J Transplant* 2004; **8**(suppl 8): 595.

166. Bia MJ, Ramos EL, Danovitch GM et al. Evaluation of living renal donors. The current practice of US transplant centers. *Transplantation* 1995; **60**: 322–327.

167. Spanos PK, Simmons RL, Lampe E et al. Complications of related kidney donation. *Surgery* 1974; **76**: 741–747.

168. Yasumura T, Nakai I, Oka T et al. Experience with 247 living related donor nephrectomy cases at a single institution in Japan. *Jpn J Surg* 1988; **18**: 252–258.

169. D'Alessandro AM, Sollinger HW, Knechtle SJ et al. Living related and unrelated donors for kidney transplantation: a 28-year experience. *Ann Surg* 1995; **222**: 353–362.

170. Shaffer D, Sahyoun AI, Madras PN, Monaco AP. Two hundred one consecutive living-donor nephrectomies. *Arch Surg* 1998; **133**: 426–431.

171. Ottelin MC, Bueschen AJ, Lloyd LK et al. Review of 333 living donor nephrectomies. *South Med J* 1994; **87**: 61–64.

172. Johnson EM, Remucal MJ, Gillingham KJ et al. Complications and risks of living donor nephrectomy. *Transplantation* 1997; **64**: 1124–1128.

173. Duraj F, Tyden G, Blom B. Living-donor nephrectomy: how safe is it? *Transplant Proc* 1995; **27**: 803–804.

174. Wiesel M, Carl S, Staehler G. Living donor nephrectomy: a 28-year experience at Heidelberg University. *Transplant Proc* 1997; **29**: 2769.

175. Olsson LE, Swana H, Friedman AL, Lorber MI. Pleurotomy, pneumothorax, and surveillance during living donor nephroureterectomy. *Urology* 1998; **52**: 591–593.

176. Bayazit Y, Aridogan IA, Tansug Z, Unsal I, Erken U. Morbidity of flank incision in 100 renal donors. *Int Urol Nephrol* 2001; **32**: 709–711.

177. Kumar S, Duque JL, Bae R, O'Leary MP, Loughlin KR. Morbidity of flank incision for renal donors. *Transplant Proc* 2000; **32**: 779–780.

178. DeMarco T, Amin M, Harty JI. Living donor nephrectomy: factors influencing morbidity. *J Urol* 1982; **127**: 1082–1083.

179. Schostak M, Wloch H, Muller M et al. Living donor nephrectomy in an open technique; a long-term analysis of donor outcome. *Transplant Proc* 2003; **35**: 2096–2098.

180. Gardner GP, Josephs LG, Rosca M et al. The retroperitoneal incision. An evaluation of postoperative flank 'bulge'. *Arch Surg* 1994; **129**: 753–756.

181. Chatterjee S, Nam R, Fleshner N, Klotz L. Permanent flank bulge is a consequence of flank incision for radical nephrectomy in one half of patients. *Urol Oncol* 2004; **22**: 36–39

182. Fehrman-Ekholm I, Brink B, Ericsson C et al. Kidney donors don't regret: follow-up of 370 donors in Stockholm since 1964. *Transplantation* 2000; **69**: 2067–2071.

183. Johnson EM, Anderson JK, Jacobs C et al. Long-term follow-up of living kidney donors: quality of life after donation. *Transplantation* 1999; **67**: 717–721.

184. Duque JL, Loughlin KR, Kumar S. Morbidity of flank incision for renal donors. *Urology* 1999; **54**: 796–801.

185. Petersen S, Schuster F, Steinbach F et al. Sublay prosthetic repair for incisional hernia of the flank. *J Urol* 2002; **168**: 2461–2463.

186. Lennerling A, Blohme I, Ostraat O et al. Laparoscopic or open surgery for living donor nephrectomy. *Nephrol Dial Transplant* 2001; **16**: 383–386.

187. Blohme I, Gabel H, Brynger H. The living donor in renal transplantation. *Scand J Urol Nephrol Suppl* 1981; **64**: 143–151.

188. Jones KW, Peters TG, Walker GW. Anterior-retroperitoneal living donor nephrectomy: technique and outcomes. *Am Surg* 1999; **65**: 197–204.

189. Baptista-Silva JC, Poli de Figueiredo LF, Camara AL et al. Outcome of 605 consecutive living donor nephrectomies through an anterior subcostal retroperitoneal approach. *Transplant Proc* 2002; **34**: 451–452.

190. Peters TG, Repper SM, Vincent MC et al. One hundred consecutive living kidney donors: modern issues and outcomes. *Clin Transplant* 2002; **16**(suppl 7): 62–68.

191. Baier PK, Pisarski P, Wimmenauer S, Kirste G. Kidney donation by living donors. Surgical procedure. *Zentralbl Chir* 1999; **124**: 729–733.

192. Redman JF. An anterior extraperitoneal incision for donor nephrectomy that spares the rectus abdominis muscle and anterior abdominal wall nerves. *J Urol* 2000; **164**: 1898–1900.

193. Yang SC, Ko WJ, Byun YJ, Rha KH. Retroperitoneoscopy assisted live donor nephrectomy: the Yonsei experience. *J Urol* 2001; **165**: 1099–1102.

194. Yang SC, Park DS, Lee DH, Lee JM, Park K. Retroperitoneal endoscopic live donor nephrectomy: report of 3 cases. *J Urol* 1995; **153**: 1884–1886.

195. Yang SC, Lee DH, Rha KH, Park K. Retroperitoneoscopic living donor nephrectomy: two cases. *Transplant Proc* 1994; **26**: 2409.

196. Watanabe R, Saitoh K, Kurumada S, Komeyama T, Takahashi K. Gasless laparoscopy-assisted live donor nephrectomy. *Transplant Proc* 2002; **34**: 2578–2580.

197. Suzuki K, Ishikawa A, Ushiyama T et al. Gasless laparoscopy-assisted live donor nephrectomy: the initial 23 cases. *Transplant Proc* 2000; **32**: 788–789.

198. Suzuki K, Ushiyama T, Ishikawa A, Mugiya S, Fujita K. Retroperitoneoscopy assisted live donor nephrectomy: the initial 2 cases. *J Urol* 1997; **158**: 1353–1356.

199. Yang SC, Rha KH, Kim YS, Kim SI, Park K. Retroperitoneoscopy-assisted living donor nephrectomy: 109 cases. *Transplant Proc* 2001; **33**: 1104–1105.

200. Ishikawa A, Suzuki K, Saisu K et al. Endoscopy-assisted live donor nephrectomy: comparison between laparoscopic and retroperitoneoscopic procedures. *Transplant Proc* 1998; **30**: 165–167.

201. Mourad M, Malaise J, Squifflet JP. Laparoscopy-assisted living donor nephrectomy in combination with minilaparotomy. *Transplant Proc* 2000; **32**: 488–490.

202. Suzuki K, Ishikawa A, Ushiyama T, Fujita K. Retroperitoneoscopic living donor nephrectomy without gas insufflation: the five-year Hamamatsu University experience. *Transplant Proc* 2002; **34**: 720–721.

203. Kuo PC, Johnson LB, Sitzmann JV. Laparoscopic donor nephrectomy with a 23-hour stay: a new standard for transplantation surgery. *Ann Surg* 2000; **231**: 772–779.

204. Ashcraft EE, Baillie GM, Shafizadeh SF et al. Further improvements in laparoscopic donor nephrectomy: decreased pain and accelerated recovery. *Clin Transpl* 2001; **15**(suppl 6): 59–61.

205. Thomas JA, McIntosh JM. Are incentive spirometry,

intermittent positive pressure breathing, and deep breathing exercises effective in the prevention of postoperative pulmonary complications after upper abdominal surgery? A systematic overview and meta-analysis. *Phys Ther* 1994; **74**: 3–10.

206. Smith GC, Trauer T, Kerr PG, Chadban SJ. Prospective psychosocial monitoring of living kidney donors using the SF-36 health survey. *Transplantation* 2003; **76**: 807–809.

Long-term risks after living kidney donation

7

Ingela Fehrman-Ekholm, Gilbert T Thiel

INTRODUCTION

With more and more living kidney donors worldwide, knowledge regarding long-term risk for kidney donors is of increasing importance. Unfortunately, although many reports of early and late complications after donor nephrectomy have been published, most are retrospective analyses with substantial gaps in data. Nonetheless, one can learn important lessons from published data, to which in this chapter we will add our own experience. The chapter therefore focuses on five key issues, each of which is related to the others:

- renal function
- proteinuria and albuminuria
- hypertension
- occurrence of end-stage renal disease (ESRD) in donors
- general health and causes of death in donors.

RENAL FUNCTION

Accurate assessment of renal function is an essential component of donor evaluation. The gold standard is measurement of the glomerular filtration rate (GFR) by inulin clearance. However, inulin clearance is time-consuming and expensive for clinical purposes and most centres use more easily

performed techniques to measure or estimate GFR. These include 24-hour urine collection for creatinine clearance (CCr), iothalamate clearance, chromium-51-labelled ethylenediaminetetra-acetate (Cr^{51}-EDTA) or a calculated estimate using the Cockcroft–Gault formula or the Levey formula.

Cockcroft–Gault formula†

$$CCr = \frac{1.22\ (140 - age) \times weight}{serum\ creatinine}\ (men)$$

$$CCr = \frac{1.04\ (140 - age) \times weight}{serum\ creatinine}\ (women)$$

Levey formula*

GFR [ml/min/1.73m^2] = $170 \times$ (serum creatinine [µmol/l]/88.4)$^{-0.999} \times$ (age)$^{-0.176}$ × (serum urea [mmol/l] ×2.75$^{-0.170} \times$ (serum albumin [g/l]/10)$^{0.318} \times$ (0.762 if female) × (1.180 if black)

More recently, measurement of cystatin C, also an endogenous substance in blood, has been proposed to estimate GFR.[1,2] Using this technique, GFR can be estimated from a single blood sample and the outcome reflects average GFR over time independent of muscle mass, gender, and tubular excretion. Although data appear promising, there is currently little experience worldwide with this technique.[3]

†CCr = Creatinine Clearance (ml/min). In these two formulae serum creatinine is expressed in µmol/l. The resulting CCr is given in ml/min, and is thus not yet corrected for body surface area (ml/min/1.73m^2).

*In this formula serum creatinine is expressed in µmol/l; serum urea in mmol/l; serum albumin in g/l; age in years; weight in kg; height in m. The Levey Formula estimates GFR (not CCr) already in ml/min/1.73m^2. No correction for body surface area is needed.

Table 7-1 Comparison of techniques for measuring renal function

Method	Measure	Advantages	Disadvantages
Inulin clearance	GFR	Gold standard	Expensive and time consuming
Iohexol	GFR	Simple	Time consuming
Iothalamate Cr-EDTA	GFR	Well-standardized GFR estimate	Expensive Radioisotope handling for labelled iothalamate, Cr-EDTA
24-hour urine	Creatinine clearance	Simple and cheap	May under- or overestimate GFR Adequate urine collection is difficult
Cystatin C	GFR	Simple	Uncertain results
Calculations of GFR based on different formulae	GFR	Simple The most accurate method requires blood tests and information regarding height, weight, age, sex and race	Various methods Levey's is probably the best; Cockroft–Gault may under- or overestimate GFR, depending on the assay used for serum creatinine determination

GFR, glomerular filtration rate; Cr-EDTA, chromium-labelled ethylenediaminetetra-acetate.

Table 7-2 Key components of annual or biannual examination after donor nephrectomy

General	Clinical biochemistry	Physical examination	Urinary status
• Donor check-up • Anamnesis • Medications • Smoking habit • Current status • Listen to experiences • Thank them	• Serum urea • Serum creatinine • Serum albumin • Serum urate • Blood glucose • Blood haemoglobin • Lipids	• Blood pressure • Weight • Height • Abdomen, (scar)	• Urinalysis • Urinary albumin and creatinine • Microalbuminuria

It is important to recognize that each of these simplified methods has its own limitations (Table 7-1) and only provides reliable estimates if all variables, time intervals, volumes and techniques are performed exactly as stipulated. Indeed, even minor deviations from the prescribed protocol may result in significant errors.

During follow-up, knowledge regarding the chemical method used to determine creatinine is imperative, since results of different methods will be different. For example, the results from Jaffé's method are typically 15% higher than those obtained using an enzymatic technique.[4] Thus, if meaningful follow-up data are to be obtained, it is essential that creatinine levels are measured at the *same* laboratory using the *same* technique as that used for the initial determination. Age, body weight, sex and height should also be recorded (Table 7-2) to adapt creatinine clearance to a standard body surface area of $1.73\,m^2$. In addition, serum urea and albumin need to be estimated to apply Levey's formula.[5] This is important because a recent study in the elderly (>70 years) showed that GFR was more strongly correlated to serum urea than to serum creatinine.[6] Urea clearance, however, increases proportional to water intake, in contrast to creatinine and inulin clearance. Some elderly people with a high water intake have a higher urea clearance and lower serum urea level despite unchanged GFR.

After donor nephrectomy, serum creatinine levels increase by approximately 25% and creatinine clearance (or GFR) falls by approximately the same percentage. Several studies indicate that functional adaptation occurs rapidly after uninephrectomy, with GFR remaining stable over many years. Indeed, data from the Swiss Organ Living Donor Health Registry (SOL-DHR) showed stable (or improved) serum creatinine levels in donors followed for up to 10 years after donation (Figure 7-1). The SOL-DHR registry data indicate a slow improvement for measures of serum creatinine and creatinine clearance. This finding is in contrast with the expected physiological decline in GFR associated with ageing (i.e., approximately 1 mL/min/year).[7] Thus, the effect of nephrectomy in terms of increasing GFR by hyperfiltration *outweighs* the effect of normal renal ageing, at least during the first decade. The as-yet-unanswered questions are whether this trend will continue beyond the first decade after nephrectomy and whether it may, over time, result in adverse changes (e.g. glomerulosclerosis, interstitial fibrosis) within the remaining kidney.

Most long-term data are limited by incomplete information. Nevertheless, a recent report from Sweden showed no statistical evidence of a more rapid decline in GFR than expected in the general population. In addition, the ratio of observed-to-predicted GFR remained stable at 0.72 in a cross-sectional study of 348 donors when estimated 2–33 years after nephrectomy (Figure 7-2).[8] This study provides valuable data as it included 87% of all donors in the Stockholm region over that period. Similar findings have been observed in US centres. At the Cleveland Clinic, data on 70 persons who had undergone donor nephrectomy at least 25 years previously indicated that creatinine clearance was stable at 72% of pre-donation levels. However, the study only included data from 40% of cases over this period, a factor that may have masked the expected age-dependent decline in creatinine clearance over the observation period.[9] Another recent study included data from 464 of 773 donors (60%)

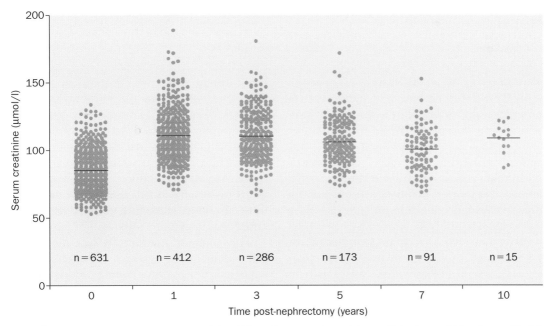

Figure 7-1 Serum creatinine values from living kidney donors registered in the Swiss Organ Living Donor Health Registry since 1993. Donors were followed-up continuously at 1, 3, 5, 7 and 10 years (April 1993 to November 2003) after nephrectomy. The initial increase in serum creatinine after nephrectomy was followed-up by a slight reduction until 10 years' post-nephrectomy. (All serum creatinine values were measured in the same laboratory, using Jaffé's assay.)

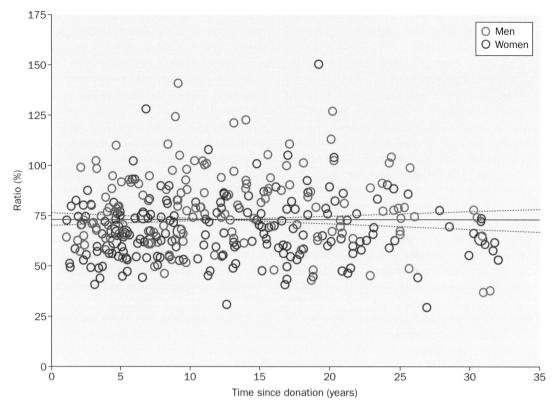

Figure 7-2   Renal function after nephrectomy. The ratio of estimated-to-predicted glomerular filtration rate showed no correlation with time since donation, indicating no accelerated loss of renal function after donation. Redrawn from Fehrman-Ekholm I et al[8] with permission from Lippincott Williams & Wilkins.

who were at least 20 years post-nephrectomy.[10] Of these, 84 had died (at least three of whom had renal failure), but renal function appeared stable in 375 of the remaining 380 (99%) donors. Although these data appear reassuring, the gaps in reporting mean that caution is needed in their interpretation. They also highlight the need for prospective data collection or registries. Even fewer data are available beyond 40 years' post-nephrectomy. One study in veterans of the US military (men) approximately 45 years after uninephrectomy due to accidents showed acceptable serum creatinine levels and no increased risk for ESRD.[11]

The individual risk of developing ESRD and its overall impact on life expectancy remains unknown. Kiberd and Clase analysed data from the USA and showed the cumulative lifetime risk of ESRD for a 20-year-old

black woman was 7.8%.[12] Equivalent risks for black men, white men and white women were 7.3%, 2.5% and 1.8%, respectively. Lost years of life attributable to ESRD were 1.09, 1.10, 0.40 and 0.32 years for black women, black men, white men and white women, respectively. Any determination of long-term morbidity associated with donor nephrectomy must, therefore, take into account the differential risks associated with sex and ethnicity.

The relevant question is whether ESRD will occur at a greater frequency than expected in living renal donors. Clearly, from available data, particularly concerning 'very late' long-term risk, we can draw only limited conclusions. The counselling of young potential kidney donors (18–30 years) has no solid evidence base regarding very late renal outcome. Likewise, there is little guidance for an individual with borderline low renal function $(<80\,\mathrm{mL/min/1.73\,m^2})$ and a life expectancy greater than 40 years. Caution is indicated in such cases.

ALBUMINURIA AND PROTEINURIA

Most progressive renal disease and all advanced glomerular diseases are accompanied by proteinuria and albuminuria. Albuminuria may be the better variable to follow in the context of donor nephrectomy. First, albumin is a single, relatively small protein, which can be measured fairly accurately by the use of a specific antibody. In contrast, proteinuria reflects a less specific mixture of different size proteins, with less reliable chemical measurements that are influenced by the presence of very small proteins (i.e. α1-microglobulin, retinol-binding protein) or the rather large Tamm–Horsfall glycoprotein (produced in the ascending limb of the loop of Henle), thought to be of little or no clinical significance. Second, although the excretion of larger proteins such as immunoglobulin is a characteristic of advanced glomerular damage (unselective proteinuria), small amounts of albumin (microalbuminuria) appear at a much earlier stage than would be otherwise detectable.

Early detection of glomerular injury in potential donors and in donor follow-up is critical since treatments are available that may limit progression. If, for economic reasons, monitoring has to be restricted, the detection of albuminuria (rather than proteinuria) is preferred. Some contend that if dipstick testing (specific for albumin) is negative, no further evaluation for proteinuria is indicated. However, consensus is emerging that simple dipstick evaluation for proteinuria is, in itself, inadequate for evaluation and surveillance of living donors, primarily due to the insensitivity of such a measurement in detecting microalbuminuria. To illustrate the difficulties encountered with interpretation of urine protein excretion, the results of 1577 urinary samples from donors in the SOL-DHR are summarized in Figure 7-3. All assays were undertaken at the same laboratory (Viollier AG, Basel), using

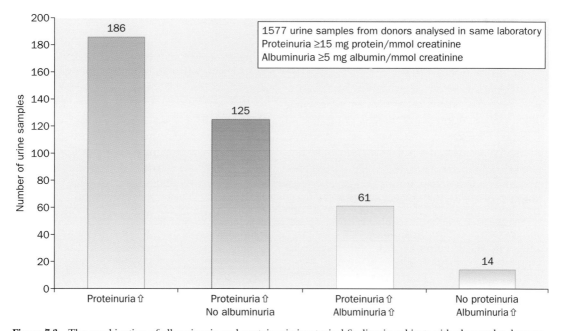

Figure 7-3 The combination of albuminuria and proteinuria is a typical finding in subjects with glomerular damage. Isolated albuminuria is an early sign for glomerular lesions, whereas isolated proteinuria has a 'post-glomerular' origin or is an artefact of the sensitive method of measurement (i.e. benzethonium chloride). Data from SOL-DHR, 2003.

identical techniques (benzamethonium chloride precipitation for urinary protein and a specific antibody for albumin). In 186 samples (12%), proteinuria was present in excess of 15 mg/mmol creatinine, while only 61 of those had significant albuminuria (≥5 mg/mmol creatinine). Additionally, 14 patients (1%) had microalbuminuria without measurable proteinuria. Thus, proteinuria in two-thirds of patients studied was unlikely to be clinically significant. Microalbuminuria may be not only a better predictor of subsequent renal disease (being more sensitive and more specific), but also a more reliable indicator for intervention with angiotensin-converting enzyme inhibitors (ACEI) or angiotensin receptor blockers (ARBs) to prevent further damage.[13]

Albuminuria (and proteinuria) should be expressed in mg per mmol urinary creatinine rather than in mg/L or dL of urine, otherwise different degrees of water diuresis may significantly distort the results. The urinary albumin to creatinine ratio is increasingly used in modern studies for the quantification of albuminuria.[14] In the SOL-DHR registry albuminuria (>5 mg albumin/mmol creatinine) was elevated before donation in 3% of donors, and the proportion of affected patients tripled over seven years to 9% (Figure 7-4). Using an upper limit of 2 mg albumin/mmol creatinine (as applied in the recently published HOPE (Heart Outcomes Prevention Evaluation) trial), the number would have risen to 18%.[14] Since by seven years post-nephrectomy nearly 20% of kidney donors were receiving ACEI or ARBs, the observed rate of albuminuria might have been much higher without such treatment.

There are few reports about microalbuminuria after donor nephrectomy in the literature.[15-17] In a retrospective study, seven of 29 kidney donors (24%) developed microalbuminuria after a mean follow-up of 11.1 years.[15] In another prospective study, two of 23 living donors developed microalbuminuria within one year of donation.[17] In most other studies, dipstick measurement has been used

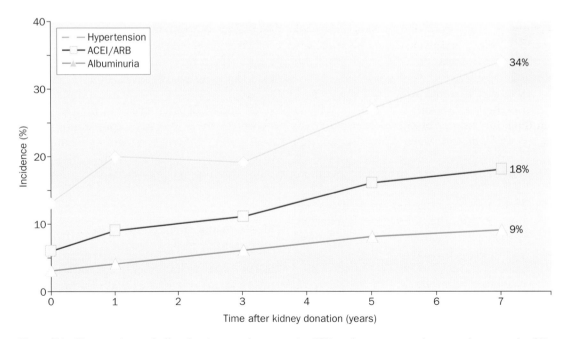

Figure 7-4 Hypertension and albuminuria at nephrectomy (n=631) and at seven years' post-nephrectomy (n=91). The percentage of donors with hypertension or albuminuria progressively increases over seven years post-nephrectomy. The rate of albuminuria tripled (but would be higher if angiotensin-converting enzyme inhibitor (ACEI) or angiotensin receptor blocker (ARB) treatment had not been applied). Data from SOL-DHR, November 2003.

as the standard test. Nonetheless, we recommend that albuminuria should be measured *before donation*, and an ideal potential donor should not have *any* microalbuminuria (<3 mg albumin/mmol creatinine).

More long-term data are available concerning proteinuria. In 1983, Vincenti and colleagues published a study of renal variables measured at a mean of 15.8±0.3 years after uninephrectomy in 20 former donors.[18] One donor developed glomerulonephritis, and mean urinary protein excretion was 141±20 mg/day compared with 74±3 mg/day in controls. Renal function remained stable (78±2% of pre-donation creatinine clearance) and only one donor developed mild hypertension.

Another early analysis of proteinuria after kidney donation from Brigham and Women's Hospital examined 52 donors at least 10 years after nephrectomy.[19] Thirteen (25%) donors excreted in excess of 250 mg urinary protein over 24 hours and four excreted more than 500 mg/day (maximum 1012 mg/day). Significant proteinuria was commoner in those donors (n=11) examined 15 or more years after donation than in those investigated at less than 15 years, but the study was too small to assess the significance of this finding. Similarly, a Japanese study found increasing proteinuria with duration of post-nephrectomy follow-up, but without impact on renal function or blood pressure.[20] Finally, a report from the Mayo Clinic found that seven of 90 donors (8%) at 10–20 years post-nephrectomy excreted urinary protein in excess of 150 mg/day (maximum 1334 mg/day).[21] In the latter studies, proteinuria was more commonly noted in males than females. Unfortunately, all these studies examined changes in protein excretion in only a subset of donors (perhaps those not experiencing complications), thereby limiting broad applicability of the findings.[19,21] The SOL-DHR donors (all of whom were followed prospectively, with fewer than 20% lost to follow-up) with proteinuria (defined as >15 mg/mmol creatinine) at seven years after donation showed no male preponderance. Restricting the analysis to donors who developed both proteinuria and albuminuria above three times the defined limit (i.e. >45 mg/mmol for protein and >15 mg/mmol for albumin) within seven years identified four male and two female subjects, which is a reversal of the gender ratio seen in the whole SOL-DHR population. If the prevalence of very high albuminuria (>20 mg/mmol) is examined (ignoring coexisting proteinuria), the preponderance of males is even higher (five males and two females) (see Chapter 5).

The Swedish experience in 1984 from donors followed-up for 10–20 years after donation showed that eight of 34 had protein excretion in the range of 0.2–1.5 g/L and nine had microproteinuria <0.1 g/L.[22] In another larger Swedish study of 348 donors who had donated 2–33 years previously, 40 of the 331 (12%) studied had proteinuria and 25% of these (10 donors) had proteinuria in excess of 1 g/day.[8] The majority of donors had undergone nephrectomy more than 16 years earlier. The most important finding was that the donors with proteinuria were more prone to hypertension and had a lower GFR than donors without proteinuria (GFR 62% vs 73% of the age-predicted value, respectively). Therefore, these data appear to indicate that although most donors do not develop significant proteinuria over time, some do, probably in excess of what might be expected in the general population. Ultimately, the consequences and implications of this proteinuria remain uncertain. Microalbuminuria, however, is recognized as a risk factor for cardiovascular disease.[23]

Mechanisms and treatment of albuminuria and proteinuria

Slight increase of glomerular intracapillary pressure or minimal glomerular hypertension' is believed by us as being the 'normal state' after unilateral nephrectomy, even in donors with normal systemic blood pressure. As glomerular injury progresses, systemic and glomerular hypertension may worsen and accelerate renal damage. While clinically significant renal injury, hypertension and albuminuria affect only a minority of donors, close surveillance with aggressive intervention to control blood pressure is warranted after unilateral nephrectomy. Since microalbuminuria is a sign of glomerular injury, its recognition and treatment are important if progressive damage is to be avoided. We believe that documented albuminuria should be treated *even before* hypertension develops (see below) and thus, kidney donors should be evaluated for microalbuminuria at 1- or 2-year intervals after nephrectomy.

Today, renoprotective drugs such as ACEIs and ARBs are widely available. Albuminuria can be eliminated, or at least attenuated, by adequate treatment. Although not yet supported by experimental data in kidney donors, we find data from other populations sufficient to support early and aggressive intervention. However, we do not share the opinion of some that these drugs should be administered to all donors prophylactically, for the following reasons:

- only a fraction of donors develop microalbuminuria despite the occurrence of some degree of hyperfiltration in donors following nephrectomy
- if surveillance occurs at regular intervals, incipient glomerular disease will be evident in time for appropriate intervention
- ACEIs and ARBs can be costly with unpleasant adverse effects.

In Switzerland, donors who develop albuminuria are advised to consult their family physicians who are well versed in appropriate therapies.

HYPERTENSION

Whether or not the occurrence of hypertension is increased after kidney donation remains unresolved. The observed incidence of hypertension in the donor population is variable and reflects age, time since nephrectomy, sex, ethnicity and definitions/methods used to detect hypertension. Yasumura et al

reported a low rate of hypertension (2.4%) in a questionnaire-based study in 1988.[24] However, most investigators have reported hypertension in 17–33% of former donors.[25–28] Others have found that the overall incidence of hypertension was comparable to that in the age-matched general population.[8–10,29] However, all these studies were retrospective and sometimes involved as few as 40% of those who had donated kidneys at a given location. Two similar analyses performed in Sweden (Figure 7-5) and Switzerland (Figure 7-6) compared the incidence of hypertension after kidney donation to that in the general population.[8,30,31] Both studies arrived at a similar conclusion: the prevalence of hypertension is not increased compared with age-matched controls.

The frequency of hypertension was remarkably similar in renal donors in Sweden and Switzerland, reaching 50% among those over the age of 65 years in both countries. The main differences were seen in the control groups, with a higher incidence of hypertension in Sweden than in Switzerland. Both studies used the same definition for hypertension (i.e. diastolic blood pressure >90 mmHg or the need for patients to take antihypertensive therapy). The mean time after donation was longer in Sweden (12±8 years) than in Switzerland (5.9±1.3 years). Thus, these studies offer no evidence of increased risk for hypertension as a direct consequence of donor nephrectomy.

Hypertension does, however, remain an issue of concern in kidney donors. Untreated hypertension is a known risk factor for nephrosclerosis and renal failure in the general population. It is possible that this risk is enhanced in those with a solitary kidney. Renal reserve is reduced even if serum creatinine remains within normal levels.[32] It seems reasonable that glomeruli of uninephrectomized donors are exposed to greater systemic blood pressure than are those of hypertensive individuals with two kidneys. So, in essence, hypertension, although perhaps not caused or accelerated by kidney donation, may predispose donors to more adverse

(A)

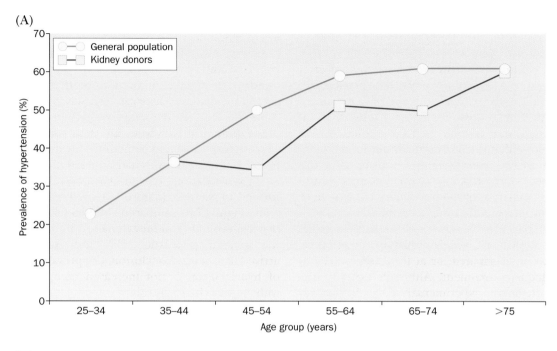

(B)

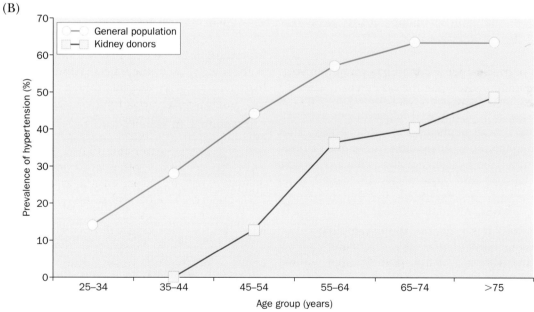

Figure 7-5   Hypertension in Swedish (A) male and (B) female kidney donors compared with the general population. Redrawn from Fehrman-Ekholm et al[8] with permission from Lippincott Williams & Wilkins.

renal consequences. Again, aggressive treatment appears indicated. It seems reasonable to advise potential donors of the need for screening for hypertension at the time of evaluation, even before the operation occurs.

Although controlled trials of individual antihypertensive agents after donor nephrectomy do not exist, it seems reasonable that ACEIs or ARBs should be included in treatment regimens.

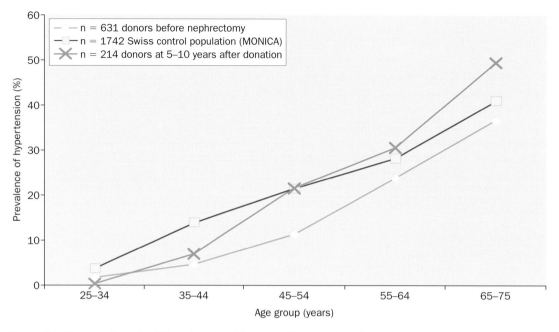

Figure 7-6   Hypertension after kidney donation. The rate of hypertension observed at 5–10 years after kidney donation did not differ from an age-matched Swiss control population (MONICA study[30,31]). The same definition for hypertension was used in both the SOL-DHR analysis and the MONICA study. MONICA data were provided by V
Wietlisbach (Institute of Social and Preventive Medicine, University of Lausanne, Switzerland).

OCCURRENCE OF ESRD IN DONORS

As opposed to living liver donation, where at
least 80% of removed hepatic tissue regener-
ates, new nephrons do not appear after
nephrectomy. Adaptation to the loss of renal
mass, both functionally (haemodynamic
changes) and anatomically (increased renal
size), is accomplished by the remaining
nephrons. Ablation of renal mass in experimental models is known to cause hyperfiltration, albuminuria and, ultimately, renal
insufficiency.[33] It is possible that similar
events may occur in human kidney donors.
Although minimal data exist regarding
glomerular haemodynamics in humans, it
seems likely that reduced pre-glomerular
vascular resistance is responsible for the
glomerular hyperfiltration that occurs rapidly
after nephrectomy, with increases in glomerular capillary pressure.[34,35]

Without hyperfiltration, serum creatinine
levels would double as clearance decreases by
50% when half the total renal mass is

removed. As noted earlier, adaptive hyperfiltration rapidly stabilizes clearance at 70–80%
of pre-donation values. The appearance of
albuminuria in donors with or without systemic hypertension may reflect the impact of
increased glomerular capillary pressure on
the selectivity of glomerular permeability,
ultimately resulting in injury. Over years this
may lead to slow attrition of nephron
numbers, commonly termed 'hyperfiltration
injury', but likely reflecting a more complicated pathogenesis. These processes may
ultimately lead to focal and then global
glomerulosclerosis in the remnant kidney.
Fortunately, for most people who have
undergone uninephrectomy, this process
evolves quite slowly, is variable from person to
person, and may be mitigated by renoprotective interventions, such as ACEIs and ARBs.

The exact number of donors who develop
ESRD is unknown, but the incidence appears
to be quite low. In 2002, a United Network
for Organ Sharing (UNOS) database analysis

of 47996 living donors showed that just 20 donors (0.04%) had been listed for cadaveric kidney transplantation.[36] Another 36 donors had been transplanted before UNOS was started in 1987. The appropriate denominator for these findings is uncertain so the incidence/prevalence cannot be calculated precisely, but the estimated prevalence of 0.04% approximates to a 0.03% incidence in the general population. Interestingly, 85% of the subjects had donated to a sibling, indicating the possibility of a genetic predisposition to kidney disease. The time from donation to ESRD in these subjects ranged from 2 to 31 years. Hypertensive nephrosclerosis, focal glomerulosclerosis and chronic glomerulonephritis accounted for two-thirds of diagnoses leading to ESRD.

A study from Norway involving 1696 living donors at 1–31 years post-donation showed that 0.41% had developed ESRD.[37] A recent analysis from Minneapolis involving 773 living donors followed for at least 20 years post-nephrectomy showed that 0.64% had developed ESRD.[10] These findings underline the necessity for regular check-ups and prompt intervention when indicated.

In Sweden, of 451 donors investigated 2–33 years post-donation, one donor (0.22%) developed ESRD due to haemolytic uraemic syndrome (the same diagnosis as in the recipient).[8] Again, it seems that genetic factors are important, and given the recent increase in the number of unrelated living donors, genetic susceptibility to renal disease may become less of a problem in the future. However, cancer in the remaining kidney has recently developed in another of our donors. Therefore, only two of 737 donors (0.27%) have gone on to receive dialysis at 0–40 years post-donation (own observations). In Sweden, the incidence of ESRD (starting dialysis or having a kidney transplant) is 1.2% per million per year and the prevalence is 7.7% per million.[38] In Switzerland (SOL-DHR; including 631 donors from 1993 to 2003), no donor has developed ESRD or has become pre-uraemic to date.

Current data are inconclusive but might be interpreted to indicate that the occurrence of ESRD is higher after living donor nephrectomy than in the general population. However, since over 50% of donors are relatives of someone with kidney disease, the actual increment in risk may be difficult to calculate.[39] Furthermore, the risk may vary among different populations in different parts of the world due to dissimilar lifestyles and genetic backgrounds. Additional studies and lengthier follow-up using the existing databases will be necessary to be able to provide accurate information about the risk of developing ESRD to prospective donors.

GENERAL HEALTH AND CAUSES OF DEATH IN DONORS

Long-term extrarenal morbidity and overall mortality in living renal donors has not been well chronicled. A study of living donors in Sweden from 1964 to 1995 has shown that, in general, living donors live longer and are healthier than the age-matched general population.[40] If true, it likely reflects an appropriate selection bias in favour of healthy persons serving as donors. Over 2–31 years post-donation, 41 of 430 donors in the Swedish study died. Causes of death were predominantly cardiovascular disease (50%) and malignancy (25%), which is similar to what might be expected in the general population in Sweden.

In Switzerland, seven of 631 living kidney donors have died since 1993. The causes of death were cancer (n=3; colon, breast, brain); myocardial infarction (n=1); traffic accident (n=1); stroke (n=1); and suicide (n=1). The earliest death occurred one year after donation and none of the deaths appeared to be directly related to the procedure.

It must be restated that this rather benign picture is predicated on utilization of essentially healthy donors. The impact of pre-existing comorbidity on outcomes is documented in two studies in obese persons. With relatively short-term follow-up, Pesavento and colleagues found an increased risk of perioperative complications in obese donors, but no impact of obesity on renal functional measures despite higher systemic blood pressures.[41] In contrast, Praga and co-workers showed that a pre-nephrectomy body mass index of $>30\,kg/m^2$ multiplied the risk for hypertension, proteinuria and renal insufficiency in patients who were at least 10 years post-nephrectomy.[42] In SOL-DHR no similar trend was observed beside hypertension (see Chapter 5).

Two recent developments may prove critical in evaluating long-term health status after donor nephrectomy. First is the recently described link between reduced GFR and cardiovascular risk in the elderly and patients with chronic kidney disease (CKD).[43,44] By strict definition, after nephrectomy donor GFR falls within a range indicating stage 2 or 3 CKD (i.e. GFR 30–90 mL/min).[45] However, otherwise healthy persons whose GFR falls within this range due to uninephrectomy are specifically excluded from this classification. No existing data define cardiovascular risk in this population, and any interrelation between uninephrectomy and hyperlipidaemia is not known. Second, recent trends using donors with 'isolated medical abnormalities' may alter the perceived lack of adverse impact associated with donor nephrectomy (see Chapter 6).[46,47] Additional data are required to assess the impact of these changes on long-term donor outcomes.

CONCLUSION

In conclusion, currently available data indicate that long-term health risks associated with donor nephrectomy are quite low. This is at least partially a direct consequence of using only healthy persons as donors, and it seems important going forward to preserve this precedent.

Thus, donors should be healthy before undergoing uninephrectomy. Baseline GFR must be adequate to withstand loss of 50% of renal mass with appropriate compensatory changes. Follow-up should occur at a frequency adequate to detect changes in blood pressure, albumin excretion and renal function early

enough to institute appropriate therapy in a timely fashion (see Table 7-2). Early detection and appropriate medical or surgical intervention is of the utmost importance as it generally gives the best chance for preventing deterioration in health or ESRD. These findings and recommendations are consistent with the recent consensus statement of the Amsterdam Forum and offer our donors the best opportunity for long and healthy lives.[48]

REFERENCES

1. Hoek FJ, Kemperman FA, Krediet RT. A comparison between cystatin C, plasma creatinine and the Cockcroft and Gault formula for the estimation of glomerular filtration rate. *Nephrol Dial Transplant* 2003; **18**: 2024–2031.
2. Larsson A, Malm J, Grubb A, Hansson LO. Calculation of glomerular filtration rate expressed in mL/min from plasma cystatin C values in mg/L. *Scand J Clin Lab Invest* 2004; **64**: 25–30.
3. Davis CL. Evaluation of the living kidney donor: current perspectives. *Am J Kidney Dis* 2004; **43**: 508–530.
4. Leger F, Seronie-Vivien S, Makdessi J et al. Impact of the biochemical assay for serum creatinine measurement on the individual carboplatin dosing: a prospective study. *Eur J Cancer* 2002; **38**: 52–56.
5. Levey AS, Bosch JP, Lewis JB et al. A more accurate method to estimate glomerular filtration rate from serum creatinine: a new prediction equation. *Ann Intern Med* 1999; **130**: 461–470.
6. Fehrman-Ekholm I, Skeppholm L. Renal function in the elderly (>70 years old) measured by means of iohexol clearance, serum creatinine, serum urea; estimated clearance. *Scand J Urol Nephrol* 2004; **38**: 73–77.
7. Graneus G, Aurell M. Reference values for Cr-EDTA clearance as a measure of glomerular filtration rate. *Scand J Clin Lab Invest* 1981; **41**: 611–616.
8. Fehrman-Ekholm I, Duner F, Brink B, Tyden G, Elinder CG. No evidence of accelerated loss of kidney function in living kidney donors: results from a cross-sectional follow-up. *Transplantation* 2001; **72**: 444–449.
9. Goldfarb DA, Matin SF, Braun WE et al. Renal outcome 25 years after donor nephrectomy. *J Urol* 2001; **166**: 2043–2047.
10. Ramcharan T, Matas AJ. Long-term (20–37 years) follow-up of living kidney donors. *Am J Transplant* 2002; **2**: 959–964.
11. Narkun-Burgess DM, Nolan CR, Norman JE et al. Forty-five year follow-up after uninephrectomy. *Kidney Int* 1993; **43**: 1110–1115.
12. Kiberd BA, Clase CM. Cumulative risk for develop-

ing end-stage renal disease in the US population. *J Am Soc Nephrol* 2002; **13**: 1635–1644.

13. Berl T. Angiotensin-converting enzyme inhibitors versus AT1 receptor antagonist in cardiovascular and renal protection: the case for AT1 receptor antagonist. *J Am Soc Nephrol* 2004; **15**(suppl 1): 71–76.

14. Mann JF, Gerstein HC, Pogue J, Bosch J, Yusuf S. Renal insufficiency as a predictor of cardiovascular outcomes and the impact of ramipril: the HOPE randomized trial. *Ann Intern Med* 2001; **134**: 629–636.

15. Eberhard OK, Kliem V, Offner G et al. Assessment of long-term risks for living related kidney donors by 24-h blood pressure monitoring and testing for microalbuminuria. *Clin Transplant* 1997; **11**: 415–419.

16. Fourcade J, Labeeuw M, Demaziere J, Pozet N, Aissa AH. Compensatory hyperfunction in living kidney donors. *Nephrologie* 2002; **23**: 173–177.

17. Bock HA, Gregor M, Huser B et al. Glomerular hyperfiltration following unilateral nephrectomy in healthy subjects. *Schweiz Med Wochenschr* 1991; **121**: 1833–1835.

18. Vincenti F, Amend WJ Jr, Kaysen G et al. Long-term renal function in kidney donors. Sustained compensatory hyperfiltration with no adverse effects. *Transplantation* 1983; **36**: 626–629.

19. Hakim RM, Goldszer RC, Brenner BM. Hypertension and proteinuria: long-term sequelae of uninephrectomy in humans. *Kidney Int* 1984; **25**: 930–936.

20. Higashihara E, Horie S, Takeuchi T, Nutahara K, Aso Y. Long-term consequence of nephrectomy. *J Urol* 1990; **143**: 239–243.

21. Anderson CF, Velosa JA, Frohnert PP et al. The risks of unilateral nephrectomy: status of kidney donors 10 to 20 years postoperatively. *Mayo Clin Proc* 1985; **60**: 367–374.

22. Fehrman I, Widstam U, Lundgren G. Long-term consequences of renal donation in man. *Transplant Proc* 1986; **18**: 102–105.

23. Gerstein HC, Mann JF, Yi Q et al. Albuminuria and risk of cardiovascular events, death, and heart failure in diabetic and nondiabetic individuals. *JAMA* 2001; **286**: 421–426.

24. Yasumura T, Nakai I, Oka T et al. Experience with 247 living related donor nephrectomy cases at a single institution in Japan. *Jpn J Surg* 1988; **18**: 252–258.

25. Toronyi E, Alfoldy F, Jaray J et al. Evaluation of the state of health of living related kidney transplantation donors. *Transpl Int* 1998; **11**(suppl 1): S57–S59.

26. Torres VE, Offord KP, Anderson CF et al. Blood pressure determinants in living-related renal allograft donors and their recipients. *Kidney Int* 1987; **31**: 1383–1390.

27. Sato K, Satomi S, Ohkohchi N et al. Long-term renal function after nephrectomy in living related kidney donors. *Nippon Geka Gakkai Zasshi* 1994; **95**: 394–399.

28. O'Donnell D, Seggie J, Levinson I et al. Renal function after nephrectomy for donor organs. *S Afr Med J* 1986; **69**: 177–179.

29. Vlaovic PD, Richardson RM, Miller JA et al. Living donor nephrectomy: follow-up renal function, blood pressure, and urine protein excretion. *Can J Urol* 1999; **6**: 901–905.

30. Wietlisbach V, Barazzoni F. Outcome and analysis of participation in the 2d MONICA survey (1988–1989) of cardiovascular risks factors. *Schweiz Med Wochenschrift* 1993; **48**(suppl): 13–20.

31. Wietlisbach V, Paccaud F, Rickenbach M, Gutzwiller F. Trends in cardiovascular risk factors (1984–1993) in a Swiss region: results of three populations surveys. *Prev Med* 1997; **26**: 523–533.

32. Fastbom J, Wills P, Cornelius C, Viitanen M, Winblad B. Levels of serum creatinine and estimated creatinine clearance over the age of 75: a study of an elderly Swedish population. *Arch Gerontol Geriatr* 1996; **23**: 179–188.

33. Hostetter TH, Olson JL, Rennke HG, Venkatachalam MA, Brenner BM. Hyperfiltration in remnant nephrons: a potentially adverse response to renal ablation. *Am J Physiol* 1981; **241**: F85–F93.

34. Bock HA, Bachofen M, Landmann J, Thiel G. Glomerular hyperfiltration after unilateral nephrectomy in living kidney donors. *Transpl Int* 1992; **5**(suppl 1): S156–S159.

35. Flanigan WJ, Burns RO, Takacs FJ, Merrill JP. Serial studies of glomerular filtration rate and renal plasma flow in kidney transplant donors, identical twins, and allograft recipients. *Am J Surg* 1968; **116**: 788–794.

36. Ellison MD, McBride MA, Taranto SE, Delmonico FL, Kauffman HM. Living kidney donors in need of kidney transplants: a report from the organ procurement and transplantation network. *Transplantation* 2002; **74**: 1349–1351.

37. Hartmann A, Fauchald P, Westlie L, Brekke IB, Holdaas H. The risk of living kidney donation. *Nephrol Dial Transplant* 2003; **18**: 871–873.

38. Schön S, Ekberg H, Wilkström B, Oden A, Ahlmen J. Renal replacement therapy in Sweden. *Scand J Urol Nephrol* 2004; **38**: 332–339.

39. Williams SL, Oler J, Jorkasky DK. Long-term renal function in kidney donors: a comparison of donors and their siblings. *Ann Intern Med* 1986; **105**: 1–8.

40. Fehrman-Ekholm I, Elinder CG, Stenbeck M, Tyden G, Groth CG. Kidney donors live longer. *Transplantation* 1997; **64**: 976–978.

41. Pesavento TE, Henry ML, Falkenhain ME et al. Obese living kidney donors: short-term results and possible implications. *Transplantation* 1999; **68**: 1491–1496.

42. Praga M, Hernandez E, Herrero JC et al. Influence of obesity on the appearance of proteinuria and

renal insufficiency after unilateral nephrectomy. *Kidney Int* 2000; **58**: 2111–2118.

43. Manjunath G, Tighiouart H, Ibrahim H et al. Level of kidney function as a risk factor for atherosclerotic cardiovascular outcomes in the community. *J Am Coll Cardiol* 2003; **41**: 47–55.

44. Manjunath G, Tighiouart H, Coresh J et al. Level of kidney function as a risk factor for cardiovascular outcomes in the elderly. *Kidney Int* 2003; **63**: 1121–1129.

45. National Kidney Foundation. K/DOQI clinical practice guidelines for chronic kidney disease: evalu-ation, classification, and stratification. *Am J Kidney Dis* 2002; **39**(suppl 1): S1–S266.

46. Textor SC, Taler SJ, Driscoll N et al. Blood pressure and renal function after kidney donation from hypertensive living donors. *Transplantation* 2004; **78**: 276–282.

47. Textor SC, Taler SJ, Larson TS et al. Blood pressure evaluation among older living kidney donors. *J Am Soc Nephrol* 2003; **14**: 2159–2167.

48. The consensus statement of the Amsterdam Forum on the Care of the Live Kidney Donor. *Transplantation* 2004; **78**: 491–492.

The psychosocial impact of donor nephrectomy

8

Ingela Fehrman-Ekholm

BACKGROUND

One understands how important transplantation is. There should be more information about the fact that we who have donated feel good. More of this should be heard.

This is a comment from one of our donors. However, not all donors would agree. The objective of this chapter is to present a balanced view of both the positive and negative psychosocial effects of donor nephrectomy.

There is a steadily increasing use of living donors for kidney transplantation. Today, not only family members (including spouses), but more distant relatives, friends and even anonymous parties become live donors. It is of greatest importance for all involved that the choice of donor is correct. Not all who want to donate or those suggested by potential recipients should become donors. While thorough medical evaluation is critical, the psychological makeup of a donor is also an important component of successful outcomes in both the donor and the recipient. Adequate psychological evaluation, often including standardized instruments, may require several clinical encounters between the transplant centre and the candidate before both are comfortable proceeding. In addition, imparting knowledge before transplantation about potential psychosocial consequences is important. Ultimately, most, but not all, donors are satisfied with their decision to donate.

SHORT-TERM ISSUES: PSYCHOLOGICAL COMPLICATIONS AND ECONOMIC IMPACT

Pain, worry and depression occur in 5–23% of donors after nephrectomy.[1-4] These types of complication may prolong the duration of sick leave and even result in loss of work. However, it should be remembered that a combination of pain, depression and fatigue can occur after any abdominal operation.[5] Furthermore, depression is a common symptom in today's society, affecting around 30% of the populations of Europe and the USA.[6,7] So too is chronic pain, which has been estimated to afflict 10–55% of people in the Western world.[6,7]

Donors often report feelings of 'emptiness' after nephrectomy, and in some cases such feelings can evolve into frank depression. As many as 30% of donors in Europe and the USA report feelings of depression in the postoperative period. This eventuality is more often found in donors who have lost their recipients to early death or when grafts have failed unexpectedly a short time after transplantation.[8] Despite efforts to inform donors of adverse recipient outcomes, many donors might not understand the potential for negative outcomes in the recipient, or minimized the risk, and are relatively unprepared. To reduce the chance of miscommunication, information and support should be offered to the potential donor on more than one occasion and in an individualized manner. A standardized health and psychiatric assessment questionnaire might be helpful in identifying psychosocial impairment and is also useful in

the follow-up period.[9] After the transplantation, some donors may benefit from close
contact with the transplant centre, even if the
outcome is a successful one. A standard protocol that includes post-nephrectomy telephone calls, counselling, social services or
other support may be of benefit.[2,10]

Data regarding the economic implications
of donating remain scarce. In Scandinavia,
sick leave varies from 1 to 16 weeks (median 6
weeks) after laparoscopic nephrectomy, and
from 2 to 19 weeks (median 7 weeks) after
open surgery. The Scandinavian insurance
systems cover the cost of both the hospital
stay and income lost during recovery time, so
the incentive to resume work early may be
less than in other countries. In the USA, a
recent study found all donors to have
returned to normal activities within eight
weeks, and over half by four weeks.[11]

Economic losses, though typically not large
in amount, add to the stress involved in
donor nephrectomy. Despite great financial
benefit to recipients and the healthcare
system (estimated at €500 000 in Scandinavia
and at least US$90 000 per donor in the
USA), it remains uncommon to fully compensate donors for economic losses associated
with donor nephrectomy. This policy reflects
ongoing fear of commercialization of the
living donor process. Between 15 and 25% of
donors report substantial financial losses associated with donating a kidney, with some
claiming financial hardship as a
consequence.[12,13] In some locales, donors are
now reimbursed for out-of-pocket expenses
and even lost wages.[14]

Iran initiated a programme in 1988 to
encourage living-unrelated donations. The
donors receive financial compensation from
the government, which also pays hospital
expenses related to nephrectomy and transplantation.[15,16] The policy has resulted in
elimination of the waiting list for cadaveric
transplantation, and substantially reduced the
overall costs associated with care for end-stage
renal disease. Reports indicate that 83% of
unrelated live donors in Iran were motivated
primarily by financial considerations, but

65% of them did not receive full compensation as promised.[17] In India, a recent study
showed that 86% of those who had sold a
kidney suffered from deterioration of general
health, with as much as a 30% decline in
income after nephrectomy.[18] The experience
related to donor compensation in Iran and
India informs the ongoing debate regarding
donor compensation in the West (see
Chapter 15).

LONG-TERM OUTCOME: QUALITY OF LIFE

Quality of life (QOL) is typically assessed
using standardized questionnaire-based
instruments, such as the Short Form (SF)-36
survey. These analyses allow comparison with
other patient cohorts as well as the population at large. It is striking that the QOL of
donors in the published literature seems
better or the same as that of the general
population. Donors often demonstrate high
self-esteem, and the donation process
enhances the positive traits. Many times, the
QOL benefits are linked to excellent outcomes in the recipients, as noted in the
following quotes:

- 'I got a healthy and happy wife.'
- 'It was wonderful to see my husband
  getting his life back again.'
- 'I now live a normal family life with chil-
  dren and grandchildren.'
- 'It was a great experience. Among the hap-
  piest things I have done.'
- 'I feel greater gratitude.'
- 'This is the best thing I have ever done.'
- 'I am so happy because my brother feels
  good.'
- 'I got a healthy man and our daughter a
  dad who does not need dialysis.'

However, some donors (1–5%) look back on
the procedure with regret, most commonly
due to a bad outcome in the recipient or
chronic pain or discomfort related to the
nephrectomy scar (Table 8-1). Indeed,
chronic peri-incisional discomfort, reported

Table 8-1   Quality of life after donation in living kidney donors

	Source			
	Westlie et al 1993[1]	*Johnson et al 1999[2]*	*Fehrman-Ekholm et al 2000[3]*	*Isotani et al 2002[4]*
No. of donors	494	979	370	104
Response rate	87%	60%	91%	66%
Quality of life	Better	Better	Better	Same
Regretted donation	5%	4%	1%	3%
Problems among donors				
Early recipient death or graft loss	Yes	Yes	–	–
Pain* and/or worry	–	1%	5%	3%
Economic loss	–	17%	25%	16%

*Sometimes severe or long term.

most commonly with flank incisions, can contribute to feelings of regret, especially related to the realization that often little can be done to repair the defect. It now seems apparent that chronic postoperative pain may be less common with laparoscopic approaches, particularly in the immediate perioperative period, with less use of narcotic and non-narcotic analgesia. However, a recent survey found no difference in physical activity and physical or mental energy in the long term based on surgical approach.[19] Interestingly, older donors may tolerate the procedure better than younger donors, an unexplained but commonly observed phenomenon.

The QOL of our own donors, as assessed by the SF-36 survey, was compared with the SF-36 results of kidney recipients and dialysis patients from a Japanese study. The greatest difference is in general health. Compared with transplant recipients and dialysis patients, the scores in the donors are higher, and therefore better, even if they are older (Figure 8-1).[3,20]

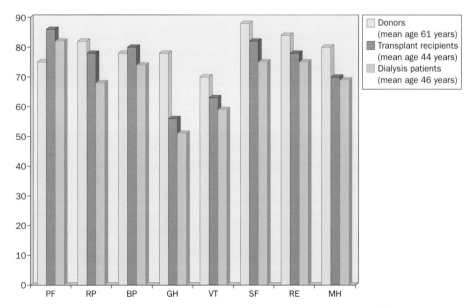

Figure 8-1   SF-36 scores in living kidney donors, transplant recipients and dialysis patients.[3,20] PF, physical functioning; RP, role physical functioning; BP, bodily pain; GH, general health; VT, vitality; SF, social functioning; RE, role emotional functioning; MH, mental health.

LONG-TERM OUTCOME: MEDICAL AND PSYCHOSOCIAL ISSUES

The issue of long-term follow-up of living donors remains controversial, but most series document about 5% of the donor population with chronic pain or other problems directly related to nephrectomy.[21] Some countries, particularly in Scandinavia and Europe, have established prospective registries based on regular clinical encounters, and it has been noted that donors appreciate the associated health services offered. In contrast, in other countries, such as the USA, there is no prescribed or even recommended standard of post-nephrectomy care. This discrepancy reflects the variability in terms of resources available to transplant physicians and surgeons in different countries.

There is also a dilemma resulting from the fact that donors generally consider themselves to be healthy. On the one hand, we inform them that the procedure is associated with a very low risk of adverse, long-term medical complications. Indeed, a recent survey of private insurers in the US documented that 19 out of 20 donors did not consider kidney donation to adversely affect longevity.[22] On the other hand, it is well recognized that there are medical complications associated with donor nephrectomy about which we need more information and which may be more effectively managed if detected early. As it becomes more commonplace to use donors with isolated medical abnormalities (hypertension, haematuria, hyperlipidaemia or microalbuminuria), follow-up becomes of even greater importance.[21,23]

In line with this thinking, current trends indicate growing support for mandatory long-term donor follow-up, a policy that if more widely implemented might help assuage donor concerns regarding safety. Such an approach would also foster greater insight into psychosocial and economic issues.

There is less support for long-term psychological follow-up/care. Indeed, most donors lead normal lives after nephrectomy. In many locales, psychological issues after donation are addressed by recognition of a donor's sacrifice (for example, by presentation of a token such as a medal or small gift), and with services such as support groups. A broader 'donor association' was recently initiated in Switzerland. Such programmes may help foster positive feelings in the donor and minimize the risk of depression. Most donors, however, remain 'silent heroes', as highlighted by the comment: 'More should be heard about how good we feel!'

INSURANCE FOR DONORS

Donor insurance is an important consideration and coverage varies widely from country to country. In Sweden, new insurance coverage aimed specifically at living donors has been created. This will give €25 000 to any donor who develops end-stage renal disease within 15 years after donation. Occasionally, donors have encountered difficulty when applying for life insurance. However, in a recent survey in the USA, almost all companies surveyed offered policies at standard rates to people who had donated kidneys.[22]

SUMMARY

Perhaps because of the extensive screening donors undergo during the evaluation process, the vast majority recover from the procedure and go on to live normal, even enhanced, lives. At a maximum, 5% suffer psychosocial long-term problems related to chronic pain or depression. Interactive follow-up and generosity after nephrectomy is always appropriate. As selection criteria become less restrictive, with donor–recipient relationships moving well beyond traditional family boundaries, new types of psychosocial problems may be encountered, emphasizing the need for improving psychosocial assessment tools and ongoing data collection. Ultimately, we must ensure that the donation process imposes as little psychological or economic stress as possible on these selfless persons that we now depend so heavily upon.

REFERENCES

1. Westlie L, Fauchald P, Talseth T, Jacobsen A, Flatmark A. Quality of life in Norwegian kidney donors. *Nephrol Dial Transplant* 1993; **8**: 1146–1150.

2. Johnson E, Anderson J, Jacobs C et al. Long-term follow-up of living kidney donors: quality of life after donation. *Transplantation* 1999; **67**: 717–721.

3. Fehrman-Ekholm I, Brink B, Ericsson C et al. Kidney donors don't regret. Follow-up of 370 donors in Stockholm since 1964. *Transplantation* 2000; **69**: 2067–2071.

4. Isotani S, Fujisawa M, Ichikawa Y et al. Quality of life of living kidney donors: the short-form 36-item health questionnaire survey. *Urology* 2002; **60**: 558–592.

5. Zalon ML. Correlates of recovery among older adults after major abdominal surgery. *Nurs Res* 2004; **53**: 99–106.

6. Jacobi F, Wittchen HU, Holting C et al. Prevalence, co-morbidity and correlates of mental disorders in the general population: results from the German Health Interview and Examination Survey (GHS). *Psychol Med* 2004; **34**: 597–611.

7. Alonso J, Amgermeyer MC, Bernert S et al. Prevalence of mental disorders in Europe: results form the European Study of Epidemiology of Mental disorders (ESEMeD) project. *Acta Psychiatr Scand* 2004; **420**(suppl): 21–27.

8. Haljamäe U, Nyberg G, Sjöström B. Remaining experiences of living kidney donors more than 3 yr after early recipient graft loss. *Clin Trans* 2003; **17**: 1–8.

9. Smith GC, Trauer T, Kerr PG, Chadban SJ. Prospective psychosocial monitoring of living kidney donors using the SF-36 health survey. *Transplantation* 2003; **76**: 807–809.

10. Jacobs C, Johnson E, Anderson K et al. Kidney transplants from living donors: how donation affects family dynamics. *Adv Renal Replace Ther* 1988; **5**: 89–97.

11. El-Galley R, Hood N, Young CJ, Deierhoi M, Urban DA. Donor nephrectomy: a comparison of techniques and results of open, hand assisted and full laparoscopic nephrectomy. *J Urol* 2004; **171**: 40–43.

12. Schover LR, Streem SB, Boparai N, Duriak K, Novick AC. The psychosocial impact of donating a kidney: long-term followup from a urology based center. *J Urol* 1997; **157**: 1596–1601.

13. Smith MD, Kappell DF, Province MA et al. Living-related kidney donors: a multicenter study of donor education, socioeconomic adjustment, and rehabilitation. *Am J Kidney Dis* 1986; **8**: 223–233.

14. Jacobs CL, Thomas C. Financial consideration in living organ donation. *Prog Transplant* 2003; **13**: 130–136.

15. Ghods AJ. Renal transplantation in Iran. *Nephrol Dial Transplant* 2002; **17**: 222–228.

16. Al-Khader AA. The Iranian transplant programme: comment from an Islamic prespective. *Nephrol Dial Transplant* 2002; **17**: 213–215.

17. Ghods AJ, Nasrollahzadeh D. Gender disparity in a live donor renal transplantation program: assessing from cultural perspectives. *Transplant Proc* 2003; **35**: 2559–2560.

18. Goyal M, Metha RL, Schneiderman LJ, Sehgal AR. Economic and health consequences of selling a kidney in India. *JAMA* 2002; **288**: 1589–1593.

19. Lennerling A, Blohmé I, Östraat Ö et al. Laporascopic or open surgery for living donor nephrectomy. *Nephrol Dial Transplant* 2001; **16**: 383–386.

20. Fujisawa M, Ichikawa Y, Yoshiya K et al. Assessment of health-related quality of life in renal transplant and hemodialysis patients using the SF-36 health survey. *Urology* 2000; **56**: 201–206.

21. The consensus statement of the Amsterdam Forum on the Care of the Live Kidney Donor. *Transplantation* 2004; **78**: 491–492.

22. Spital A, Jacobs C. Life insurance for kidney donors: another update. *Transplantation* 2002; **74**: 972–973.

23. Textor SC, Taler SJ, Larson TS et al. Blood pressure evaluation among older living kidney donors. *J Am Soc Nephrol* 2003; **14**: 2159–2167.

Overcoming ABO incompatibility

9

Kazunari Tanabe, Gunnar Tydén

INTRODUCTION

The supply of cadaveric kidneys is currently not sufficient to satisfy the increasing number of patients requiring renal transplantation. Expansion of the donor pool by overcoming immunological barriers, such as ABO incompatibility and positive crossmatches, would expand the availability of organs considerably and ultimately reduce mortality in patients with end-stage renal failure.

ABO-incompatible renal transplantation has been attempted since the early 1970s.[1,2] Today, Japan has the largest experience of ABO-incompatible renal transplantation in the world due to the serious shortage of deceased donor kidneys in that country. However, even in countries with well-developed deceased-donor procurement activities, as many as 15–20% of potential living donors are excluded because of ABO incompatibility. In this chapter, we will review clinical practices for dealing with ABO incompatibility and evaluate the outcomes achieved to date.

BLOOD GROUP ANTIGENS AND THEIR DISTRIBUTION IN THE KIDNEY

Blood group A is characterized by the terminal trisaccharide GalNAcα-3[Fucα 1-2] Galβ-, blood group B by the terminal trisaccharide Galα1-3[Fucα1-2] Galβ-, and blood group O by the disaccharide Fucα1-2 Galβ-.[3,4] The basic core structures of carrier or precursor chains have been classified into four different types:

- Type 1 chain – Galβ1-3GlcNAcβ1-R
- Type 2 chain – Galβ1-4GlcNAcβ1-R
- Type 3 chain – Galβ1-3GalNAcα1-R
- Type 4 chain – Galβ1-3GalNAcβ1-R

Blood group A can be further divided into A1 and A2 subgroups. The A2 subgroup constitutes about 20% of the European blood group A population, but only 0.15% of the Japanese population.[5] The glycosyltransferase of A1 individuals adds the terminal *N*-acetyl-galactosamine sugar residue to the H-epitope, using all the four chain types, whereas the A2 transferase can only use the type 1 and 2 chains. Thus, both a quantitative and a qualitative difference in A antigen expression has been noted in individuals with A1 and A2 subtypes. The β-transferase, with the addition of the terminal galactose sugar residue, is probably restricted to the type 1 and 2 chains, which means that individuals with blood group B express a smaller amount of B antigens.[6]

The ABH antigens are expressed in the vascular endothelium and in the distal convoluted tubules and collecting tubules, whereas Lewis blood group antigens are expressed in the epithelial cells of the distal convoluted and collecting tubules, but not in the vascular endothelium. The glycosyltransferase activity necessary for the synthesis of ABH and Lewis antigens is found in the cortex, medulla and glomeruli of the kidney. All the vascular endothelia have ethanol-soluble ABH antigens in both secretors and non-secretors, but the blood group antigens in the epithelial cells of the collecting tubules and the calyceal epithelium are water-soluble and are expressed only in secretors.[5–8] In ABO-incompatible recipients, preformed anti-A/B antibodies react with blood group A/B antigens in the vascular endothelium of the ABO-incompatible grafts; this results in immediate loss of graft function due to what is now termed antibody-mediated rejection.

EARLY EXPERIENCE OF ABO-INCOMPATIBLE RENAL TRANSPLANTATION

Early experience with ABO-incompatible renal transplantation antedated much of the scientific knowledge outlined above. Attempts to cross the ABO barrier almost uniformly resulted in rapid graft failure, with histopathological changes (thrombosis, necrosis and immune complexes) indicating aggressive antibody-mediated rejection. The generally accepted clinical dogma was that ABO-incompatible transplantation should not be performed.[6] However, there were exceptions to this rule.

In the 1970s, due to a serious shortage of blood group O donor kidneys, Rydberg et al started transplanting A2-incompatible kidneys into incompatible blood group O recipients. Using conventional immunosuppression, long-term graft survival was obtained in 60% of recipients.[1] At the same time, several immunomodulating techniques such as plasmapheresis and immunoadsorption were being developed to extend the availability of renal transplantation. Both ABO-incompatible and crossmatch-positive renal transplantation, formerly contraindicated, have been performed successfully by removing blood group A/B antibodies or preformed Anti-HLA antibodies using plasmapheresis prior to grafting.

In 1981, Slapak et al[9] reported a favourable effect of plasmapheresis on hyperacute rejection in a patient who happened to receive a kidney from an ABO-incompatible donor. After transplantation, four sessions of plasmapheresis were performed to remove anti-A/B antibodies and the graft was successfully rescued. Four years later, Alexandre et al[10] reported the first successful case of ABO-incompatible living donor renal transplantation, performed deliberately after removal of the recipient's isoagglutinins by plasmapheresis.

A2-incompatible renal transplantation

Economidou et al[11] demonstrated that the expression of A2 antigens on erythrocytes was much weaker than that of A1 antigens. Other investigators[12,13] reported that skin grafts from blood group A2 to O individuals survived for almost the same period as skin grafts from blood group O to O (whereas skin grafts from A1 or B to O individuals were rejected immediately). Based on these findings, it was speculated that solid organ transplantation from blood group A2 to O might be possible.[12,13]

In 1974, Rydberg et al started A2-incompatible renal transplantation using conventional immunosuppression without pretransplant conditioning. Among 20 A2-incompatible renal transplant recipients, eight lost their graft within one month of surgery, whereas the remaining 12 grafts functioned long term.[1,2]

Due to the extended waiting time of blood group B and O transplant candidates, more recent organ transplant programmes in the USA and Europe have preferentially allocated blood group A2 and A2B cadaveric kidneys to type O and B individuals.[14–16] Nelson et al[17] reported that between 1994 and 2000, 41 of 121 end-stage renal disease patients with blood group B who underwent cadaveric renal transplantation received either an A2 or an A2B kidney. These recipients (all of whom demonstrated low anti-A2 antibody titres) underwent A2-incompatible renal transplantation without pretransplant treatment or splenectomy. The 1- and 5-year graft survival rates for the recipients of A2 or A2B kidneys were 91% and 85%, respectively, not significantly different from 91% and 80% graft survival rates for the recipients of B or O kidneys. The authors concluded that allocation of A2 and A2B kidneys to blood group B candidates on the waiting list would increase their access to renal transplantation.

Recently, several investigators have attempted A2-incompatible living donor renal transplantation. Gloor et al[18] reported that eight cases of A2-incompatible living renal transplantation were successfully performed using an immunosuppressive regimen comprising rabbit antithymocyte globulin induction, tacrolimus, mycophenolate mofetil (MMF) and prednisone, combined with pretransplant plasmapheresis, intravenous immunoglobulin and splenectomy. Thus, A2-incompatible transplantation from deceased and living donors has increased, with results that appear to be acceptable (Table 9-1).

Non-A2-incompatible renal transplantation

Unfortunately, non-A2-incompatible renal transplantation poses more of a problem. In the 1980s, Slapak et al[24] reported three successful cases of A1 to O renal transplantation with pretransplant immunoadsorption and plasmapheresis treatment. In total, 16 cases of ABO-incompatible renal transplantation were undertaken using 14 cadaveric and two living donors. Five of the 16 patients underwent splenectomy. One-year graft survival was 87% and did not appear to be related to splenectomy. Subsequently, Alexandre et al[25]

reported their first experience of ABO-incompatible renal transplantation in 26 cases. Their immunosuppressive treatment included corticosteroids, azathioprine, ciclosporin, antilymphocyte globulin, donor-specific platelet transfusion and splenectomy in 21/24 cases.

Shortly thereafter, Japanese transplant centres began performing ABO-incompatible renal transplantation in an attempt to overcome the severe shortage of cadaveric donors. Toma et al[26] reported the largest series of ABO-incompatible renal transplantation from a single centre, with short-term results (up to four years after transplantation) significantly poorer than those of ABO-compatible cases. However, there appeared to be little difference in outcomes as follow-up increased over time. The same group recently reported the updated outcomes of ABO-incompatible renal transplantation using more modern immunosuppression, documenting excellent patient and graft survival that was not significantly different from ABO-compatible cases.[27] Among the 34 patients enrolled in the study, 1- and 3-year graft survival were both 97%. Furthermore, the 23% incidence of rejection in these patients was comparable to that of ABO-compatible recipients, and most cases (80%) were due to antibody-mediated rejection.

Recently, the Mayo Clinic group[28] reported updated results of ABO-incompatible living

Table 9-1 A2-incompatible renal transplantation

Authors	N	Cad	Living	Donor blood type		Recipient blood type		Graft loss at 1 month
				A2	A2B	O	B	
Rydberg et al[1]	20	20	0	20	0	20	0	8
Welsh et al[19]	16	16	0	16	0	20	0	5
Shapira et al[20]	5	2	3	4	1	4	1	0
Mendez et al[21]	9	9	0	3	6	2	7	0
Nelson et al[22]	50	46	4	47	3	31	19	10
Alkhunaizi et al[14]	15	15	0	15	0	6	9	1
Sorensen et al[23]	11	0	11	11	0	10	1	0
Nelson et al[17]	41	41	0	4	37	0	41	7
Gloor et al[18]	10	0	10	10	0	8	2	1

Cad, cadaveric donor.

Table 9-2   Non-A2-incompatible renal transplantation

Authors	Cad/living	N	Pretreatment			1-year graft survival (%)
			PEX	IA	Spx	
Alexandre et al[25]	19/5	24	Y	Y	21	75
Bannett et al[29]	0/6	6	Y	Y	6	83
Slapak et al[30]	14/2	16	Y	Y	5	81
Ota et al[31]	0/51	51	Y	Y	51	84
Aswad et al[32]	0/6	6	N	Y	6	83
Aikawa et al[33]	0/40	40	Y	Y	40	85
Karakayali et al[34]	0/21	21	Y	N	9	67
Kobayashi et al[35]	0/25	25	Y	Y	25	96
Gloor et al[28]	0/30	30	Y	N	26	93
Toma et al[26]	0/141	141	Y	Y	140	82
Tyden et al[36]	0/8	8	N	Y	0	100

Cad, cadveric donor; PEX, plasmapheresis; IA, immunoadsorption; Spx, splenectomy; Y, yes; N, no.

donor renal transplantation, again with excellent outcomes (Table 9-2).

PRETRANSPLANT MANAGEMENT

Since it is well known that pre-existing anti-A/B reactivity causes antibody-mediated rejection, removal of these antibodies before transplantation is mandatory to prevent allograft injury in the immediate perioperative period. Several procedures to remove anti-A/B antibodies have been described, but plasmapheresis and immunoadsorption are the two most commonly employed.[5]

Plasmapheresis (using either filter or centrifugation techniques) can rapidly remove large amounts of blood proteins in a relatively brief period of time. Volume losses are replaced with albumin and saline, or in certain situations (e.g. thrombotic microangiopathy) with plasma or immunoglobulin. To reduce the unselective loss of plasma proteins, the plasma obtained after the initial separation can be further treated with double-filtration plasmapheresis (DFPP). DFPP was designed to selectively remove the immunoglobulin fraction from the serum and thus, to minimize the volume of substitution fluid required. In this process the plasma is separated by a plasma separator and the gamma-globulin fraction is removed by a plasma fractionator as a second filter. DFPP

removes the concentrated serum globulin fraction, which includes anti-A/B antibodies, from the filtered plasma. The amount of globulin removed in one session of DFPP is equivalent to that concentrated in 5 L of plasma, but only 1 L of substitution fluid is necessary to replace the deficiency.[37,38]

Complications associated with this procedure are usually few, but include haemorrhage and infection, with some increased risk of viral infections if volume is replaced with plasma.

The technique of immunoadsorption involves the specific removal of targeted proteins, and does not require replacement of large volumes of plasma proteins or fluids. The immunoadsorbent used to remove anti-A/B antibodies in the 1980s was a Biosynsorb column (Chembiomed Ltd, Edmonton, Canada), which contained chemically synthesized human blood-group ABO antigens covalently linked to crystalline silica.[38-40] However, this product disappeared from the market in the 1990s. Recently, a low-molecular carbohydrate column with A or B blood-group antigen linked to a sepharose matrix (Glycosorb ABO, Glycorex Transplantation, Lund, Sweden) that specifically depletes anti-A or anti-B antibodies was registered in Europe.[41]

Unfortunately, immunoglobulin removal appears to stimulate resynthesis of the antibody repertoire, so plasmapheresis and immunoadsorption both require concomitant measures to inhibit antibody synthesis. Traditionally, this has implied splenectomy, and its potential for short- and long-term complications. Alexandre and colleagues[25] emphasized that splenectomy is a prerequisite for successful ABO-incompatible renal transplantation. In their series, the three patients who were not splenectomized showed hyperacute graft rejection in the first week after transplantation, whereas 10 of 11 patients who underwent splenectomy retained functioning grafts. Toma[5] reviewed 155 ABO-incompatible renal transplant recipients reported in the literature. Of these, 103 had undergone splenectomy, with 81% of grafts surviving more than a year. Conversely, of the 52 transplants performed without splenectomy, only 17 (33%) survived. However, significant controversy accompanied this analysis, since most of the non-

splenectomized patients did not undergo preconditioning with plasmapheresis or immunoadsorption. Among the 22 patients who did, graft survival after one year was 73%, which was not significantly different from that achieved in splenectomized patients. In our series (from Tokyo), all but one patient underwent splenectomy. This particular patient lost his graft due to severe antibody-mediated rejection.[5]

In more recent years, a humanized anti-CD20 antibody, rituximab, in combination with potent immunosuppression (tacrolimus, MMF, corticosteroids) has become an accepted alternative to splenectomy.

THE TOKYO EXPERIENCE

At the Tokyo Women's Medical University (TWMU), we usually employ immunosuppression for seven days prior to transplantation. Currently, this includes tacrolimus

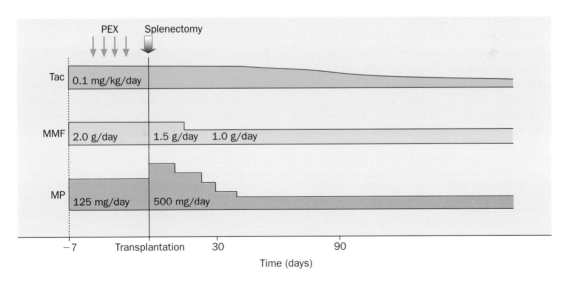

Figure 9-1 Immunosuppressive regimen at the Tokyo Women's Medical University.[27] To remove anti-A and/or anti-B antibodies, the recipient receives three or four sessions of double-filtration plasmapheresis and/or some sessions of regular plasmapheresis (PEX), starting from seven days prior to renal transplantation. All three drugs, including tacrolimus (Tac), mycophenolate mofetil (MMF) and methylprednisolone (MP) are started seven days pretransplantation. Tacrolimus is started at a dose of 0.1 mg/kg and reduced according to the target trough levels, which are around 10 ng/mL before surgery. MMF is started at a dose of 1–2 g/day and the same dose is continued until surgery unless adverse events occur. MP is started at a dose of 80–125 mg/day and increased to 500 mg/day on the day of renal transplantation. The recipients undergo splenectomy at the time of renal transplantation.

(0.1 mg/kg, with a target trough blood level of 10 ng/mL), MMF (1–2 g daily) and methyl-prednisolone (80–125 mg/day, increased to 500 mg on the day of transplantation). This is accompanied by two to four sessions of con-comitant plasmapheresis or DFPP to remove anti-A and/or anti-B antibodies[27] (Figure 9-1). In addition, all recipients undergo splenectomy at the time of renal transplanta-tion.

Both the Mayo Clinic[28] and Johns Hopkins teams[42] employ a similar protocol, namely, a pretransplant conditioning regimen of plasmapheresis, followed by administration of low-dose (100 mg/kg) intravenous immunoglobulin, with or without splenec-tomy at the time of transplantation. More specifically, at the Mayo Clinic, rituximab (375 mg/m²) is given one week prior to trans-plantation rather than performing splenec-tomy (Table 9-3).

In our early experience, we employed quin-tuple drug treatment, comprising ciclosporin, azathioprine, methylprednisolone, antilym-phocyte globulin and deoxyspergualin.[43] In the ciclosporin era, graft survival was signifi-cantly poorer in ABO-incompatible than in ABO-compatible recipients in the early post-transplantation period, but over the longer term survival was comparable: 79% and 95%

at one year; 79% and 92% at three years; 75% and 83% at five years; and 73% and 80% at eight years. These findings were recently reconfirmed by our group and also by Japan-ese multicentre data.[44,45] One hundred and forty-one patients underwent ABO-incompati-ble renal transplantation between 1989 and 2001. The 1-, 5- and 13-year graft survival rates for ABO-incompatible recipients were 82%, 76% and 56%, respectively.[26] The correspon-ding graft survival rates for ABO-compatible recipients were 96%, 85% and 58%, respec-tively (log-rank test, p=0.007). Again, the dif-ference in graft survival between the two ABO groups occurred early after transplantation, and the ABO-incompatible recipients who retained their allografts during the first years post-transplantation did relatively well over the long term. Patient survival rates for ABO-incompatible and ABO-compatible recipients were 94% and 98%, respectively, at one year; 94% and 97% at five years; and 84% and 91% at 13 years.

Since 1998, graft survival has improved markedly with tacrolimus or ciclosporin microemulsion-based immunosuppression in combination with MMF. Five-year graft sur-vival was almost 90% and no difference was noted between the ABO-compatible and -incompatible groups. Thirty-four patients

Table 9-3   Recent outcomes of ABO-incompatible renal transplantation

	TWMU[27] (n=34)	Huddinge[36] (n=8)	Mayo clinic[28] (n=30)
Pretransplant management			
Plasmapheresis	Y	N	Y
Immunoadsorption	N	Y	N
Intravenous immunoglobulin	N	Y	Y
Tacrolimus	Y	Y	Y
MMF	Y	Y	Y
Corticosteroids	Y	Y	N
Splenectomy	Y	N	Y/N
Rituximab	N	Y	N/Y
Post-transplant immunosuppression			
Tacrolimus	Y	Y	Y
MMF	Y	Y	Y
Corticosteroids	Y	Y	Y
Rejection	23%	–	30%
1-year graft survival	97%	100%	93%

TWMU, Tokyo Women's Medical University Hospital; Y, yes; N, no; MMF, mycophenolate mofetil.

have been treated with our current regimen (as outlined above).[27] Three-year graft survival was 97%, and during the observation period only one graft was lost due to humoral rejection. Furthermore, only seven patients (23%) experienced acute rejection and of these, six were cases of antibody-mediated rejection. No severe infectious complications were reported.

THE STOCKHOLM EXPERIENCE

Facing an ever-increasing shortage of cadaveric organs, our group at Huddinge University Hospital decided to implement a programme of ABO-incompatible living donor transplantation using preoperative antigen-specific immunoadsorption (Glycosorb ABO treatment), rituximab (instead of splenectomy) and conventional immunosuppression. The protocol consisted of a 10-day pretransplantation conditioning period, beginning with a single dose of rituximab ($375 mg/m^2$) followed by full-dose tacrolimus (0.2 mg/kg), aiming at target trough levels of 15–20 ng/mL, MMF (2 g), with a target area under the curve of $200 \mu mol/h/L$ and prednisolone (30 mg). Postoperatively, a standard triple-drug immunosuppressive regimen was followed, with the objective of achieving tacrolimus trough levels of 15 ng/mL during month 1, 10 ng/mL during month 2 and 5 ng/mL thereafter. MMF was administered at 2 g/day during the first three months and 1 g/day thereafter. The prednisolone dose was increased to 100 mg on the first postoperative day, and then decreased by 10 mg every day until 20 mg, which was maintained for the first month, 15 mg during the second month and 10 mg thereafter.

Glycosorb ABO apheresis was performed on pretransplant days –6, –5, –2 and –1. At each session, between one-and-a-half and two plasma volumes were processed. The IgM and IgG titres against donor erythrocytes were measured before and after each apheresis using standard direct and indirect agglutination techniques. More apheresis sessions were performed if there was a rebound of antibody titres between pretransplant days –3 and –1 or if the titres following the last session exceeded 1:8. Following the last session, 0.5 g/kg of intravenous immunoglobulin was administered.

Postoperatively, three additional apheresis sessions were given routinely every third day for a total time of nine days. At each of these sessions, one plasma volume was processed. Again, if there was a significant increase in the antibody titres (two steps), extra sessions were considered. The protocol was approved by the local ethics committee at Huddinge University Hospital.

To date, 11 patients have been included in the study and all have had successful transplantations (Table 9-4). Since blood groups A2 and B express lower amounts of antigen than blood group A1,[2] we decided to start with an A2–O donor–recipient combination. The recipient had anti-A2 titres of IgM 1:32 and IgG 1:64, but the antibodies were readily absorbed and there was no post-transplantation rebound. Since no major complications associated with the treatment were observed, we decided to try the procedure in two patients with blood group B donors. Again, the antibodies were readily removed and the postoperative course was completely uneventful. We then decided to embark on a donor A1–recipient O combination, where the pretransplantation anti-A1 antibody levels in the recipient were comparatively high (IgM 1:16, IgG 1:64). In this patient, a strong rebound of antibodies was observed following the first of four aphereses, and the transplantation was therefore postponed for one week and another four aphereses were undertaken. Following this, the titres decreased (IgM 1:1, IgG 1:1) and transplantation was successfully undertaken. Postoperatively, however, the antibodies tended to recur. Since the apheresis sessions were completely without side effects, we decided not to wait for three days between every postoperative session, and gave one session every day for a total of 16 postoperative sessions. Following this pioneering series,[41] another seven patients have been included in the protocol, and all have had successful transplantations.

Table 9-4   ABO-incompatible renal transplantation at the Huddinge University Hospital: donor and recipient characteristics, effect of antigen-specific immunoadsorption and current recipient serum creatinine

Case	Donor		Recipient		Blood group	Anti-A or -B titres				Follow-up (months)	Serum creatinine (μmol/L)
	Sex	Age (years)	Sex	Age (years)	Donor/ recipient	Before adsorption		At transplantation			
						IgM	IgG	IgM	IgG		
1	M	47	F	20	A2/O	1:32	1:64	1:2	1:2	31	75
2	F	64	M	24	B/O	1:16	1:32	1:1	1:4	19	159
3	M	67	F	58	B/A	1:16	1:16	1:1	1:1	19	108
4	F	48	F	19	A1/O	1:16	1:64	1:1	1:1	17	113
5	M	65	M	32	A2/O	1:32	1:64	1:2	1:4	12	154
6	M	36	F	13	A1/O	1:64	1:128	1:2	1:2	10	89
7	M	56	F	54	A2/O	1:32	1:64	1:1	1:1	8	99
8	F	41	M	43	B/A	1:4	1:8	1:1	1:1	8	120
9	M	28	M	1	B/O	1:2	1:2	1:2	1:2	2	8
10	M	43	M	52	A1B/B	1:16	1:16	1:1	1:1	2	175
11	F	40	M	38	A1/O	1:16	1:16	1:2	1:2	1	103

M, male; F, female.

This small series of blood group-incompatible living donor transplantations using Glycosorb ABO blood group antibody adsorption, anti-CD20 monoclonal antibody infusion and conventional immunosuppression is very promising. The results demonstrate that with a modern protocol, neither splenectomy nor the excessively enhanced immunosuppressive protocols that are usually required, are necessary. The Glycosorb ABO carbohydrate column effectively adsorbed blood group antibodies, lowering the antibody titres from four to two steps for each session. Also, no side effects were apparent. Because of the mobilization of antibodies between the adsorptions, at least four pre-transplantation sessions seem to be necessary. For donors with a low amount of antigen (A2 and B), it is probably sufficient to monitor recipient antibody titres postoperatively and employ Glycosorb ABO treatment only if the titre increases significantly. For recipients of A1 kidneys, however, we presently propose a programme of postoperative apheresis sessions every second day for approximately two weeks until accommodation has occurred.

All peripheral CD20-positive cells were effectively removed following administration of a single dose of rituximab. In the patient with the longest follow-up (almost three years), the CD20-positive cells were not detectable until 12 months post-transplantation. Additionally, rituximab treatment could not be related to any observable side effects and there were no serious infections.

REJECTION AND CLINICOPATHOLOGICAL FINDINGS

There are few reports on the pathological findings of ABO-incompatible renal transplantation. The Tokyo group reported the largest clinicopathological series of ABO-incompatible renal transplantation.[44,46,47] A total of 380 biopsy specimens were taken from 125 ABO-incompatible renal allografts at our institute. Among these, 128 specimens were 0- or 1-hour biopsies taken from 122 grafts, and 252 additional biopsies were performed at the time of acute rejection in 85 patients. Pathological analysis of the histological specimens obtained during the rejection episodes demonstrated humoral rejection alone in 62 specimens (27%, from 25 patients), cellular rejection alone in 67 specimens (29%, from 27 patients), humoral rejection combined with cellular rejection in 30 specimens (13%, from eight patients) and chronic rejection in 31 specimens (13%, from 12 patients).

Some patients demonstrated evidence of calcineurin inhibitor nephrotoxicity and/or transplant glomerulopathy.[44] Thus, the incidence of humoral rejection was extremely high; 12 patients lost their graft due to humoral rejection within one year after renal transplantation. Most humoral rejections occurred within one month after ABO-incompatible transplantation.[44]

During the ciclosporin era, episodes of acute rejection were significantly more frequent among recipients of ABO-incompatible grafts (85 of 141, 60%) than among recipients of ABO-compatible grafts (377 of 777, 49%). Early graft loss caused by antibody-mediated rejection was the main reason for the poor short-term outcome. In most cases, humoral rejection occurred within two weeks after renal transplantation and the patients lost the graft immediately. In many cases, injury of the vascular endothelium was manifest by accompanying changes indicating thrombotic microangiopathy (TMA), an often irreversible finding.[48] However, since we started using more potent immunosuppression (tacrolimus, MMF), antibody-mediated rejection is much less common (23%) and the resulting incidence of TMA has been significantly reduced. Nonetheless, most of these rejections retain a humoral component, similar to findings noted by the Mayo team.[27,28]

Currently, the significance of C4d staining in renal tissue after ABO-incompatible renal transplantation remains controversial.[42,49–51] Our experience with C4d positivity in Tokyo is informative. Although C4d positivity of the peritubular capillaries is usually considered a good indicator of rejection in ABO-compatible renal transplantation, C4d was positive in 70% of the specimens showing no signs of rejection.[42,51] Conversely, glomerular capillaries appeared not to stain for C4d in the non-rejection specimens, but were strongly positive for C4d during rejection episodes. Thus, in our experience, C4d positivity of glomerular capillaries may be a good marker of humoral rejection after ABO-incompatible renal transplantation.[51]

ACCOMMODATION

After ABO-incompatible renal transplantation, the anti-A/B antibody titre often remains at low levels for some time.[44] However, in most patients, no significant rejection occurs despite the presence of these antibodies, allograft expression of blood group A/B antigens (in vascular endothelium and tubular cells) and an intact complement system. In fact, some investigators have reported that the A/B antigens in ABO-incompatible grafts are expressed for many years after transplantation.[52,53] This phenomenon has been described as 'accommodation' by Platt and Bach.[54] The titres of anti-A/B antibody sometimes increase to much higher levels than before transplantation, but in most cases, no significant rejection occurs. Park et al[55] reported that accommodation in ABO-incompatible renal transplantation might be caused by alterations in signal transduction, cell–cell adhesion, T cell activation pathways and the prevention of apoptosis. However, the exact mechanisms for this phenomenon have not yet been elucidated.

CONCLUSIONS AND FUTURE EXPECTATIONS

Short-term and long-term outcomes of ABO-incompatible renal transplantation seem to be excellent according to recent reports from not only our centres,[26,27,41,43] but also others in the USA[18,28] and Europe.[36,41] A2-incompatible renal transplantation can be successfully performed in recipients with low titres of anti-A/B antibodies, without pretransplant plasmapheresis and splenectomy.[17] For non-A2-incompatible renal transplant recipients, the anti-CD20 antibody, rituximab, may provide a useful alternative to splenectomy.[41] For patients with high titres of anti-A/B antibody, the removal of these antibodies by plasmapheresis remains necessary in order to prevent hyperacute rejection. However, immunoadsorption seems to be a very promising alternative with potentially fewer adverse effects.[41] These advances are making ABO-incompatible renal transplantation an increasingly attractive option in the effort to make transplantation available to a greater number of potential recipients.

REFERENCES

1. Rydberg L, Breimer ME, Samuelsson BE, Brynger H. Blood group ABO-incompatible (A2 to O) kidney transplantation in human subjects: a clinical, serologic, and biochemical approach. *Transplant Proc* 1987; **19**: 4528–4537.
2. Rydberg L. ABO-incompatibility in solid organ transplantation. *Transfus Med* 2001; **11**: 325–342.
3. Clausen H, Levery SB, Nudelman E, Tsuchiya S, Hakomori S. Repetitive A epitope (type 3 chain A) defined by blood group A1 specific monoclonal antibody TH-1: Chemical basis of a qualitative A1 and A2 distinction. *Proc Nat Acad Sci* 1985; **82**: 1199–1203.
4. Clausen H, Levery SB, Dabelsteen E, Hakomori S. Blood group ABH antigens: a new series of blood group A-associated structures (genetic regulation and tissue distribution). *Transplant Proc* 1987; **19**: 4408–4412.
5. Toma H. ABO-incompatible renal transplantation. *Urol Clin North Am* 1994; **21**: 299–310.
6. Samuelsson BE, Breimer ME. ABH antigens: some basic aspects. *Transplant Proc* 1987; **19**: 4401–4404.
7. Bariety J, Oriol R, Hinglais N et al. Distribution of blood group antigen A in normal and pathologic human kidneys. *Kidney Int* 1980; **17**: 820–826.
8. Oriol R, Cartron JP, Cartron J et al. Biosynthesis of ABH and Lewis antigens in normal and transplanted kidneys. *Transplantation* 1980; **29**: 184–188.
9. Slapak M, Naik RM, Lee HA. Renal transplant in a patient with major donor-recipient blood group incompatibility. *Transplantation* 1981; **31**: 4–7.
10. Alexandre GPJ, Squifflet JP, De Bruyere M et al. Splenectomy as a prerequisite for successful human ABO-incompatible renal transplantation. *Transplant Proc* 1985; **17**: 138–141.
11. Economidou J, Hugh-Jones N, Gardner B. Quantitative measurements concerning A and B antigen sites. *Vox Sang* 1967; **12**: 321–328.
12. Visetti M, Leigheb G, Scudeller G, Ceppellini R. Importanza dei sottogruppi A1-A2 e delle reazioni crociati A-B per la sopravvivenza di alloinnesti di cute. *Minerva Dermatol* 1967; **42**: 563–569.
13. Ceppellini R, Bigliani S, Curtoni ES, Leigheb G. Experimental allotransplantation in man: II. The role A1, A2 and B antigens; III. Enhancement by circulating antibody. *Transplant Proc* 1969; **1**: 390–394.
14. Alkhunaizi AM, de Mattos AM, Barry JM et al. Renal transplantation across the ABO barrier using A2 kidneys. *Transplantation* 1999; **67**: 1319–1324.

15. Bryan CF, Shield CF, Nelson PW et al. Transplantation rate of the blood group B waiting list is increased by using A2 and A2B kidneys. *Transplantation* 1998; **66**: 1714–1717.
16. Schnuelle P, van der Woude FJ. Should A2 kidneys be transplanted into B or O recipients? *Lancet* 1998; **351**: 1675–1676.
17. Nelson PW, Shield III CF, Muruve NA et al. Increased access to transplantation for blood group B cadaveric waiting list candidates by using A2 kidneys: time for a new nation system. *Am J Transplant* 2002; **2**: 94–99.
18. Gloor JM, Lager DJ, Moor SB et al. ABO-incompatible kidney transplantation using both A2 and non-A2 living donors. *Transplantation* 2003; **7**: 971–977.
19. Welsh KI, van Dam M, Koffman CG et al. Transplantation of blood group A2 kidneys into O or B recipients: the effect of pretransplant anti-A titers on graft survival. *Transplant Proc* 1987; **19**: 4546–4547.
20. Shapira Z, Yussim A, Shmueli D, Nakache R. Experience with blood group A2 renal grafts in ABO-incompatible recipients. *Transplant Proc* 1987; **19**: 4562–4564.
21. Mendez R, Sakhrani L, Chaballout A, Mendez RG. ABO incompatible transplants involving A2 donors. *Transplant Proc* 1991; **23**: 1738–1741.
22. Nelson PW, Landreneau MD, Luger AM et al. Ten-year experience in transplantation of A2 kidneys into B and O recipients. *Transplantation* 1998; **65**: 256–260.
23. Sorensen JB, Grant WJ, Fuller TC et al. Transplantation of blood group A2 kidney from living donors into non-A recipients [abstract]. *Transplantation* 1999; **67**: S615.
24. Slapak M, Evans P, Trickett L et al. Can ABO-incompatible donors be used in renal transplantation? *Transplant Proc* 1984; **16**: 75–79.
25. Alexandre GPJ, Squifflet JP, De Bruyere M et al. Present experiences in a series of 26 ABO-incompatible living donor renal allografts. *Transplant Proc* 1987; **19**: 4538–4542.
26. Toma H, Tanabe K, Tokumoto T et al. Excellent long-term outcome of ABO-incompatible renal transplantation. A single center experience [abstract]. *Am J Transplant* 2004; **4**: 402.
27. Tanabe K, Tokumoto T, Ishida H et al. Three-year outcome of ABO-incompatible kidney transplantation under pretransplant one-week immunosuppression with tacrolimus, mycophenolate mofetil, and steroid [abstract]. *Am J Transplant* 2004; **4**: 402.
28. Gloor JM, Larson TS, Lager DJ et al. ABO incompatible kidney transplantation with and without splenectomy using non-A2 blood group donors [abstract]. *Am J Transplant* 2004; **4**: 307.
29. Bannett AD, McAlack R, Raja R, Baquero A, Morris M. Experiences with known ABO-mismatched renal transplants. *Transplant Proc* 1987; **19**: 4543–4546.
30. Slapak M, Digard N, Ahmed M, Shell T, Thompson F. Renal transplantation across the ABO-barrier. A

9-year experience. *Transplant Proc* 1990; **22**: 1425–1428.

31. Ota K, Takahashi K, Agishi T et al. Multicenter trial of ABO-incompatible kidney transplantation. *Transpl Int* 1992; **5**(suppl 1): S40–43.

32. Aswad S, Mendez R, Mendez RG et al. Crossing the ABO blood barrier in renal transplantation. *Transplant Proc* 1993; **25**: 267–270.

33. Aikawa A, Ohara T, Hasegawa A et al. ABO-incompatible kidney transplantation on triple drug therapy compared with quadruple therapy. *Transplant Proc* 1998; **30**: 1337–1338.

34. Karakayali H, Moray G, Demirag A et al. Long-term follow-up of ABO-incompatible renal transplant recipients. *Transplant Proc* 1999; **31**: 256–257.

35. Kobayashi T, Yokohama I, Nagasaka T et al. Comparative study of antibody removed before pig-to-baboon and human ABO-incompatible renal transplantation. *Transplant Proc* 2000; **32**: 1097.

36. Tyden G, Kumlien G, Fehrman I. ABO-incompatible kidney transplantation without splenectomy using antigen-specific immunoadsorption and rituximab [abstract]. *Am J Transplant* 2004; **4**: 401.

37. Agishi T, Kaneko I, Hasuo T et al. Double filtration plasmapheresis. *Trans Am Soc Artif Intern Organs* 1980; **26**: 406–411.

38. Tanabe K, Takahashi K, Agishi T, Toma H, Ota K. Removal of anti-A/B antibodies for successful kidney transplantation between ABO blood type incompatible couples. *Transfus Sci* 1996; **17**: 455–462.

39. Bensinger WI, Bruckner CD, Clift RA. Whole blood immunoadsorption of anti-A or anti-B antibodies. *Vox Sang* 1985; **48**: 357–361.

40. Bensinger WI, Buckner CD, Thomas ED et al. ABO-incompatible marrow transplants. *Transplantation* 1982; **33**: 427–429.

41. Tyden G, Kumlien G, Fehrman I. Successful ABO-incompatible kidney transplantations without splenectomy using antigen-specific immunoadsorption and rituximab. *Transplantation* 2003; **76**: 730–743.

42. Simpkins CE, Warren DS, Sonnenday CJ et al. Accommodation of ABO-incompatible renal allografts is associated with persistent C4d staining [abstract]. *Am J Transplant* 2004; **4**: 490.

43. Tanabe K, Takahashi K, Sonda K et al. Long-term results of ABO-incompatible living kidney transplantation. *Transplantation* 1998; **65**: 224–248.

44. Tanabe K, Tokumoto T, Ishida H et al, ABO-incompatible renal transplantation at Tokyo Women's Medical University. In: Cecka JM, Terasaki PI (eds) *Clinical Transplants*. Los Angeles, California: UCLA Immunogenetics Center, 2003: 175–181.

45. Takahashi K, Saito K, Takahara S et al. Excellent long-term outcome of ABO-incompatible living donor kidney transplantation in Japan. *Am J Transplant* 2004; **4**: 1089–1096.

46. Toma H, Tanabe K, Tokumoto T. Long-term outcome of ABO-incompatible renal transplantation. *Urol Clin North Am* 2001; **28**: 769–780.

47. Tanabe K, Takahashi K, Sonda K et al. Clinicopathological analysis of rejection episodes in ABO-incompatible kidney transplantation. *Transplant Proc* 1996; **28**: 1447–1448.

48. Tanabe K, Tokumoto T, Ishida H et al. Prospective analysis and successful treatment of thrombotic microangiopathy in renal allografts under tacrolimus immunosuppression. *Transplant Proc* 2001; **33**: 3688–3690.

49. Onitsuka S, Yamaguchi Y, Tanabe K, Takahashi K, Toma H. Peritubular capillary deposition of C4d complement fragment in ABO-incompatible renal transplantation with humoral rejection. *Clin Transplant* 1999; **3**(suppl 1): 33–37.

50. Fidler ME, Gloor JM, Lager DJ et al. Histologic findings of antibody-mediated rejection in ABO blood-group-incompatible living-donor kidney transplantation. *Am J Transplant* 2004; **4**: 101–107.

51. Tanabe K, Ishida H, Tokumoto T et al. Correlation between humoral rejection and C4d attaining in ABO-incompatible renal transplantation [abstract]. *Am J Transplant* 2004; **4**: 164.

52. Bannett AD, McAlack RF, Morris M, Chopek MW, Platt JL. ABO-incompatible renal transplantation: a qualitative analysis of native endothelial tissue ABO antigens after transplantation. *Transplant Proc* 1989; **21**: 783–785.

53. Yamashita M, Aikawa A, Ohara T et al. Local immune states in ABO-incompatible renal allografts. *Transplant Proc* 1993; **25**: 274–276.

54. Platt JL, Bach FH. The barrier to xenotransplantation. *Transplantation* 1991; **52**: 937–947.

55. Park WD, Grande JP, Ninova D et al. Accommodation in ABO-incompatible kidney allografts, a novel mechanism of self-protection against antibody-mediated injury. *Am J Transplant* 2003; **3**: 952–960.

Overcoming MHC incompatibility 10

Robert A Montgomery, Christopher E Simpkins, Daniel S Warren

INTRODUCTION

Renal transplantation is clearly the optimal therapy for eligible patients with end-stage renal disease (ESRD).[1] Unfortunately, due to the growing disparity between the number of patients waiting for renal transplantation and available organs, only a fraction of patients each year enjoy the benefits of transplantation. Patients who have become sensitized to human leukocyte antigen (HLA) molecules, whether this be due to previous transplants, blood transfusions or pregnancies, are disproportionately disadvantaged and comprise 30% of the patients on the waiting list in the USA.[2] The situation is particularly desperate for the subgroup of highly sensitized (panel reactive antibody (PRA) >80%) patients who, on average, wait 6.7 years for a compatible organ or, indeed, never receive a transplant.[2]

It has been known for nearly 40 years that patients whose antibodies react with donor lymphocytes are at risk of developing hyperacute or acute antibody-mediated rejection (AMR).[3–5] Once it had been established that the presence of preformed anti-HLA donor-specific antibody (DSA) placed the recipient at substantial risk of early graft loss, pretransplant crossmatching (XM) with donor lymphocytes became the standard of practice, with a positive cytotoxicity XM considered a contraindication to renal transplantation.[4] As more sensitive techniques for detecting lower levels of donor-reactive antibody were developed (e.g. anti-human globulin enhanced and flow cytometric XMs), the incidence of humoral rejection decreased but so did the likelihood of undertaking transplan-

tations in sensitized patients, heightening the inequality in access to donor organs.[6,7]

Dramatic technological advances in the ability to identify and track DSA and diagnose AMR have allowed a renaissance in thinking about the significance of a positive (+) XM. In this chapter we will discuss techniques and clinical approaches that have been developed for modifying risk among patients who harbour donor-reactive anti-HLA antibody. The discussion is based principally on the Johns Hopkins' experience. The results of the initial Hopkins' series are summarized in Table 10-1. Most medically eligible patients evaluated to date have been considered candidates for desensitization. The one exception is that patients who have a DSA titre >256 by anti-human globulin enhanced lymphocytotoxicity crossmatch (AHG-CDC XM) are now placed into a paired-kidney exchange pool in order to identify a more immunologically favourable donor rather than directly undergo desensitization. Ninety-seven per cent of the patients who have been enrolled in the Hopkins' protocol have had successful transplantations.

CURRENT PRACTICES

Pretransplant assessment

Immunological profile

On initial evaluation, sensitized patients should undergo an in depth interrogation of sensitizing events (Table 10-2). If they have received transplants in the past, the identity of mismatched HLA antigens must be sought from the patient's medical records. Early graft losses should be characterized by obtaining pathology

Table 10-1 Outcomes and characteristics of live donor renal transplantation following PP/CMVIg desensitization for an anti-HLA antibody incompatibility at the Johns Hopkins Hospital (n = 62)

Outcomes and characteristics	
Age (years)	45.6 ± 13.7
HLA mismatch (range)	3 (1–6)
Rate of transplantation	97%
Follow-up (months)	28.2 ± 20.2
Pretransplant PP/CMVIg treatments	4.2 ± 4.4
Post-transplant PP/CMVIg treatments	4.4 ± 3.8
Anti-class I HLA Ab	31 (50%)
Anti-class II HLA Ab	35 (56.5%)
CDC XM (−), flow XM (+) at initiation of PP/CMVIg	33 (53.2%)
Initial AHG-CDC XM titre (range)	6 (1–4096)
Flow XM (+) at transplant	19 (30.6%)
CDC XM (+) at transplant	18 (29.0%)
CDC XM titre at transplant (range)	4 (1–16)
Antibody-mediated rejection	25 (40.3%)
Recurrent antibody-mediated rejection	4 (6.5%)
Median days to antibody-mediated rejection (range)	13 (4–196)
Current serum creatinine (mg/dL)	1.3 (0.7–4.2)
Death-censored allograft survival*	88.7%

PP, plasmapheresis; CMVIg, cytomegalovirus hyperimmune globulin; AHG-CDC, anti-human globulin enhanced lymphocytotoxicity; XM, crossmatch. *Overall death-censored allograft survival for patients transplanted between 2/98 and 1/04.

reports. Early vascular thromboses labelled as technical errors will frequently have histological features of acute AMR. A detailed history of previous pregnancies, including the HLA profile of the biological father, should be obtained. Historical sera are tested to determine the evolving status of relevant antibodies over time. If the antibody titre appears to be decreasing, it might, in some cases, be advantageous to observe for further spontaneous decline before initiating desensitization. If the patient has undergone transfusion, it is important to discover when and to obtain information on the transfusion as well as its impact on the antibody titres.

Once the historical immunological profile has been assembled the focus turns to the proposed transplantation (Table 10-2). The number and character of repeat HLA mismatches in the donor should be determined. A cytotoxic XM using recipient serum and donor lymphocytes is performed. At our centre, we use an AHG-CDC XM with T cells and a one-wash CDC (1wCDC) with B cells. Isoagglutinin titres are determined by doubling dilutions of serum using standard serological techniques. A flow cytometric assay is performed in sensitized

patients who have a negative (−) AHG-CDC XM in order to detect lower levels of DSA.[8,9] An autologous XM should be completed to rule out autoantibody as the cause of the (+) XM (it must be recognized that patients with autoimmune disorders or hypercoagulable states can have false (+) XMs). A variety of tests are available to further detect and characterize DSA, including solid-phase assays that use purified HLA molecules as targets and have a high level of sensitivity and specificity.[10,11] Desensitization should only be performed if donor-specific IgG is present, since third party anti-HLA antibodies are irrelevant and the significance of non-HLA antibodies is unclear.

The importance of B cell XM has been the subject of debate for some time probably because much of the data in existence are uninterpretable: many (+) B cell XMs do not reflect the presence of anti-HLA antibody.[12] Our view is that if the (+) B cell XM is due to the presence of documented donor-specific class II antibody, desensitization is strongly advised.

Titration of antibody in the cytotoxicity XM helps to determine the strength of reactivity with the donor lymphocytes. The strength of

Table 10-2   Pretransplant assessment of the sensitized patient

Immunological profile

Historical

Nature and number of sensitizing events

Transplants

- Number of previous transplants
- Early graft losses
    - Are there pathology reports available from explants? (Reviewing pathology reports often reveals that graft losses labelled as 'technical' were actually due to antibody-mediated rejection)
- Identity of mismatched HLA antigens from previous grafts
- Is the graft(s) still in place?
    - DSA may rebound when transplant nephrectomy is performed

Pregnancies

- How many (including miscarriages and terminations)?
- HLA of partner(s)
- Is the strength of HLA antibodies decreasing?

Transfusions

- How many and when?
- What is the antibody titre doing over time (transfusion-induced HLA antibody will often decrease with time)?

Current

General antibody characteristics

- Breadth of anti-HLA antibodies (can be estimated by PRA)
- Known repeat mismatches with current donor (repeat mismatches even in the absence of detectable DSA increases risk)

Donor-specific antibody characteristics

- Sensitivity of XM utilized
- Class I vs class II DSA
- What is the titre?
- A (+) XM does not ensure that DSA is present
    - Autoantibody may cause a false (+) XM
    - Autoimmune and hypercoagulable disorders can also result in a (+) XM
    - Non-HLA or third party anti-HLA antibody
- Identify the specificity of the DSA so it can be tracked
- Is historical sera or XM information available to determine current trend in DSA levels (are DSA levels increasing or falling)?

DSA, donor-specific antibody; PRA, panel reactive antibody; XM, crossmatch.

antibody reactivity is measured during desensitization by a variety of cell-based and solid-phase assays. Ultimately, the safety of proceeding with the transplantation is determined by a final XM. While the goal is for conversion to a (–) cytotoxic XM, 30% of the patients in the Hopkins' series have a low titre (+) AHG-CDC XM at the time of transplantation. Patients who start out with high levels of DSA will frequently plateau at a low-titre DSA that is recalcitrant to further reduction (Figure 10-1).

Risk profile

Once the immunological profile has been established, the patient is assessed for risk of AMR or graft loss after transplantation. The immunological and risk profiles can then be interpreted together to generate a rational treatment plan. For instance, not all patients will require splenectomy or anti-CD20, and a one-size-fits-all approach will result in over-immunosuppression for some patients and inadequate therapy for others.

The starting DSA titre accurately predicts the degree of difficulty of reducing the antibody to a safe level, but is only one factor that contributes to the risk of AMR and graft loss (Table 10-3). Perhaps the single most significant risk factor is the number of previous transplants, inasmuch as risk seems to increase incrementally with each subsequent

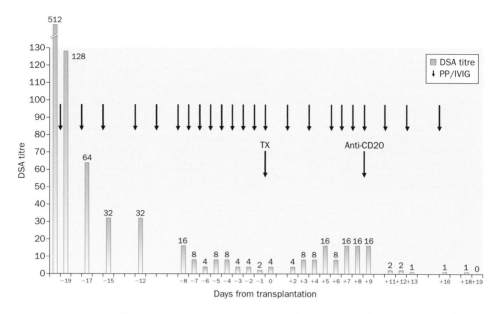

Figure 10-1   Plasmapheresis (PP)/cytomegalovirus hyperimmune globulin (CMVIg) treatment timeline (example case). The patient had a class I HLA-specific antibody titre of 512 at the initiation of PP/CMVIg desensitization therapy. Following several PP/CMVIg treatments, the donor-specific antibody (DSA) titre reached a plateau of 4 and the patient underwent transplantation with a positive cytotoxic crossmatch. Postoperatively, PP/CMVIg was continued and a single dose of anti-CD20 was administered in response to an episode of antibody-mediated rejection. The patient has since eliminated DSA. All titers were determined using AMG-CDC.

transplant. In our experience, it is rare to lose a primary graft to AMR in a patient sensitized by blood transfusions or pregnancy. While PRA itself is of limited utility in the context of

Table 10-3   Assignment of risk of antibody-mediated rejection or graft loss for patients with a (+) XM

Risk assessment

- Number of previous transplants (risk seems to increase incrementally with each subsequent transplantation)
- Early graft losses
- Repeat mismatches with earlier grafts
- Breadth of anti-HLA antibody
- Nature and number of sensitizing events (antibody response to each)
- High-risk donor–recipient pair (child-to-mother, spousal)
- Increasing titre at time of initiation of desensitization
- Rebounding titre between treatments
- High-titre donor-specific antibody
- Intravenous immunoglobulin (IVIg) non-responders
- The presence of DRw52 or DRw53 donor-specific antibody

a live donor transplant, it does give a rough estimate as to the breadth of antibody reactivity and this seems to correlate positively with risk. Also, the number of previous early graft losses and repeat mismatches are factors that portend a heightened risk of AMR. DSA against repeat mismatches not detectable in the initial characterization of the XM can appear suddenly during an AMR (spreading specificities). High-risk donor–recipient combinations, such as child-to-mother or spousal transplantations, can also contribute to the overall likelihood of AMR. Moreover, DSA that increases at the onset of desensitization or rebounds between treatments seems to be associated with added risk. Finally, we have observed that antibody against some HLA molecules (e.g. DRw52 and DRw53) can be resistant to elimination.

Desensitization protocols

It should be noted that current desensitization techniques are empirical and were ini-

Table 10-4 Desensitization regimens for renal transplantation in patients with an anti-HLA antibody incompatibility with their donor

	Authors	N*	Donor†	IVIg dose	Induction therapy	Splenectomy
IVIg	Tyan et al[24]	1	Deceased	2 g/kg	Not reported	No
	Glotz et al[22]	13	Both	2 g/kg/month for 3 months	Polyclonal antihuman thymocyte Ab	No
	Jordan et al[23]	42	Both	2 g/kg single dose	Anti-IL-2R	No
PP/IVIg	Montgomery et al[20]	4	Live	100 mg/kg after PP	Anti-IL-2R	No
	Schweitzer et al[25]	11	Live	500 mg/kg over 7 days	Anti-human CD3	No
	Sonnenday et al[26]	18	Live	100 mg/kg after PP	Anti-IL-2R	No
	Gloor et al[19]	14	Live	100 mg/kg after PP	(i) Anti-CD20 (ii) Polyclonal anti-human thymocyte Ab	Yes

*Number of patients in study who underwent desensitization for a positive crossmatch with their donor.
†Deceased, deceased donor renal transplantation; Live, living donor renal transplantation; Both, both deceased and live donors were included in the series.

tially developed to treat established de novo AMR, which historically was associated with an incidence of graft loss as high as 80%.[13–15] The advent of protocols using plasmapheresis (PP) or intravenous immunoglobulin (IVIg) made this a treatable form of rejection, generating graft survival rates of >80% at three years (see Table 10-1).[16–18]

There are two main protocols with proved efficacy for desensitizing patients with a (+) XM to a live donor: these are PP plus low-dose IVIg,[19–21] and high-dose IVIg.[22,23] In the PP/CMVIg protocol, patients receive PP every other day followed by CMVIg (Cytomegalovirus Immune Globulin) administered at a dose of 100 mg/kg. High-dose IVIg (1–2 g/kg) can be administered to precondition a patient with a (+) XM prior to live donor transplantation. Studies utilizing these approaches are summarized in Table 10-4.

High-dose IVIg

Not all patients treated with IVIg respond with a reduction in PRA or abrogation of a (+) XM to a live donor. An IVIg XM test has been developed whereby patient serum is incubated in vitro with IVIg to determine the degree of inhibition of XM. This test correlates well with the in vivo efficacy of IVIg and identifies patients most likely to benefit from IVIg therapy.[23] Patients who show no in vitro

inhibition of XM or reduction in PRA are not good candidates for IVIg desensitization therapy and should be considered for PP-based protocols.

IVIg interferes with assays that employ anti-human globulin, including the AHG-CDC XM test, the flow cytometric XM and all solid-phase immunoassays. The use of these assays is possible after serum levels of IVIg decrease but most patients administered high-dose protocols are monitored using a CDC XM. Once it is established that a patient will respond to IVIg, a 2 g/kg dose of IVIg is given monthly for a maximum of four doses. After each dose a CDC XM is performed. When the XM becomes negative, the patient receives a kidney transplant from the living donor within 24–72 hours. At one month post-transplantation the patient receives an additional IVIg infusion (2 g/kg).[22,23]

The mode of action of IVIg may be neutralization of DSA by anti-idiotypic antibodies and suppression of endogenous antibody synthesis.[27] IVIg may also work by inhibiting complement-mediated endothelial cell injury by binding C3b and C4b.[28]

As a note of caution, patients receiving high- or low-dose IVIg can exhibit isometric vacuolization on biopsy, which may be indistinguishable from the histological appearance of calcineurin inhibitor nephrotoxicity.[29] IVIg preparations that are hypertonic or contain high concentrations of sucrose may cause reversible acute renal failure at high doses (>500 mg/kg).[30–34]

PP/CMVIg

The kinetics of antibody reduction by PP are predictable and the number of treatments needed to bring the patient to a level that is safe for transplantation can be estimated from the starting titre.[35] The date of transplantation is then set and the start date for treatment established by the duration of preconditioning. The Hopkins protocol uses a centrifuge-driven cell separator to remove 1.0–1.5 plasma volumes and replaces 100% with each treatment using crystalloid and/or 5% albumin. The patient's coagulation status and proximity of therapy to invasive procedures determines the need for fresh frozen plasma.

Immunoglobulin preparations may vary widely depending on the donor pool. CMVIg as a source of immunoglobulin may have some advantages because it is produced from a stable professional pool of donors and the product is enriched for antimicrobial antibodies. Tacrolimus and mycophenolate mofetil (MMF), known to have T and B cell antiproliferative properties, are started simultaneously with PP/CMVIg, and steroids and an anti-interleukin-2-receptor induction agent are given on the day of transplant. The Mayo group has reported good results using antithymocyte globulin as the induction agent.[19,36]

PP/CMVIg is continued on an alternate day basis after the transplantation. The total number of post-transplantation treatments is dependent on the starting DSA titre and on the presence or absence of DSA at the time of transplant. In the Hopkins' series an average of four and five treatments are used pre- and post-transplantation (see Table 10-1). Patients with a positive flow cytometric, negative cytotoxic crossmatch receive two preconditioning and two post-transplantation PP/CMVIg treatments. Maintenance immunotherapy consists of tacrolimus (or rapamycin), MMF and steroids. DSA monitoring can be main-

tained throughout desensitization using all cell-based and solid-phase immunoassays because low-dose CMVIg does not interfere with these assays. We have found a close correlation between the return of DSA, graft dysfunction and histological/immunohistological features of AMR.[37]

The mechanism of long-term engraftment in patients treated with this regimen is unclear. Therapeutic immunoglobulin is known to activate anti-idiotypic networks, suppress endogenous antibody secretion and immunomodulate. PP is very effective at lowering DSA, however, the effect is short-lived and a vigorous rebound occurs when PP is discontinued. The combination of these two modalities produces durable DSA suppression provided the donor kidney is in place. PP/CMVIg appears to induce a donor-specific unresponsiveness insomuch as DSA remains undetectable by sensitive assays while third party anti-HLA antibody and antibody to nominal antigens return.[37] DSA will return if the transplantation is not performed, often at higher levels than prior to desensitization (Figure 10-2).

Immunoabsorption

Extracorporeal immunoabsorption (IA) with protein A columns has several advantages over conventional PP for therapeutic antibody removal. Most importantly, because protein A selectively depletes IgG, several plasma volumes can be treated during a single IA session without the depletion of coagulation factors that occurs with plasma exchange. Thus, much higher amounts of antibody, perhaps >90% of circulating IgG, can be safely removed over several hours in a single session of IA. Protein A IA columns have been used to remove HLA-specific antibodies prior to transplantation in highly sensitized patients (see Chapter 9).[38,39]

Splenectomy and anti-CD20

Splenectomy is known to reduce B cell mass and incapacitate immune surveillance and

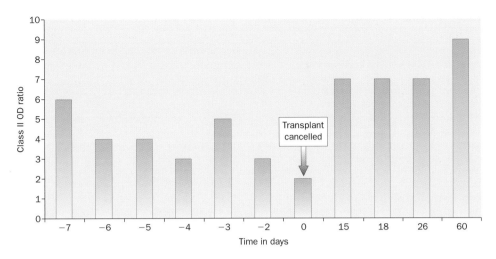

Figure 10-2 Donor-specific antibody rebound in a patient who discontinued plasmapheresis (PP)/cytomegalovirus hyperimmune globulin (CMVIg) therapy. ELISA readings of total anti-class II HLA antibody in a patient who was treated with PP/CMVIg desensitization therapy for a positive crossmatch with their donor. The transplantation procedure was cancelled prior to the operation as a result of a medical complication with the donor. The potential recipient's anti-class II HLA antibody titres were followed after cessation of PP/CMVIg and found to rebound.

antigen presentation. The spleen contains a significant number of plasma cells and removing it may 'debulk' the antibody-producing capacity of the humoral immune system. The evidence supporting splenectomy for crossing immunological barriers comes from ABO-incompatible transplantation.[40] Because the effect on the immune system is permanent, disadvantages of splenectomy include a lifelong increased risk of over-whelming infection as well as altered immunoregulatory function.[41,42]

The chimeric humanized mouse anti-human CD20 monoclonal antibody (rituximab) produces a highly effective ablation of the B cell compartment and has been considered as a possible agent for treating or preventing antibody-mediated processes in solid organ transplantation.[19,43–45] CD20 is a trans-membrane polypeptide that is expressed on the majority of pre-B cells and mature B cells but not on most plasma cells. It is a good target for monoclonal antibody therapy because it is not expressed on stem cells and does not circulate in a soluble form.[46] The monoclonal antibody binds with high affinity

to CD20, initiating antibody-dependent cell-mediated cytotoxicity, complement-mediated cell death and apoptosis in vivo.[47] Anti-CD20 has the potential to reduce the pool of pre-cursor cells responsible for the rapid clonal expansion that occurs during an AMR. The plasma cells that are actively producing DSA are unlikely to respond to anti-CD20 and must be dealt with by PP or IVIg. However, a single dose of anti-CD20 (375 mg/m²) appears to enhance the efficacy of PP/CMVIg, and when given during pre-conditioning may reduce the risk of AMR.[19,44,45] Therapeutic efficacy is monitored weekly by tracking CD20 and CD19 levels. The effect of anti-CD20 on the immune system is temporary, with the re-emergence of B cells beginning at around three months after a single dose. At our centre, we use splenectomy and/or anti-CD20 in desensitization protocols for high-risk patients and as rescue therapy for severe AMR after transplantation (Table 10-5).

Table 10-5   Determining the appropriate treatment protocol from the immunological profile and risk assessment

Risk level

Highest

- Plasmapheresis/IVIg with splenectomy and anti-CD20
- Timing of splenectomy and anti-CD20 may vary according to starting titre
  - High titre: Splenectomy and anti-CD20 prior to initiation of PP/IVIg treatments may facilitate a more responsive and rapid desensitization
  - Moderate to low titre: Splenectomy and anti-CD20 at time of transplantation may reduce the incidence or severity of AMR

High

- Plasmapheresis/IVIg with splenectomy
- Splenectomy at time of transplant may reduce the incidence or severity of AMR

Moderate

- Plasmapheresis/IVIg and anti-CD20
- A single dose of anti-CD20 ($375\,mg/m^2$) administered on the day before or day of transplantation

Low

- Plasmapheresis/IVIg
- Primary transplantations with transfusion- or pregnancy-induced sensitization rarely need splenectomy or anti-CD20

IVIg, intravenous immunoglobulin.

Diagnosis and treatment of AMR after desensitization for a positive crossmatch

The incidence of AMR is 40.3% in the Hopkins' series. Most of these rejections are mild and respond to reinitiation of PP/CMVIg and pulse steroids, with serum creatinine concentrations returning to baseline values. Early AMR is usually accompanied by graft dysfunction, triggering a renal allograft biopsy.[48] The biopsy is evaluated for characteristic immunohistological and histological features consistent with AMR, including: (i) glomerulitis/capillaritis; (ii) margination of neutrophils in the peritubular capillaries; (iii) severe or necrotizing vasculitis; (iv) interstitial haemorrhage; (v) fibrin thrombi; and (vi) diffuse, linear, C4d staining in the peritubular capillaries.[49]

The advent of sensitive assays to detect and characterize anti-HLA antibody has made it possible to differentiate DSA from antibody directed against non-HLA or third party HLA antigens and track it in real time. Response to therapy can be monitored and endpoints for treatment established.[11,50,51]

FUTURE DIRECTIONS

PP/CMVIg desensitization of patients with HLA incompatibilities and willing live donors adds about US$29 000 to Medicare costs in the first year of transplantation. The cost of maintaining a highly sensitized patient on the deceased-donor list for the median time to transplantation (currently 6.7 years) is approximately US$394 000.[2] Substantial savings to the healthcare system could be realized if these patients were desensitized and underwent transplantation expeditiously. Even greater cost savings would be generated if some of these patients received transplants in paired-kidney exchanges (PKE) (see Chapter 11). We have estimated that an optimized algorithm for a national exchange pool in the USA could result in 14% of the highly sensitized recipients finding a (–) XM exchange donor.[53] The remainder of the patients with live donors could opt for desensitization. If the requirement for a negative crossmatch were removed from exchange algorithms, patients could trade up to a better immunological compatibility or a lower titre DSA. PKE combined with lower risk desensitization could produce a substantial improvement in the rate and results of incompatible transplantation.[52] The barriers to wider application of PKE are primarily administrative, logistical and financial.

SUMMARY AND CONCLUSIONS

It has been known since the early years of renal transplantation that the presence of DSA prior to transplantation greatly increases the risk of graft loss due to AMR. A (−) XM with a potential donor became a prerequisite for proceeding with transplantation and patients broadly sensitized to common HLA molecules had little chance of ever finding a compatible donor. An explosion in technology in both histocompatibility testing and renal pathology has facilitated a major paradigm shift insomuch as a (+) XM has gone from being an absolute contraindication to a modifiable risk of transplantation.

Two major classes of desensitization protocol are PP/IVIg and high-dose IVIg, with both approaches achieving similarly good results. An immunological profile should be generated for patients undergoing evaluation for desensitization based on their previous HLA exposure. The risk to the patient posed by the live donor can be assessed in the context of their previous sensitizing events. Once their risk has been stratified, an appropriate treatment plan can be designed to match both the degree of difficulty of desensitization and the risk of graft loss. Interventions and therapies such as splenectomy, anti-CD20 and conventional induction agents can enhance the efficacy of PP or IVIg and so modify risk.

Finally, in the future recipients may choose to acquire a more immunologically compatible donor by means of PKE, improving the costs, feasibility and the results of desensitization.

REFERENCES

1. Wolfe RA, Ashby VB, Milford EL et al. Comparison of mortality in all patients on dialysis, patients on dialysis awaiting transplantation, and recipients of a first cadaveric transplant. *N Engl J Med* 1999; **341**: 1725–1730.
2. United Network for Organ Sharing. Data retrieved November 2004 from http://www.unos.org.
3. Kissmeyer-Nielsen F, Olsen S, Petersen VP, Fjeldborg O. Hyperacute rejection of kidney allografts, associated with pre-existing humoral antibodies against donor cells. *Lancet* 1966; **2**: 662–665.
4. Patel R, Terasaki PI. Significance of the positive crossmatch test in kidney transplantation. *N Engl J Med* 1969; **280**: 735–739.
5. Williams GM, Hume DM, Hudson RP Jr et al. 'Hyperacute' renal-homograft rejection in man. *N Engl J Med* 1968; **279**: 611–618.
6. Fuller TC, Phelan D, Gebel HM, Rodey GE. Antigenic specificity of antibody reactive in the antiglobulin-augmented lymphocytotoxicity test. *Transplantation* 1982; **34**: 24–29.
7. Johnson AH, Rossen RD, Butler WT. Detection of alloantibodies using a sensitive antiglobulin microcytotoxicity test: identification of low levels of preformed antibodies in accelerated allograft rejection. *Tissue Antigens* 1972; **2**: 215–226.
8. Hoffman R. In Robinson JP, Dean PN et al (eds) *Current Protocols in Cytometry*. New York: John Wiley & Sons, 2000: 1.3.1–1.3.19.
9. Bray RA. Flow cytometry in the transplant laboratory. *Ann N Y Acad Sci* 1993; **677**: 138–151.
10. Pei R, Lee JH, Shih NJ, Chen M, Terasaki PI. Single human leukocyte antigen flow cytometry beads for accurate identification of human leukocyte antigen antibody specificities. *Transplantation* 2003; **75**: 43–49.
11. Zachary AA, Bias WB, Johnson A, Rose SM, Leffell MS. Characterization of HLA class I specific antibodies by ELISA using solubilized antigen targets: I. Evaluation of the GTI QuikID assay and analysis of antibody patterns. *Hum Immunol* 2001; **62**: 228–235.
12. Gebel HM, Bray RA, Nickerson P. Pre-transplant assessment of donor-reactive, HLA-specific antibodies in renal transplantation: contraindication vs risk. *Am J Transplant* 2003; **3**: 1488–1500.
13. Lobo PI, Spencer CE, Stevenson WC, Pruett TL. Evidence demonstrating poor kidney graft survival when acute rejections are associated with IgG donor-specific lymphocytotoxin. *Transplantation* 1995; **59**: 357–360.
14. Martin S, Dyer PA, Mallick NP et al. Posttransplant antidonor lymphocytotoxic antibody production in relation to graft outcome. *Transplantation* 1987; **44**: 50–53.
15. Trpkov K, Campbell P, Pazderka F et al. Pathologic features of acute renal allograft rejection associated with donor-specific antibody. Analysis using the Banff grading schema. *Transplantation* 1996; **61**: 1586–1592.
16. Casadei DH, del C Rial M, Opelz G et al. A randomized and prospective study comparing treatment with high-dose intravenous immunoglobulin with monoclonal antibodies for rescue of kidney grafts with steroid-resistant rejection. *Transplantation* 2001; **71**: 53–58.
17. Jordan SC, Quartel AW, Czer LS et al. Posttransplant

therapy using high-dose human immunoglobulin (intravenous gammaglobulin) to control acute humoral rejection in renal and cardiac allograft recipients and potential mechanism of action. *Transplantation* 1998; **66**: 800–805.

18. Luke PP, Scantlebury VP, Jordan ML et al. Reversal of steroid- and anti-lymphocyte antibody-resistant rejection using intravenous immunoglobulin (IVIG) in renal transplant recipients. *Transplantation* 2001; **72**: 419–422.

19. Gloor JM, DeGoey SR, Pineda AA et al. Overcoming a positive crossmatch in living-donor kidney transplantation. *Am J Transplant* 2003; **3**: 1017–1023.

20. Montgomery RA, Zachary AA, Racusen LC et al. Plasmapheresis and intravenous immune globulin provides effective rescue therapy for refractory humoral rejection and allows kidneys to be successfully transplanted into cross-match-positive recipients. *Transplantation* 2000; **70**: 887–895.

21. Warren DS, Zachary AA, Sonnenday CJ et al. Successful renal transplantation across simultaneous ABO incompatible and positive crossmatch barriers. *Am J Transplant* 2004; **4**: 561–568.

22. Glotz D, Antoine C, Julia P et al. Desensitization and subsequent kidney transplantation of patients using intravenous immunoglobulins (IVIg). *Am J Transplant* 2002; **2**: 758–760.

23. Jordan SC, Vo A, Bunnapradist S et al. Intravenous immune globulin treatment inhibits crossmatch positivity and allows for successful transplantation of incompatible organs in living-donor and cadaver recipients. *Transplantation* 2003; **76**: 631–636.

24. Tyan DB, Li VA, Czer L et al. Intravenous immunoglobulin suppression of HLA alloantibody in highly sensitized transplant candidates and transplantation with a histoincompatible organ. *Transplantation* 1994; **57**: 553–562.

25. Schweitzer EJ, Wilson JS, Fernandez-Vina M et al. A high panel-reactive antibody rescue protocol for cross-match-positive live donor kidney transplants. *Transplantation* 2000; **70**: 1531–1536.

26. Sonnenday CJ, Ratner LE, Zachary AA et al. Preemptive therapy with plasmapheresis/intravenous immunoglobulin allows successful live donor renal transplantation in patients with a positive crossmatch. *Transplant Proc* 2002; **34**: 1614–1616.

27. Toyoda M, Pao A, Petrosian A, Jordan SC. Pooled human gammaglobulin modulates surface molecule expression and induces apoptosis in human B cells. *Am J Transplant* 2003; **3**: 156–166.

28. Marsh JE, Farmer CK, Jurcevic S et al. The allogeneic T and B cell response is strongly dependent on complement components C3 and C4. *Transplantation* 2001; **72**: 1310–1318.

29. Haas M, Sonnenday CJ, Cicone JS, Rabb H, Montgomery RA. Isometric tubular epithelial vacuolization in renal allograft biopsy specimens of patients receiving low-dose intravenous immunoglobulin for a positive crossmatch. *Transplantation* 2004; **78**: 549–556.

30. Ahsan N, Wiegand LA, Abendroth CS, Manning EC. Acute renal failure following immunoglobulin therapy. *Am J Nephrol* 1996; **16**: 532–536.

31. Cantu TG, Hoehn-Saric EW, Burgess KM et al. Acute renal failure associated with immunoglobulin therapy. *Am J Kidney Dis* 1995; **25**: 228–234.

32. Gupta N, Ahmed I, Nissel-Horowitz S et al. Intravenous gammglobulin-associated acute renal failure. *Am J Hematol* 2001; **66**: 151–152.

33. Rault R, Piraino B, Johnston JR, Oral A. Pulmonary and renal toxicity of intravenous immunoglobulin. *Clin Nephrol* 1991; **36**: 83–86.

34. Winward DB, Brophy MT. Acute renal failure after administration of intravenous immunoglobulin: review of the literature and case report. *Pharmacotherapy* 1995; **15**: 765–772.

35. Montgomery RA, Zachary AA. Transplanting patients with a positive donor-specific crossmatch: A single center's perspective. *Pediatr Transplant* 2004; **8**: 1–8.

36. Gloor JM, DeGoey S, Ploeger N et al. Persistence of low levels of alloantibody after desensitization in crossmatch-positive living-donor kidney transplantation. *Transplantation* 2004; **78**: 221–227.

37. Zachary AA, Montgomery RA, Ratner LE et al. Specific and durable elimination of antibody to donor HLA antigens in renal-transplant patients. *Transplantation* 2003; **76**: 1519–1525.

38. Bevan DJ, Carey BS, Lea CK et al. Antibody removal and subsequent transplantation of a highly sensitised paediatric renal patient. *Transpl Int* 1996; **9**: 155–160.

39. Palmer A, Taube D, Welsh K et al. Removal of anti-HLA antibodies by extracorporeal immunoadsorption to enable renal transplantation. *Lancet* 1989; **1**: 10–12.

40. Alexandre GP, Squifflet JP, De Bruyere M et al. Present experiences in a series of 26 ABO-incompatible living donor renal allografts. *Transplant Proc* 1987; **19**: 4538–4542.

41. Eibl M. Immunological consequences of splenectomy. *Prog Pediatr Surg* 1985; **18**: 139–145.

42. Lynch AM, Kapila R. Overwhelming postsplenectomy infection. *Infect Dis Clin North Am* 1996; **10**: 693–707.

43. Becker YT, Becker BN, Pirsch JD, Sollinger HW. Rituximab as treatment for refractory kidney transplant rejection. *Am J Transplant* 2004; **4**: 996–1001.

44. Sonnenday CJ, Warren DS, Cooper M et al. Plasmapheresis, CMV hyperimmune globulin, and anti-CD20 allow ABO-incompatible renal transplantation without splenectomy. *Am J Transplant* 2004; **4**: 1315–1322.

45. Tyden G, Kumlien G, Fehrman I. Successful ABO-incompatible kidney transplantations without splenectomy using antigen-specific immunoadsorption and rituximab. *Transplantation* 2003; **76**: 730–731.

46. Johnson P, Glennie M. The mechanisms of action of

rituximab in the elimination of tumor cells. *Semin Oncol* 2003; **30**(suppl 2): 3–8.

47. Reff ME, Carner K, Chambers KS et al. Depletion of B cells in vivo by a chimeric mouse human monoclonal antibody to CD20. *Blood* 1994; **83**: 435–445.

48. Montgomery RA, Hardy MA, Jordan SC et al. Consensus opinion from the antibody working group on the diagnosis, reporting, and risk assessment for antibody-mediated rejection and desensitization protocols. *Transplantation* 2004; **78**: 181–185.

49. Racusen LC, Colvin RB, Solez K et al. Antibody-mediated rejection criteria – an addition to the Banff 97 classification of renal allograft rejection. *Am J Transplant* 2003; **3**: 708–714.

50. Lucas DP, Paparounis ML, Myers L, Hart JM, Zachary AA. Detection of HLA class I-specific antibodies by the QuikScreen enzyme-linked immunosorbent assay. *Clin Diagn Lab Immunol* 1997; **4**: 252–257.

51. Zachary AA, Ratner LE, Graziani JA et al. Characterization of HLA class I specific antibodies by ELISA using solubilized antigen targets: II. Clinical relevance. *Hum Immunol* 2001; **62**: 236–246.

52. Montgomery RA. ABO incompatible transplantation: to B or not to B. *Am J Transplant* 2004; **4**: 1011–1012.

53. Seger DL, Gentry SE, Warren DS et al. Kidney paired donation and optimizing the use of live donor organs. *JAMA* 2005; **293**: 1883–1890.

Paired-exchange in living donor kidney transplantation

11

Kiil Park, Jong Hoon Lee

INTRODUCTION

Despite the advantages of kidney transplantation in treating end-stage renal disease (ESRD), the shortage of available organs limits its application and is now the major barrier to transplantation worldwide. Even in countries with well-developed programmes to procure kidneys from cadavers, there is increasing reliance on live donors.[1] In Korea, a country with limited cadaveric donation despite a social and legal consensus regarding brain death, there is a widening discrepancy between the number of kidneys available and the increasing number of patients awaiting transplantation. The number of patients requiring renal replacement therapy in Korea, reported as 642.3 per 10^6 population in 2001, had increased to 700.6 per million in 2002 (Figure 11.1). In 2002, the annual incidence of patients newly requiring renal replacement therapy was 129.5 per 10^6, of whom only 15.2 per 10^6 underwent kidney transplantation.[2]

Approximately 800 kidney transplants are performed each year in Korea. According to the annual report of the Korean Network for Organ Sharing (KONOS), the majority of patients (44.3%) received a kidney from a living-related donor (LRD), followed by a living-unrelated donor (LURD; 40.3%), and a cadaveric donor (15.4%).[3]

EFFORTS TO INCREASE ORGAN DONATION

Various efforts have been made to increase the number of kidneys available for transplantation in Korea. For cadaveric donation, it was proposed to use non-heart-beating donors and to undertake a donor action promotion, while attempts to increase the number of living donor organs have included the use of kidneys from marginal donors and unrelated donors. In addition, several trials of renal transplantation between ABO- and major histocompatibility complex (MHC)-incompatible donors and recipients using desensitization protocols have produced reasonable results. However, this approach has not gained wide acceptance due to excessive cost and medical risks.

HISTORICAL BACKGROUND OF PAIRED-EXCHANGE LIVING DONOR KIDNEY (LDK) TRANSPLANTATION

In the early period of kidney transplantation, living donors and recipients were genetically related. Kidneys from genetically unrelated but emotionally motivated donors (LURD), such as spouses, close relatives, common law partners, close friends and well-motivated voluntary donors were discouraged because of relatively poor results and the fear of commercialization. Now, however, such donors are commonly used, and excellent short- and long-term results have been achieved.[4,5] Nevertheless, ABO incompatibility and other problems of histocompatibility, such as poor human leukocyte antigen (HLA) match and/or positive cross-matches, make some donations unacceptable under current standards of care.

In 1986, Rapaport et al proposed the idea of paired-kidney exchanges in an attempt to increase the availability of organs for transplantation.[6] The proposal was to use kidneys from living donors that were incompatible

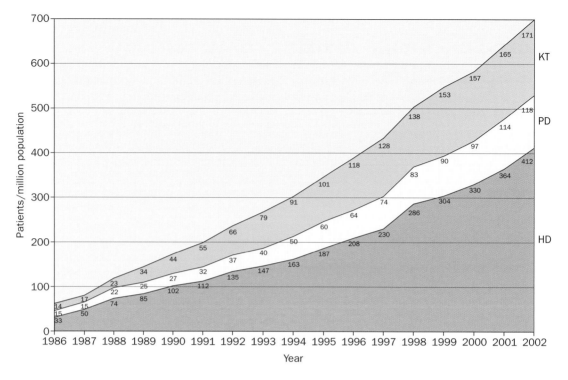

Figure 11-1 Point prevalence of renal replacement therapy in Korea (patient numbers per million population (PMP)). HD, haemodialysis, PD, peritoneal dialysis, KT, kidney transplantation. Redrawn from the Korean Society of Nephrology, with kind permission.[2]

with their designated recipients through an exchange arrangement between two donor–recipient pairs. Such an approach has seemed attractive to many transplant centres, but has not been widely implemented due to social, legal, cultural and/or financial issues. Given the emergence of satisfactory results obtained with LURD, an exchange donor programme was developed in Korea in 1991.[7] Initiated by Park and colleagues at Severance Hospital in Seoul, this programme has resulted in excellent patient and graft survival and gained increasing acceptance. A collaborative study involving three Korean transplant centres documented that the number of LURD transplants performed under the exchange donor programme has increased from 4/184 (2.2%) in 1991 to 38/124 (31%) in 1997. They reported that the main reasons for donor exchange were ABO blood type incompatibility (76%), poor HLA match in

cases of transplantation between spouses (2%) and a positive lymphocyte cross-match (22%).[8]

CURRENT PRACTICE MODELS

Swap (direct donor exchange) and swap-around (indirect donor exchange)

A donor exchange (swap) was offered to patients who had a family member willing to donate, but was incompatible with the recipient due to positive lymphocyte cross-matching and/or incompatible ABO blood groups. The first swap between two families in Korea was successfully performed in 1991. The reason for donor–recipient incompatibility was a positive cross-match, and these ESRD patients exchanged their donor kidneys with satisfactory results.

The second phase of the programme was prompted by this initial success. This was the so-called swap-around scheme in which many kinds of potential living donors, such as close friends, spouses, distant relatives and emotionally motivated volunteers were listed in the database after careful screening. Groups of two or more donor–recipient pairs were assembled within this pool, according to the degree of HLA match and ABO compatibility. Potential donors and recipients were then informed of availability for exchange donation.

List-paired exchange

Another variant of paired exchange is termed 'list pairing'. Again, a potential living donor, incompatible with their chosen recipient, agrees to donate a kidney to a suitable transplant candidate identified from the waiting list. In return, the original recipient is given priority on the waiting list for the next available, ABO-compatible, deceased donor kidney. Such a programme was recently instituted in the USA, within the domain of the New England Organ Bank, and resulted in 17 living donor kidneys being added to the pool between 2001 and 2003.[9] List pairing, at least within the USA, requires the consent of all transplant programmes within a service area, and authorization of a 'variance' in allocation procedures from the United Network of Organ Sharing policies.[10]

ADVANTAGES AND DISADVANTAGES ASSOCIATED WITH DONOR EXCHANGES

The principal advantages of donor exchange are that, after arrangements are made and consent obtained, an uncomplicated ABO-compatible transplant is performed under standard immunosuppression with excellent results.[8] Expensive interventions such as intravenous immunoglobulin and plasmapheresis are avoided. In addition, previously unusable kidneys can be used, allowing patients with ESRD to be removed from the waiting list, resulting in benefit not only for those recipi-ents, but also for those remaining on the list. Such transplants can be performed in a timely fashion, which may reduce or obviate the need for dialysis, thereby minimizing medical intervention prior to transplantation. Other potential advantages include:

- Alleviation of the donor supply problem.
- The attainment of short- and long-term patient and graft survival rates comparable to those achieved with HLA haplo-identical LRD kidney transplantation.
- The short time on dialysis or pre-emptive transplantation, associated with improved patient and graft survival.
- The ability to schedule transplants for medical and personal convenience.
- Emotional benefit for donor and recipient families.
- Removal of the need for or consideration of commercial transplantations.

With a large enough pool of willing donors and recipients, even highly sensitized patients, such as those with positive cross-matches with multiple donors or elevated panel reactive antibody, may be candidates for exchange LDK transplantation.

Psychological benefit for the donor is an additional feature of living donor exchange transplantation. Even if the transplantation fails, the donor knows that he or she did everything possible to help a loved one. Since the donation is indirect in exchange donor kidney transplantation, the psychological benefit may be more diffuse. In the Korean programme, almost all the families knew each other, especially in the case of direct exchange. In fact, donor exchange must be managed carefully to avoid interfamilial conflicts, and it is essential to explain the entire procedure and expected results of the kidney transplantation before the operation so that expectations are realistic. Nonetheless, there is no reason to believe that the psychological benefits of donating would vary substantially from those documented in more standard schemes.[11–13]

On the other hand, there are potential disadvantages in donor exchange. These include: psychological stress to donor and family; possible conflicts between donor's or recipient's families, especially in the event of significant discrepancies in transplant results; less opportunity for blood group O recipients to find exchange donors; and general risks assumed by all living donors.

As mentioned above, it is possible that patients of ABO blood type O have fewer chances of obtaining exchange donors. In Korea, blood group O is the second commonest blood type in the general population and in patients with ESRD waiting for a cadaveric kidney donor.[3] Blood group O recipients require a blood group O donor, but blood group O donors can give to any ABO-type recipient. Since ABO incompatibility is the commonest reason underlying paired-exchange transplantation, it is likely that blood type O recipients will rarely find themselves eligible for kidney paired-exchange transplantation (except in the case of positive cross-match with the intended donor).

Another disadvantage is the ethical and logistic complexity of the transaction.[14] Informed consent requires greater explanation of risks and benefits for multiple parties and documentation of thorough understanding by many different people. The requirement for simultaneous donor nephrectomy and allograft implantation may also pose a problem at many centres.

While paired-exchange between live donors and their corresponding recipients impacts on only those involved, list pairing has substantially greater implications. In this transaction, one patient receives a kidney from a living donor, while the other gets a cadaveric kidney, and the quality of results may differ accordingly. Additionally, even though the 'system' benefits from another kidney added to the pool, the burden may be substantially greater for candidates on the list with blood type O. Most list-paired exchanges are performed for ABO incompatibility where the potential recipient is ABO type O, and the donor A or B. The net impact is a kidney from the limited pool of O cadaveric kidneys going to the originally intended O recipient, further depleting the pool of O kidneys, and placing the remaining O candidates at relative disadvantage.[15] In fact, Ross and Zenios have written extensively on the implications of this imbalance, and have recently advocated discontinuation of the New England programme.[16] Its proponents, however, maintain that the impact of these discrepancies in access will dissipate over time.[9]

EXCHANGE DONOR SELECTION AND EVALUATION

Selection of appropriate donors and recipients for an exchange programme is of critical importance. However, before proceeding with exchange donation, additional factors must be considered with both donor and recipient candidates. These include first exploring all options for traditional HLA and ABO compatible donors. A thorough investigation regarding the urgency of need for transplantation and likelihood of receiving a cadaveric kidney is also warranted. In addition, those who elect to proceed with donor exchange must be fully informed and able to comprehend the risk, benefits and nuances of such a programme, including the potential for unequal benefits should graft failure ensue for one recipient, but not the other.

Under current standards, it is essential to ensure that no commercial transaction is involved, especially in the face of substantial socioeconomic differences. A team of social workers under the guidance of an ethics committee meets with both donor and recipient to evaluate the possibility of commercial exchange. Routine psychiatric evaluation of both is also recommended to help evaluate the level of commitment of those involved, and document the absence of perceived coercion. Medical evaluation of donors and recipients for exchange transplantation is otherwise identical to that of any other potential donor and recipient.

A hesitant donor is usually given many opportunities to withdraw consent. However, concern about coercion may be heightened for paired kidney exchanges, because a reluctant donor cannot invoke ABO incompatibility or positive cross-match as the reason for not proceeding with the donation. Psychiatric evaluation in the exchange living donor programme should help ensure that coercion is minimized and that the donor's decision is voluntary. The potential kidney exchange donor should be able to opt out of the process at any time, right up until the perioperative period. To ensure donor autonomy, a healthcare professional not involved in the care of the recipient, an independent donor advocate, confirms the decision to donate.[17]

The problem of reneging could occur in living donor exchange. Obviously, donors must be given the opportunity to change their minds. The only way to ensure that both recipients in a paired-exchange receive their grafts (i.e. that neither donor withdraws from the exchange agreement) is to perform the transplantations simultaneously.[20] In Korea, swaps are arranged to preferentially facilitate HLA matching, so that donor and recipient share at least two class I and one class II alleles if possible. In other programmes, the principal goal of minimizing the risk for different outcomes between recipients focuses attention on sex, age, socioeconomic status, renal function and body habitus in addition to HLA match.[10]

CURRENT RESULTS WITH PAIRED-EXCHANGE TRANSPLANTATION

Given selection criteria that included HLA matching, graft survival following exchange LDK transplantation was comparable with that obtained for LURD or HLA haplo-identical LRD kidney transplants.[19] Park et al have reported upon their experiences of exchange LDK transplantation at Severance Hospital.[20] They retrospectively studied 876 kidney transplants between 1995 and 2002, divided into donor types: 546 LRD kidney transplants (89 HLA identical, 454 HLA haplo-identical, 3 HLA zero match); 90 LURD kidney transplants (swap programme); 240 LURD kidney transplants (without swap programme). As shown in Figure 11-2, 5-year patient and graft survival rates were 92.1% and 90.6%, respectively, for exchange donor kidney transplantation, 94.3% and 90.0% for LURD kidney transplantation and 94.5% and 90.7% for HLA haplo-identical LRD kidney transplantation. HLA-identical LRD transplantation was associated with a higher patient survival (100%) and graft survival (97.8%) than that achieved with the other procedures. No

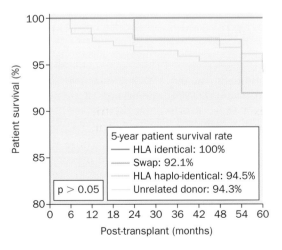

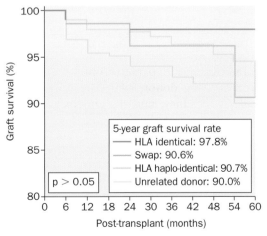

Figure 11-2 Patient and graft survival of exchange living donor kidney transplantation (1995–2002): experience from Severance Hospital, Korea.[21]

difference in the frequency and severity of acute rejection was observed between exchange donor transplants (31%) and other LURD transplants (33%) or HLA haplo-identical LRD transplants (27%).[20]

According to the results of a collaborative study in three Korean transplant centres, 44.5% of patients experienced acute rejection within the first year of transplantation.[8] Two lost their kidney graft due to irreversible acute rejection, and there were seven cases of late-onset acute rejection, which developed one year after transplantation (Table 11-1). Graft failures totalled 14.5% during the study period (which had a mean follow up of 35.2 ± 23.74 months; range 12–95 months), and the commonest cause of graft failure was chronic rejection (31%).

Data regarding outcomes in list-paired exchange are more limited.[9] In the New England Organ Bank experience, recipients of living donor kidneys appeared to do well. However, two of the 17 patients receiving kidneys from deceased donors lost their grafts and required re-transplantation, emphasizing the potential discrepancy in outcomes when grafts from live and cadaveric donors are exchanged.

SUMMARY

Exchange donor transplantation facilitates the utilization of kidneys that would otherwise be unavailable for transplantation, an especially important point in countries without well-developed cadaveric organ procurement or without established brain death statutes. A variety of living donors (including relatives, friends, spouses) are potential participants in paired-exchange programmes. With appropriate screening, ethics and informed consent, the net result is a relatively uncomplicated transplantation from an immunological perspective, with outcomes comparable to other, more standard, living donor allografts. In fact, it is possible to facilitate donor–recipient combinations that demonstrate favourable profiles for successful long-term outcomes (e.g. HLA matching, body habitus, etc.). Nonetheless, some controversy remains, especially with list pairing, indicating that a cautious approach to implementation of such programmes may be warranted.

Table 11-1 Summary of outcomes in exchange donor kidney transplantation. Adapted from Park et al[8] with kind permission from Lippincott Williams & Wilkins

Outcome	Number (%) patients (n = 110)
Early acute rejection*	
One episode	40 (36.4)
Two episodes	8 (7.3)
Three episodes	1 (0.9)
Total	49 (44.5)
Late acute rejection[†]	
One episode	6 (5.5)
Two episodes	1 (0.9)
Three episodes	(0)
Total	7 (6.4)
Cause of graft failure	16 (14.5)
Chronic rejection	5 (31.3)
Patient death	4 (25.0)
Acute rejection	2 (12.5)
Recurrent disease	1 (6.3)
Other	4 (25.0)

*Within first year.
[†]>1 year post-transplantation.

REFERENCES

1. Rosendale JD. The UNOS renal transplant registry. In: JM Cecka, PI Terasaki, (eds) *Clinical Transplants 2003*. Los Angeles: UCLA immunogenetics Center, 2004: 65–76.
2. The Korean Society of Nephrology Registry. Renal replacement therapy in Korea. *Korea J Nephrol* 2003; **22s**: S353–368.
3. Annual reports of Korean Network for Organ Sharing (KONOS) registration, 2003.
4. Spital A. Unrelated living kidney donors. An update of attitudes and use among US transplant centers. *Transplantation* 1994; **57**: 1722–1726.
5. Spital A. Unconventional living kidney donors – attitudes and use among transplant centers. *Transplantation* 1989; **48**: 243–248.
6. Rapaport FT. The case for a living emotionally related international kidney donor exchange registry. *Transplant Proc* 1986; **18**(suppl 2): S5–9.
7. Kwak JY, Kwon OJ, Lee KS et al. Exchange-donor program in renal transplantation: a single-center experience. *Transplant Proc* 1999; **31**: 344–345.
8. Park K, Moon JI, Kim SI, Kim YS. Exchange donor

program in kidney transplantation. *Transplantation* 1999; **67**: 336–338.

9. Delmonico FL. Exchanging kidneys – advances in living donor transplantation. *N Engl J Med* 2004; **350**: 1812–1814.

10. Delmonico FL, Morrissey PE, Lipkowitz GS et al. Donor kidney exchanges. *Am J Transplant* 2004; **4**: 1628–1634.

11. Jacobs C, Johnson E, Anderson K, Gillingham K, Matas A. Kidney transplants from living donors: how donation affects family dynamics. *Adv Ren Replace Ther* 1998; **5**: 89–97.

12. Johnson EM, Anderson JK, Jacobs C et al. Long-term follow-up of living kidney donors: quality of life after donation. *Transplantation* 1999; **67**: 717–721.

13. Smith MD, Kappell DF, Province MA et al. Living-related kidney donors: a multicenter study of donor education, socioeconomic adjustment, and rehabilitation. *Am J Kidney Dis* 1986; **8**: 223–233.

14. Ross LF, Rubin DT, Siegler M et al. Ethics of a paired-kidney exchange program. *N Engl J Med* 1997; **336**: 1752–1755.

15. Ross LF, Woodle ES. Ethical issues in increasing living kidney donations by expanding kidney paired exchange programs. *Transplantation* 2000; **69**: 1539–1543.

16. Ross L, Zenios S. Practical and ethical challenges to paired exchange programs. *Am J Transplant* 2004; **4**: 1553–1554.

17. Abecassis M, Adams M, Adams P et al. Consensus statement on the live organ donor. *JAMA* 2000; **284**: 2919–2926.

18. Hiraga S, Tanaka K, Watanabe J et al. Living unrelated donor renal transplantation. *Transplant Proc* 1992; **24**: 1320–1322.

19. Park K. Donor exchange programmes: increasing organ availability. Presented at an approved ESOT satellite symposium: Living donor Kidney Transplantation 2003: Looking to the future. 21 September 2003, Venice Lido, Italy. Abstracts.

20. Park K, Kim YS, Lee EM, Lee HY, Han DS. Single-center experience of unrelated living-donor renal transplantation in the cyclosporine era. *Clin Transpl* 1992: 249–256.

Nondirected living donors[*] 12

Arthur J Matas, Cheryl L Jacobs, Catherine A Garvey, Deborah D Roman

INTRODUCTION

As discussed elsewhere in this volume, one of the most important problems in solid organ transplantation is the growing waiting list of potential recipients, along with the resulting increase in waiting time for those candidates actively placed on the list. This increased waiting time has important consequences: in the USA, about 7% of candidates die annually while waiting for a kidney,[1] and transplant outcome is adversely affected by long waits.[2] One way to address the waiting list problem is to increase the number of living donor transplants. Three recent novel attempts to do so – paired exchanges, use of ABO-incompatible donors, and use of positive crossmatch donors – have been discussed in other chapters. At the University of Minnesota, we have taken a different approach by developing a programme that enables anyone, even altruistically motivated persons without an identified recipient, to become potential donors.

We distinguish between 'nondirected donation', which involves a living person's offer to donate an organ to anyone on the deceased donor waiting list, and 'directed donation', which instead involves a living person's designation of a donor organ for a specific recipient. Since the inception of our transplant programme, we have regularly received (and refused until recently) requests from individuals wanting to be nondirected donors (NDDs). With recognition of the recent excellent outcome of living unrelated donor transplantations, we re-evaluated our former policy of refusal. We have previously reported on our initial deliberations and development of our current policy of accepting NDDs.[3]

CURRENT POLICY

Initial donor screening

When a potential NDD contacts our transplant programme, a transplant coordinator performs an initial screening interview. Since many candidates live far from our institution, the screening interview helps rule out those with obvious medical or psychosocial contraindications, which are the same as for any directed kidney donor. During the screening interview, the surgical risks are outlined, the process is described, an approximate timetable is provided, and a clear statement is made that no payment will be made for donation. In addition, if candidates do live far from our institution, we may enquire whether they have contacted a closer transplant programme that might be more convenient for them. (However, many centres do not have established NDD programmes.)

If, at the end of the screening interview, the candidate is not ruled out and remains interested, he or she is mailed a packet of donor education information (including information on surgical risks, a list of

[*]Published in part in the *American Journal of Transplantation*, 2004. Supported by NIH grant #DK13083.

previous donors to talk to, a discussion of the decision-making process, internet sites, a list of references to journal articles, and a description of travel resources). If still interested after reading the information, he or she can re-contact our programme and forward a written, more detailed medical history, including reasons for wanting to donate. Before a full evaluation at our institution, we request that a minimum number of laboratory tests be performed at the candidate's local clinic (e.g. blood typing and viral studies for hepatitis B and C, human immunodeficiency virus testing), thus preventing the expense of an unnecessary full evaluation and unnecessary visits to our institution. The tests performed at the candidate's local clinic are paid for by our transplant programme.

Detailed donor evaluation

If the candidate's written medical history and local laboratory results are acceptable, he or she must then come to our institution for a full medical and psychosocial evaluation. The candidate meets with an independent donor team, comprising a surgeon, nephrologist, coordinator, clinical social worker, and psychologist (who are not involved with recipient care). The medical evaluation does not differ greatly from that for directed donors, except for the requirements that the potential NDD must come to our institution for the medical evaluation and must also see our psychologist.

The psychosocial evaluation of the potential NDD is more extensive than that for directed donors. Both a designated clinical social worker and a psychologist routinely evaluate potential NDDs. In contrast, our directed donors do not see a psychologist, unless we have concerns about cognitive deficits or other psychological risk factors. Both our social worker and psychologist assess each potential NDD's psychosocial stability, ability to comprehend information, and reasons for donating.[4] We feel that this more extensive evaluation is warranted because the psychosocial consequences for NDDs are not yet fully understood.

We explore each potential NDD's motives for donating, to obtain a better understanding of what influenced the desire to donate to a complete stranger. We assess whether the decision to be a donor was made impulsively and whether any unrealistic or ulterior motives exist, such as individual or societal approval, compensation, atonement, redemption, or media attention. In such instances, the offer would be declined.

Potential NDDs who are found ineligible for any reason are sent a note thanking them for their interest, and if appropriate, recommendations or referrals for additional care. They are also informed about other transplant programmes if they desire another opinion.

Waiting interval

If, after the evaluation, the potential NDD is accepted, we require a waiting period of at least three months before surgery to allow time for reflection and adequate preparation.

Recipient selection

We select recipients using the same algorithm as for allocating deceased donor kidneys (United Network for Organ Sharing [UNOS]). With NDDs, one advantage (over deceased donation) is the opportunity for the recipient to schedule a preoperative clinic visit and undergo re-evaluation. After all, many prospective recipients have been on the waiting list for many years. Problems can thus be identified and addressed before scheduling the transplant. During this preoperative clinic visit, the prospective recipient is informed of the requirements of our non-directed donation programme, including the need to respect the NDD's anonymity.

Donor costs

NDDs are required to pay for any non-medical expenses, including the cost of two trips to our institution, but they may be eligible for an institutional donor grant. Such grants – which require financial screening by a social worker – are made available to all potential organ donors and may only be used to help defray donor-related costs (e.g., travel, lodging, other expenses incurred as a direct result of donation). However, the maximum limit of such grants rarely covers all donor-related costs.

Donor and recipient communication

The prospective NDD and recipient are not permitted to meet before surgery. Meeting the recipient could make the NDD feel a greater sense of obligation or even coercion. Alternatively, the NDD might renege because of an undisclosed or underlying bias against the recipient's personal situation, religion, or ethnic group.

After the transplant, we encourage the recipient to write and thank the NDD. The letter is sent via our transplant programme. Both parties may wish to continue to communicate in writing (again, via our transplant programme). After six months, if mutually desired, the NDD and the recipient can communicate directly or meet. If they wish, we can help facilitate the meeting; otherwise they are free to meet on their own. Either way, we urge them to consider the potential consequences of meeting and require each of them to sign a release form before learning each other's identity.

RESULTS

Between 1 October 1997 and 1 March 2003, we received 397 enquiries about our nondirected donation programme, mostly (64%) from individuals who lived outside Minnesota. A similar number of enquiries came from men (n=200) and women (n=197). Their average age was 42 years (range 18–64).

Of the 397 enquirers, 73 (18%) were deemed ineligible after the preliminary telephone screening interview: 37 (51%) because of medical reasons, 13 (18%) because of psychosocial reasons, nine (12%) because they requested compensation, eight (11%)

because of their age (three <21 years; two >78 years), and six (8%) because of other reasons (e.g., stipulations on the surgery or desire to direct the kidney to a certain subgroup of recipients). Individuals who were turned down were given the option of contacting another transplant programme.

The remaining 324 enquirers were sent information about donation. Of these, 263 (82%) have made no further contact. Of the remainder, 56 have come to our institution for at least partial or full evaluation. Of these 56 individuals, 26 (46%) were accepted as NDDs, 24 (43%) were denied for either medical (n=16) or psychosocial (n=8) reasons, and six (11%) did not complete the full evaluation. The motivations of those individuals who underwent full evaluation have been described elsewhere.[5]

To date, at our institution, 24 transplants have now been performed using NDDs: 23 grafts continue to function, but one failed secondary to recurrent disease. Although follow-up time remains short (three months to three years), all 24 NDDs continue to be pleased with their decision to donate.

DECISION PROCESSES

When establishing a nondirected donation programme, each transplant center must address a number of practical, logistical and ethical issues. First, should the kidney be allocated to that programme's list, to a regional list, or, in the case of a 6-antigen match, to a national list? Good logistical reasons exist for considering only that programme's list. For example, other programmes within the area may not be willing to use NDDs (as was the case when we started our programme), or NDDs may prefer to come to a specific programme. One of the advantages of any living donor kidney transplant is the short ischaemic time; this advantage would be eliminated if the kidney needed to be transported. However, allocation to a regional list allows for the potential for a better human leukocyte antigen (HLA) match, and may lead to a more equitable allocation of organs. Some regional organ procurement organizations have worked out the logistical issues and have successfully developed a system to share kidneys from NDDs within a designated geographic area.[6]

Second, should the kidney be allocated to the number one person on the waiting list, without regard for recipient morbidity or mortality risk factors (with or without a transplant)? In establishing our programme, we felt that the balance between efficacy and equity had been established (after years of discussion) in the UNOS allocation system for deceased donor transplants. We elected to use the same system.

Third, should NDDs be allowed to at least direct the kidney to a specific subgroup? When we established our programme, we initially identified specific subgroups (e.g., children) that we could possibly imagine defending as socially acceptable for such directives. We have had five NDDs who would have preferred that their kidney go to a child, two who wanted to direct their kidney to an African American (citing the increased waiting time for minorities), and two who asked about designating their kidney to a single mother raising a family. However, in creating the actual protocol for our programme, we could not satisfactorily determine how to allow directives in what we determined to be acceptable situations without creating problems when faced with the possibility of directives in socially unacceptable situations (e.g., directives based on religious or racial bigotry or discrimination). So we elected to allocate the kidneys of all NDDs solely according to the established UNOS algorithm. Most of our potential NDDs were still willing to donate after learning of that policy.

Other transplant programmes have allowed subgroup directives by their allegedly 'nondirected' donors. In a national telephone survey conducted by Spital on whether NDDs should or should not be allowed to direct their kidney, most respondents thought that a donor should be permitted to insist that their gift go to a child but not to a member of a specific religious or racial group.[7] We believe that programmes permitting subgroup directives need to find a consistent system so as to eliminate potential discrimination. Importantly, each programme's policy for allocation must be described to all its potential NDDs.

DISTINCTIVE ASPECTS

Our nondirected donation programme differ in two key ways from our directed donation programme. First, with regard to donor family interactions, we have found absolutely no family pressure on NDDs to donate. Potential NDDs have unlimited time to consider whether or not to proceed, without having the regular reminder of a loved one or family member doing poorly with end-stage renal disease. In contrast, we have also seen, in some cases, a lack of family member involvement or support. In fact, when many of our potential NDDs first suggested the idea of donation, family members were opposed.

Second, the NDD process is anonymous. Although we tell both the NDD and the recipient that there might not be any contact posttransplant, some of our NDDs became concerned when they did not hear from the recipient. They enquired about their recipient's status while the latter was in hospital and they liked knowing how the recipient was doing long after surgery. Some of our NDDs have contacted our transplant programme to ask about their recipient (and sometimes assumed he or she was not well when they did not automatically hear from us on a regular basis). Programmes must decide how much information will be communicated, and when, to NDDs, since most do want to hear about the effects of their donation.

Both directed donors and NDDs do require long-term follow-up. Long-term studies of directed donors have shown quality of life equal to or better than the agematched general population.[8] Similar studies of NDDs (who do not necessarily have the benefit of seeing the result of their act) are needed. Importantly, studies of directed donors have shown that they wish that the transplant team would show more concern for them after donation.[9,10] NDDs are likely to feel similarly and may require even more support, especially if they have no recipient feedback or family support. Further research is needed to help identify NDDs and family members who may be at risk for psychosocial morbidity and to determine the types of interventions needed to prevent or mitigate these problems.

REFERENCES

1. Wolfe RA, Ashby VB, Milford EL et al. Comparison of mortality in all patients on dialysis, patients on dialysis awaiting transplantation, and recipients of a first cadaveric transplant. *N Engl J Med* 1999; **341**: 1725–1730.

2. Meier-Kriesche H-U, Port FK, Ojo AO et al. Effect of waiting time on renal transplant outcome. *Kidney Int* 2000; **58**: 1311–1317.

3. Matas AJ, Garvey CA, Jacobs CL, Kahn JP. Nondirected donation of kidneys from living donors. *N Eng J Med* 2000; **343**: 433–436.

4. Abecassis M, Adams M, Adams P et al. Consensus statement on live organ donation. *JAMA* 2000; **284**: 2919–2926.

5. Jacobs CL, Roman D, Garvey C, Kahn J, Matas AJ. Twenty-two nondirected kidney donors: An update on a single center's experience. *Am J Transplant* 2004; **4**: 1110–1116.

6. Washington Regional Transplant Consortium, 8110 Gatehouse Rd, Suite 101 W, Falls Church, VA 22042 (www.wrtc.org).

7. Spital A. Should people who donate a kidney to a stranger be permitted to choose their recipients? Views of the United States public. *Transplantation* 2003; **76**: 1252–1256.

8. Johnson EM, Anderson JK, Jacobs CJ et al. Long-term follow-up of living kidney donors: quality of life after donation. *Transplantation* 1999; **67**: 717–721.

9. Jacobs C, Johnson E, Anderson K, Gillingham K, Matas A. Kidney transplants from living donors: how donation affects family dynamics. *Adv Ren Replace Ther* 1998; **5**: 89–97.

10. de Graaf Olson W, Bogetti-Dumlao A. Living donors' perception of their quality of health after donation. *Prog Transplant* 2001; **11**: 108–115.

Legal and ethical dilemmas in living donor kidney transplantation

13

David PT Price

INTRODUCTION

Statute laws pertaining to living donor organ transplantation date back to the 1960s and even before. These were typically sketchy, highlighting the infancy of the field and as-yet-undeveloped ethical and legal reflection on such a novel ethical as well as clinical procedure. Even today, these statutes are invariably broad frameworks, largely facilitative and permissive in nature.[1] They vary relatively little despite considerable cultural differences among jurisdictions and the attitudes of clinicians within them. There are some common proscriptive provisions found in such legislation. The most widespread and homogeneous relate to prohibitions on commercial dealings. Some jurisdictions restrict organ donation by minors and adults without decision-making capacity, or place legal impediments upon organ donation by those lacking a genetic tie with the recipient, or alternatively perhaps, an emotional bond with him or her, but such provisions are very far from universal.[1,2]

There are few international instruments in this sphere. Policy directives have generally emanated from within Europe, although the influence of the European Union in this area has been marginal, limited to a Directive concerning blood and blood products, and a recent Directive relating to tissue banking. In contrast, the Council of Europe has had a longstanding interest in this sphere, reflecting the human rights dimensions of the procedure. A resolution in 1978 attempted to achieve greater unity with respect to organ and tissue transplantation, and was accompanied by a Recommendation of the Committee of Ministers to the Member States in 1979.[3,4] More recently, the Council of Europe Convention on Human Rights and Biomedicine was issued, supplemented by an associated protocol relating specifically to the transplantation of organs and tissues.[5,6] The impact of these instruments has so far been limited, though their influence may be felt through interpretation of the Council of Europe's European Convention on Human Rights, which has been ratified by all Member States and requires adherence within those jurisdictions.[7]

Unlike the World Health Organization's *Guiding Principles on Human Organ Transplantation* issued in 1991, whose emphasis is principally in relation to commerce in organ procurement and the equitable distribution of organs, the recent Council of Europe initiatives impact on living organ donation more generally and pervasively.[8] Although the mandatory impact of these statements has so far been fairly limited, their influence will certainly increase as international obligations and human rights protections are enhanced and the global character of transplantation as an activity expands.

Thus, the historical legacy largely resides in the absence of detailed legal regulation. This vacuum may limit the guidance available to clinicians, but at the same time enhances clinical discretion and autonomy. This 'light touch' enables flexibility to be preserved where new technologies and procedures are involved and has allowed the transplant community to 'expand' and 'contract' living donor kidney (LDK) transplantation in the light of clinical factors and prevailing conditions, most recently the (un)availability of cadaveric organs. Within the UK, LDK transplantation dwindled considerably in the 1980s and early 1990s when there seemed huge 'promise' in terms of cadaveric transplantation. Of late, living kidney donation has now reached around 23% of all kidney transplants in the UK due to a revised Department of Health policy to encourage LDK transplantation.[9] This has occurred in spite of, rather than because of, any legal changes. A similar phenomenon can be observed in the USA over the past decade or so, again without significant alteration in supportive legal statutes. In Germany, where supportive regulations were put in place in 1997, LDK transplantation has increased slowly, though the precise legal framework in place is now perceived as an obstacle to further growth.

LDK transplantation, by virtue of its intended benefit for the recipient as opposed to the donor, has attracted ethical and philosophical attention and scepticism from the outset. The procedure has been perceived to infringe the ethical maxim *primum non nocere* (above all do no harm) and the principle of 'non-maleficence' (do no harm). These Hippocratic notions have often been misconstrued to invoke the idea that the deliberate causing or risking of physical harm to a person is illegitimate, when they are in fact far less dogmatic and prescriptive.

First, one may benefit a patient as a whole yet inflict physical harm in an immediate sense, such as where a liver resection is performed in a patient with liver cancer. Second, if no procedure was ever permissible where no medical benefit would accrue to that individual, then bone marrow or even blood donation would be illegitimate as well. However, if harm may be done to one individual for the sake of benefit to another the spectre of utilitarianism raises its head, and the potential for respect for individual rights to be forsaken. But while such a danger is ever present in this area, living kidney donors are *not* treated merely as means to the ends of others, to invoke the Kantian doctrine, when

their autonomy is properly respected and other general ethical prerequisites are observed.

GENERAL LEGAL AND ETHICAL ISSUES

The potential legality of LDK transplantation per se is conceded in statutes and policy documents. In any individual case, clinicians need to be convinced that the risks and benefits are favourably weighted, balancing both physical and psychological factors in relation to both donor and recipient. The recipient of course usually stands to gain the most, typically from avoidance of long-term dialysis. These 'gains' will vary from patient to patient in terms of the impact of dialysis on their health and quality of life. The risks of nephrectomy for the psychological health of the donor are not extremely well known, and demand further study, although in the majority of instances it is apparent that there are psychological *gains* for the donor as well, in terms of boosted self-esteem, the restoration of one who is close to near proper health, etc.[10]

However, this is not the only legal and ethical consideration. If so, donation would be permissible even where the risks to the donor were inordinately high, wherever the potential benefit to the recipient exceeded such risks. Article 11 of the Council of Europe Protocol stipulates that 'The removal may not be carried out if there is a serious risk to the life or health of the donor'.[6] The perioperative mortality risk of nephrectomy is normally accepted as being of the order of 0.03% and the risks of major morbidity around 2%. Although uncertainties remain as to the limits of risk taking in the interests of others, LDK transplantation is properly regarded, in the light of the very substantial evidence accumulated over a considerable period of time, as generally being clearly within such acceptable limits. Living *non-renal* donation, especially involving donation of the right lobe of the liver or a lobe of lung, has more significant inherent risks and generally poses more difficulties of assessment, although the use of marginal renal donors who are at greater than normal risk generates similar issues.[11]

Although a clinician properly rejects LDK transplantation where he or she assesses the risk to a potential donor as too high or greater than the potential benefit to the recipient, where these 'risk-based' conditions are satisfied clinicians ought not to substitute their views about whether a donation is justified from the donor's point of view. Such substituted opinion partially accounts for the considerable historical diversity of LDK transplantation practice, with some centres, and indeed nations as a whole, performing very large numbers of LDK transplantations, with others doing few or even none. Exclusive emphasis on the physical aspects of the procedure, and undue adherence to a literal interpretation of the duty of non-maleficence, have led in the past, in Europe in particular, to an overly paternalistic approach. As Spital has said, clinicians are not better able to assess whether the risks are *worth taking* than the potential donor.[12] This is not of course to mandate the carrying out of a nephrectomy in all feasible instances where the donor so wishes. A nephrologist or surgeon is entirely justified in refusing to participate in any such instance, but this reflects personal reservation or conscience and should usually result in a referral to another centre or clinician.

There is one further prerequisite to be satisfied. In view of the potential risk to a living donor, it is generally accepted that *all things being equal* it is preferable to use a cadaveric rather than a living organ donor. Moreover, other options are usually available to sustain life following end-stage renal failure. Article 19 of the Council of Europe Convention on Biomedicine stipulates that: 'living organ donation is only permissible where there is no suitable cadaveric organ available and no other alternative therapeutic method of comparable effectiveness', and some laws have explicit provisions to the same effect.[5] However, a cadaveric kidney would need to

be actually, or very shortly, available, and be able to offer prospects at least as good for the recipient. While there are differences of medical opinion, it is typically accepted that LDK transplantation offers better prospects than cadaveric donation for various reasons. There is also general consensus that dialysis is ordinarily an inferior option. Thus, in reality, things would rarely *be* equal.

All in all, in most instances, there are no substantial legal or ethical impediments, and clinical discretion to permit live kidney donation is relatively unfettered. But we have been considering the 'typical' case, and it is generally with respect to non-typical cases that problems may arise, driven in part by the pressure to expand the donor pool. However, the need for organs as a whole cannot ethically and legally justify a particular case of living organ donation. Each case needs individual assessment as even the techniques used; for example laparoscopic nephrectomy, may alter the picture at least slightly. The consent of the individual donor is necessarily also a vital constituent of legitimate LDK transplantation and is considered more fully below.

SPECIFIC LEGAL AND ETHICAL ISSUES

Age

Maximum donor age, assuming decision-making capacity has not been lost, is rarely an issue with impact beyond the general assessments noted above. Minimum donor age, on the other hand, is an issue that often attracts legal or ethical prerequisites. Although living bone marrow donation from minors to relatives is normally permitted, living kidney donation from minors is illegitimate under many laws and is contrary to the policy of many professional groups in the medical domain (e.g. British Medical Association) and of most transplant centres.[1,2] This is also viewed as unacceptable under the Council of Europe Convention on Biomedicine and the Additional Protocol on the Transplantation of Organs and Tissues.[5,6] In view of the risks involved in nephrectomy and the usual lack of immediate urgency, this is generally justified, although arguably the door should not be closed completely.[13] For such an exceptional donation to be permissible, not only would there have to be an immediate and serious need which could not be otherwise satisfied, it would have to be clearly shown that the *donor* as well as the recipient would benefit from the donation, a highly unusual circumstance. But it is conceivable that courts in some jurisdictions might exceptionally endorse an individual instance of donation from a minor where this was in the 'best interests' of that person. This principle would probably protect from infringement of the rights to liberty and to private life stipulated in Articles 5 and 8 of the European Convention on Human Rights.[14] However, it is most probable that donation would only be justified where the minor was an adolescent and possessed decision-making capacity in healthcare matters generally, for example, 17-year-old identical twins with normal maturity and understanding for their chronological age. In the USA, the commonest reason for refusing to allow minors to donate kidneys is the belief that minors are unable to grant informed consent.[15] This is an overly sweeping view. Certainly, vulnerable individuals require additional protection, but one does not automatically cease to be vulnerable at any particular 'magic age'. Nonetheless, this is an area where there is a need to be especially circumspect.

Relatedness

There has been rapid growth in the use of emotionally related donors (spouses, friends, etc.) in LDK transplantation across the world. However, in some areas, laws contain limitations regarding donations where there is a lack of a close, typically genetic, relationship between the parties.[1,2] Nonetheless, legal stipulations, ethical guidance and practice itself have all liberalized in this regard in recent years. This is mainly because the clinical justification for placing restrictions on genetically unrelated living donors has been undermined by evidence that graft and patient survival outcomes are now comparable with genetically related donors.[16] Moreover, their motivation appears transparent and beyond moral doubt, especially when the donor is one's spouse (the commonest of genetically unrelated donors). Once 'genetics' has been taken out of the equation in terms of outcomes, the relevance and definition of 'relationship' becomes increasingly arbitrary. The Human Organ Transplants Act 1989 in the UK excludes grandparents from such 'relatedness' for instance, even though they are genetically related to their grandchildren.

A principal rationale for prohibitions or additional constraints connected to relatedness is recognition of potential commercial implications. Policy limitations are clearly linked to this underlying rationale, as in the UK where the Human Organ Transplants Act 1989 was a direct response to a Turkish individual coming to Britain and selling a kidney in the mid-1980s. But while this phenomenon is a real one, policy restraints have typically addressed non-genetically related donors, when there is no reason those with an undoubted emotional relationship with the patient are motivated by anything other than a desire to help without any expectation of financial gain. However, in the UK, the 1989 Act distinguishes genetically and non-genetically related (as legislatively defined) donors, and, though not forbidding donation by the latter outright, places additional obstacles in its path. The Unrelated Live Transplants Regulatory Authority (ULTRA) oversees and scrutinizes such intended donations prospectively for evidence of financial irregularity, and is viewed by some as regulatory excess and by others as reassurance. The Council of Europe's Additional Protocol states that donation should be permissible between individuals with a 'close personal relationship as defined by law', thus allowing a margin of discretion to individual states in defining relationships for this purpose. In Germany for instance, fianc(é)es are expressly included.[17]

In some jurisdictions, relationship is not regulated explicitly by law, but is left to the discretion of each individual centre. While in theory the Council of Europe Protocol (and many laws) would allow donation by altruistic living strangers, as in the UK, such practices remain rare. However, where commerce can be ruled out and proper donor consent shown to exist (after appropriate screening and counselling), there seems no reason why such donations should be entirely ruled out. As with many other matters, where a properly controlled and regulated system can be established, potential problems recede (see Chapter 12).

Laws and policy statements to date typically treat kidney exchange programmes analogously with unrelated, stranger donations, and where legal impediments exist in this regard doubts have arisen about their legitimacy. The potential problems relate either to voluntariness of consent, in that once one has agreed, one has also attracted a donor for one's sick relative and therefore may feel inherent coercion to proceed, or stem from disparity in the level of capability of the different personnel and facilities implicated in the two removals. The former problem is potentially most acute where the other donor has already had his or her kidney removed, and it is therefore advised that such removals take place simultaneously. For myself, I believe that limited (e.g. paired) exchanges are unproblematic if properly controlled, although expansion of such schemes beyond the local level would require considerable forethought and planning.[18,19] Even though caution is advisable as potential ethical problems are evaluated in the light of accumulating experience, living exchange donation carries considerable potential and should not be forestalled by spurious arguments that this constitutes a form of 'payment in kind'.

One ironic feature of appraising unrelated donors prospectively has been that the quality of consent given by such individuals is much more closely monitored. In the UK, genetically *related* donors have no such legal safe-

Table 13-1 Key issues of relatedness

Living-unrelated donors
• Laws and official policies ordinarily fairly 'loose'
• Increasing acceptance and use of emotionally related donors
• No provisions as yet specifically directed to 'paired' (or swap) donation
• Responses should reflect the rationale underpinning the restriction

guards at present. It is noteworthy that a new Human Tissue Act expected to be fully in force by 2006 will establish an oversight body (a new Human Tissue Authority) for all living donors, along the lines of the German model.[20] The key issues surrounding relatedness are summarized in Table 13-1.

Commerce

The emphasis in legislation regarding financial issues is upon banning commerce in organ transplantation, reflecting the stance consistently taken by the World Health Organization and the general antipathy of the transplant community towards commercial dealings in organs.[8,21] The majority of jurisdictions have such laws, and Article 21 of the Council of Europe Biomedicine Convention expressly prohibits 'financial gain' being obtained from body parts. Most laws, such as the Human Organ Transplants Act 1989 in the UK and the Council of Europe Convention, permit reimbursement of expenses, including loss of earnings. While this is only a legal obligation in a small minority of cases, there is a clear moral imperative to reimburse losses sustained. These statements attempt to make a distinction between 'compensation' and 'profit'. But is modest compensation for time and inconvenience, or only a very modest financial gesture, profit making? This has sometimes been dubbed 'rewarded gifting' or 'compensated donation'. But despite the euphemisms, even modest payment over and above actual loss incurred must be distinguished from 'reimbursement'. It seeks to create an incentive to donate, as opposed to removing what might otherwise

be a disincentive to donation. It seeks to per-
suade individuals to agree to organ removal
for transplantation, who might otherwise not
have done so. It is moreover likely, and especially where the payment is relatively modest,
to only attract the interest of those from the
lowest economic strata within the relevant
(national or global) 'society'.

But whether this distinction between profit
and loss is of any moral distinction is the
more crucial matter. It is only morally relevant if one considers that donation should be
motivated wholly by non-economic factors or
reasons. However, such a view would appear
to be fairly prevalent across Europe at least,
where one finds reference in legislation such
as the UK's Human Organ Transplants Act
1989 to 'inducements' and commercial 'pressures'. Some see such payments as 'commodi-
fication' of the body, with any 'additional'
sum being viewed as a payment for the transplantable organ. But of course such a
payment could equally be regarded as
payment for the services of the donor. Many
perceive that where such commercial incentives or inducements exist, the voluntariness
of the consent to donate itself is undermined.
This is a dubious view and conflicts with our
views of fair exchange in other contexts
within society, and especially in nations where
such payments would enhance quality of life
as opposed to merely providing the basic
necessities of life themselves. If such deontological arguments can be overcome then the
imperative might instead be to ensure that
sellers of organs receive a proper level of
payment for their sacrifice (see Chapter 15
parts 1 and 2). These arguments suggest that
if there are concerns here, they are largely
consequentialist, as opposed to inherent concerns, that will alter in nature and extent with
the cultural, social and economic context
involved.

Consent

Informed voluntary consent is a vital prerequisite of a legitimate living kidney donation
assumed to reflect the autonomy of the

donor.[19] No one can be compelled to donate
an organ for transplantation; this would not
be 'donation' at all. However, it has sometimes been alleged that, considering a potential donor's status as a close relative of a very
sick patient, informed consent does not in
reality exist by virtue of the absence of con-
temporaneous knowledge of risks and effects
coupled with almost instantaneous commitment.[22] But this notion of rationalistic
decision making ignores the emotional and
relational nature of such decision making.[23]
Moreover, while informed consent is
intended as a protection for prospective
donors, as Sauder and Parker have remarked,
'such a decision may most truly fulfil the
autonomy-orientated goal of informed
consent for healthcare decision making: to
allow persons to act in medical contexts in
ways that respect their autonomy by reflecting
their deeply held values'.[24] They contend that
to reject a 'consent' on such a basis would be
to violate the spirit of informed consent in
the mistaken service of the supposed letter of
the doctrine. Moreover, it is still possible to
change one's decision right up until the
point of surgery, although recognition of the
psychological forces playing on such donors
compels a need to provide the fullest impar-
tial information at the earliest opportunity in
an easily accessible and understandable form.

Arguably, the voluntariness of decision
making is more problematic than its
informedness here, in view of the substantial
inherent pressures attendant on almost all
potential donors. Role expectations in
particular may produce ambivalence in
donors (most often siblings), which require
probing in a sensitive and flexible fashion.
Individuals should be enabled and empowered to reach a decision with the support of
healthcare professionals, which reflects their
own true wishes and values, which may
nonetheless be consistent with a sense of
(familial or other) obligation. A psychosocial
evaluation conducted by independent experts
is a very valuable additional element of an
LDK transplantation programme wherever
ambivalence or pressure may be anticipated

from the context of the decision or from evidence arising during early assessment. This is of course quite separate from the function of the healthcare professional to screen for health *risks* in the prospective donor, which would include psychological as well as physical evaluation.[25]

The existence of such a consent prevents the donor being 'used' in any way here. Utilitarians themselves concede the need for autonomy to govern involvement in various activities and where autonomy is respected there is no additional need for the clinician to decide that the donation is for the benefit of the donor. This is a matter for the donor to decide. The factors which the donor will employ to reach such a decision will be as much social and economic, and influenced by the nature of the relationship with the patient, as clinical, and are largely out of the sight of clinicians. The key issues surrounding donor consent are summarized in Table 13-2.

CONCLUDING REMARKS

LDK transplantation is becoming increasingly important around the world. This is a trend set to continue as availability of deceased donor kidneys remains inadequate to satisfy demand even in major transplantation nations in the West. LDK transplantation is now a common procedure, and legal and ethical attention has tended to shift towards non-standard renal donors as the donor pool is increasingly being widened. A proper ethical programme of LDK transplantation requires suitable legal and pragmatic support, careful consideration of individual cases, and

a commitment to enhancing donor autonomy as far as possible. Respect for the dignity of individuals is a central contemporary ethical imperative. Such respect is enhanced rather than compromised where donors are empowered to make autonomous decisions and where the additional ethical pre-requisites noted earlier are observed.[26] Such donors are ends in themselves as opposed to merely means to the ends of others. Indeed, the plight of a loved one is very often itself a threat to the interests and wellbeing of such persons. Regulation of storage and use of human tissue more broadly, for research, education and other purposes is increasing and this trend will also continue, but the principles and processes which such regulation will implement pose no threat to transplantation programmes, which generally adhere to robust and proper principles of practice.

REFERENCES

1. Price D. *Legal and Ethical Aspects of Organ Transplantation.* Cambridge: Cambridge University Press, 2000.
2. Garwood-Gowers A. *Living Donor Organ Transplantation: Key Legal and Ethical Issues.* Aldershot: Ashgate, 1999.
3. Resolution (78) 29 on harmonization of legislation of member states to removal, grafting and transplantation of human substances, 11 May 1978.
4. Recommendation No.R (79) of the Committee of Ministers to the Member States concerning international exchange and transportation of human substances.
5. Convention for the Protection of Human Rights and Dignity of the Human Being with regard to the Application of Biology and Medicine. 4 April 1997, Oviedo.
6. Additional Protocol to the Convention on Human Rights and Biomedicine, on Transplantation of Organs and Tissues of Human Origin. Council of Europe, Strasbourg, 24 January 2002.
7. European Convention on the Protection of Human Rights and Fundamental Freedoms, 1950.
8. World Health Organization. *Guiding Principles on Human Organ Transplantation, 1991.* Geneva: WHO, 1991.
9. Department of Health. *Saving Lives, Valuing Donors: A Transplant Framework for England.* London: Department of Health, 2003, para 6.4.
10. Taghavi R, Mahdavi R, Toufani H. The psychological effects of kidney donation on living kidney donors

Table 13-2 Summary of key issues of consent

- Donors should be approached 'neutrally'
- Potential donors should be fully informed about risks, benefits and alternatives as early as possible
- Coercive, inherent and external pressures should be probed for and detected wherever possible
- Independent clinicians and other healthcare professionals should be involved where possible
- An opportunity to withdraw discreetly should be offered

(related and unrelated). *Transplant Proc* 2001; **33**: 2636–2637.

11. Neuberger J, Price D. Role of living liver donation in the United Kingdom. *BMJ* 2003; **327**: 676–679.

12. Spital A. Ethical issues in living organ donation. *Am J Kidney Dis* 1998; **32**: 676–691.

13. Price D, Akveld J. Living donor organ transplantation in Europe: re-evaluating its role. *Eu J Health Law* 1998; **5**: 19–44.

14. Garwood-Gowers A. Extraction and use of body materials for transplantation and research purposes: the impact of the Human Rights Act 1998. In: Garwood-Gowers A, Tingle J, Lewis T (eds) *Health-care Law: The Impact of the Human Rights Act 1998.* London: Cavendish, 2001: 295–312.

15. Spital A. Should children ever donate kidneys? *Transplantation* 1997; **64**: 232–236.

16. Humar A, Durand B, Gillingham K et al. Living unrelated donors in kidney transplants: better long-term results than with non-HLA-identical living related donors. *Transplantation* 2000; **69**: 1942–1945.

17. Law of 5 November 1997, section 8(1).

18. Ross L, Rubin D, Siegler M et al. Ethics of a paired-kidney-exchange program. *N Engl J Med* 1997; **336**: 1752–1755.

19. Veatch R. *Transplantation Ethics.* Washington DC: Georgetown University Press, 2000.

20. Choudry S, Daar A, Radcliffe-Richards J et al. Unrelated living organ donation: ULTRA needs to go. *J Med Ethics* 2003; **29**: 169–170.

21. Council of the Transplantation Society. *Commercialisation in Transplantation: The Problems and some Guidelines for Practice.* Council of the Transplantation Society. *Transplantation* 1986; **41**: 1–3.

22. Fellner C, Marshall J. Kidney donors – the myth of informed consent. *Am J Psychiatry* 1970; **26**: 1245–1251.

23. Price D. The voluntarism and informedness of living donors. In: Price D, Akveld J (eds) *Living Organ Donation in the Nineties: European Medico-Legal Perspectives.* Leicester: EUROTOLD, 1996: 107–126.

24. Sauder R, Parker L. Autonomy's limits: living donation and health-related harm. *Cambridge Quarterly Healthcare Ethics* 2001; **10**: 399–407.

25. EUROTOLD Project Management Group. *Questioning Attitudes to Living Donor Transplantation, Report to the European Commission, 1997.* Leicester: EUROTOLD, 1997.

26. Beyleveld D, Brownsword R. *Human Dignity in Bioethics and Biolaw.* Oxford: Oxford University Press, 2001.

Financial and insurance considerations for living donors

14

Jürg Steiger, Thomas R McCune

INTRODUCTION

Living donor kidney (LDK) transplantation is an important treatment modality for end-stage renal disease (ESRD) worldwide. It is now widely accepted in the medical community that a kidney from a living donor provides the best avenue to timely transplantation, with better outcomes for recipients in terms of graft survival, renal function (with reduced cardiovascular risk) and quality of life.[1,2] In some countries, living donors now provide more than half of all transplantable kidneys. Indeed, in Switzerland in 2002, living donations (n=83) outnumbered cadaveric donations (n=75). Moreover, in the USA between 1991 and 2001, the number of cadaveric transplants increased by a factor of 1.1, the number of living-related transplants increased by 1.7, but the number of living-unrelated transplants increased by a factor of 12.4.[3] Thus, use of unrelated donors accounts for much of the noted increase in living donation, a result not only of decreasing reliance on human leukocyte antigen (HLA) matching with modern immunosuppression, but of wider acceptance of LDK transplantation on the part of potential donors and the community at large.

From the donor's perspective, the stress (and perhaps risk) of donor nephrectomy has been reduced by less invasive diagnostic procedures and minimally invasive operations (see Chapter 6). These procedures are associated with less pain, a shorter hospital stay and faster recovery.[4–7] There is also increasingly better knowledge regarding short- and long-term consequences of donor nephrectomy, as

defined in such registries as the Swiss Organ Living Donor Health Registry (SOL-DHR; Chapter 5). In addition, greater emphasis on donor autonomy and self-determination has emerged.

As a result of these changes, it is possible to identify numerous beneficiaries of LDK transplantation, beyond just the donor and designated recipient. Wait-listed patients benefit from the net addition of a kidney to the donor pool and an increased chance of transplantation. Society gains not only from reduced costs of dialysis and transplantation (compared with cadaveric transplantation), but also from the ongoing contributions (fiscal and social) of a healthy recipient.[8] Since most Western governments ban 'valuable consideration' in exchange for a donated organ, there is a tendency in the transplant community to avoid discussion of financial issues.[9] However, these statutes specifically allow reimbursement of expenses and lost wages. Because significant fiscal considerations accompany kidney donation, it is reasonable to speak about financial interests of the donor, and the responsibility of the society at large to optimize economic conditions and security for those willing to donate.

FINANCIAL ISSUES IN LIVING DONOR NEPHRECTOMY

Economic concerns have been shown to affect a potential donor's decision to step forward. Donors often list fear of financial consequences and days off work as key concerns in choosing whether or not to donate.[10]

In a study of 113 family members of potential kidney recipients, 24% refused to donate because of financial issues.[11] Given the sacrifices made by donors in terms of time and physical risk, along with the enormous benefits outlined above, it seems unreasonable to ask potential donors to also consider assuming additional economic burdens. Indeed, several surveys indicate that the majority (75–90%) do not experience significant financial outlays associated with donor nephrectomy.[12–15] Nonetheless, living kidney donation should not be associated with any financial disincentive for any donor. Discussion of fiscal issues should occur early in the donor evaluation process. The way in which this dictum is interpreted and implemented may vary from country to country. Nonetheless, some common issues exist that must be addressed:

- costs associated with medical evaluation, testing, and pre- and perioperative care
- loss of income during evaluation, hospitalization and post-nephrectomy recuperation
- costs of travel, lodging and childcare, which may occur as part of the donation process
- payment of all medical costs associated with donation-related complications
- psychosocial counselling before and after donation
- adequate donor follow-up, with a registry to compile (and make widely available) data on complications after donation, including blood pressure, kidney function, albuminuria and psychosocial issues
- insurance in case of death or disability of the donor
- difficulties in obtaining life or health insurance after donation.

In view of the economic, social and medical benefits associated with LDK transplantation, it seems reasonable that the primary financial burden should be borne either by the recipient's insurer or society (i.e. government).

Donor evaluation

It is generally accepted that the direct costs associated with evaluation of potential donors should not fall to the donors themselves. Indeed, these costs are most often borne by the recipient's insurance. However, at least two caveats must be noted. First, it may be unclear when the donor evaluation actually commences. For instance, donors may be asked to obtain initial clearance from their own primary physician. It is important to document that any such associated costs should not be the responsibility of the potential donor. Rather, all clinic visits, blood testing, or other diagnostic studies initiated by a transplant centre should be reimbursed through the transplant centre, government (in countries with socialized medicine) or the recipient's insurance. Second, all costs associated with donor evaluation, even if evaluation of multiple potential donors is required before finding someone suitable, should be appropriately reimbursed. The altruistic kidney donor programme at the University of Minnesota found that over 20 candidates began the evaluation process for each actual donor that resulted.[16] In a more typical setting, it may not be unusual to evaluate two or three potential donors for a given transplant candidate before a suitable donor is identified. While it is the responsibility of the transplant centre not to initiate frivolous evaluations, potential donors must not be expected to assume the costs of donor evaluations that do not lead to actual transplantation.

Loss of income and other costs associated with the living donor process

The evaluation of a single living donor can take several months. During this time, multiple trips to the transplant centre may be required. Currently, it is not uncommon for donors to pay for their own travel to and from the transplant centre, as well as any lodging, meals and childcare expenses. In the USA, the income tax code allows deductions for travel expenses when performing a charitable act, a provision that does not extend to the kidney donation process. Some individual transplant centres, however, provide assistance with travel expenses on a case-by-case basis.

These visits not only generate travel expenses, but also require time away from work, depleting available sick leave that may be needed during recuperation. When 100 potential donors were asked about financial considerations related to donation, half were concerned about lost wages and inadequate sick leave.[17] The greatest financial burden is probably loss of income during the normal recuperation period. In the USA, the Donor Medical Leave Act of 2000 offers government employees up to 30 days of additional sick leave to recuperate after donating a kidney or any other solid organ. Unfortunately, this provision does not cover time spent undergoing evaluation, and such benefits are not available to all workers in the USA. In a recent study, only 7% of donors were eligible for this benefit.[18] Donors not eligible for the Donor Medical Leave Act must use personal sick leave and vacation time to recuperate. On average, donors report utilizing 21 ± 23 days of sick leave and vacation time after donation, but reported needing 34 ± 19 days to actually recuperate. Thus, donors at centres participating in the Living Organ Donor Network (LODN) absorbed the cost of 13 unpaid workdays during recuperation. If a medical complication occurred, the burden was even greater. In general, return to work occurs more quickly after minimally invasive procedures.[19] In the prospective Norwegian registry, 41% of donors required sick leave for more than six weeks and 12% of donors required more than 12 weeks.[14]

Donor coverage in Europe varies from country to country, but in general greater resources are made available than in the USA. In Sweden, the government covers all costs (medical, travel, loss of income and any complications that might occur) of all potential donors (even if evaluation does not result in nephrectomy). More than 15 years ago in Switzerland, authorities acknowledged that living donation reduces healthcare costs. As transplantation saves about 50 000 CHF annually compared with dialysis for each ESRD patient, it was easily established that all medical costs and loss of income during the pre- and post-transplantation period are fully compensated, including treatment of complications.

Costs related to complications after donor nephrectomy

The largest retrospective review of complications related to donor nephrectomy reported a complication rate of 1.2%.[20] Another survey-based study identified a complication rate of 8%, most of which were considered minor.[21] The Norwegian live donor registry reported 2.1% serious perioperative complications (not including two cases of pulmonary embolism).[14] According to the SOL-DHR, which has collected data for over 10 years, the complication rate is considerably higher than that reported in the retrospective studies mentioned above (GT Thiel, personal communication). When live donors at 13 US transplant centres participating in the LODN prospective registry were surveyed, 37% reported complications.[18] In the study by Matas and colleagues noted above,[20] 26% of US programmes did not respond to the questionnaire about donor complications. In contrast, in the LODN study,[18] an attempt to catalogue all complaints may have led to over-reporting. These findings indicate that, although donors and transplant teams may interpret them differently, complications are an unavoidable consequence of donor nephrectomy.

Any medical expense incurred by the donor in seeking care for complications of nephrectomy should not be the responsibility of either the donor or their health insurance. Rather, such coverage should be an assumed element of the costs of living donor transplantation, covered in full by whatever party pays for the transplant. Whereas appropriate care may be delivered via the transplant centre or other practitioner, it is the responsibility of the transplant centre to ensure proper access. In the USA, if Medicare is the primary insurance provider covering the transplant procedure (and sometimes even if it is not), the costs of treating donor complications may be recovered as a transplant-associated expense via the Kidney Acquisition Cost Center (KACC). However, LODN data indicated that 32% of donors travel from out of state, making reimbursement for care delivered after returning home more problematic, requiring co-ordination of benefits between the treating hospital and the transplant centre.

At times, donor charges are directly linked to a recipient's insurance coverage to recover costs not reimbursed via the KACC, with payment coming via the recipient's private insurance or Medicare (Part B). Utilization of non-directed donors (when there is no direct donor–recipient relationship) may require more creative approaches.

In Switzerland, the donor is linked to the recipient's insurance for the coverage of complications, a largely successful approach despite occasional cases of denied benefits after the death of a recipient. Regardless of specific arrangements in different countries, the principle that donors should not be burdened with any cost related to treatment of complications must remain paramount.

DATA REGISTRY

Since 1993, the SOL-DHR has collected the following data prospectively from all donors in Switzerland: type of nephrectomy (open vs laparoscopic), early complications, pain, psychosocial condition, kidney function, blood pressure, albuminuria and proteinuria. In the USA, no such universal government- or insurance-funded registry exists, despite recommendations of several groups within the transplant community.[22] In 2004, a similar registry (based on the Norwegian registry that was initiated in 1997[14]) was implemented in Scandinavia. Recently, the Southeastern Organ Procurement Foundation established a voluntary registry (LODN) funded by transplant centres that voluntarily chose to participate.

INSURANCE FOR DONORS

In general, most living donors (80–90%) report few, if any, financial consequences of having completed the donation process.[23] However, invariably some problems have arisen. Advocates have proposed insurance coverage to ensure that no gaps exist. Ideally, either the transplant centre or insurer would provide some variant of classic 'term-life' policies, enabling coverage to persist over the lifetime of the donor. Currently this specific option is not available.

The aim of insuring living donors is to avoid any financial hardship that might be associated with donation, providing benefits to be paid immediately, if needed, as bridge capital. These policies are modifications of typical 'accidental death or dismemberment' coverages, which usually define an accident as 'sudden, unintentional, harmful influence of an unusual, external factor on the human body from outside'. The living donor coverage invokes a different definition specifically associated with donor nephrectomy: 'damage to health and bodily injury caused by the preliminary examination, the clinical procedure and the associated anaesthesia'. Thus, only the direct consequences of organ removal are covered. The resulting lump-sum payment is independent of individual circumstances or other insurance coverage and is also independent of the liability claims for which the hospital or the doctors may be responsible.

In Sweden, potential donors and actual donors are treated the same, with an insurance policy that covers the cost of treating complications and an accidental death benefit for adverse events that may occur at any stage in the process, including travel to and from the transplant centre (J Wadström, personal communication). Life insurance in case of death or disability in connection with donation is offered on a more limited basis in Switzerland (one of six transplant centres) and in the USA (four of 264 programmes).

In the USA, insurance is available to cover the life and health of the living kidney donor.

It is administered through the LODN and underwritten by a private company (American International Group).[18] Coverage begins at the time of hospital admission (for donor nephrectomy) and continues for two years subsequently. The LODN policy includes a death benefit (payable in case of accidental death related to the donor hospitalization or any complication-related treatment within a year of donation), disability income provision and healthcare coverage for any complications not covered by the recipient's insurance policy. The disability income benefit of the LODN policy compensates for income lost if the donor is unable to return to work after a donation-related complication, but not during the operation itself or routine recuperation. The determination of a donation-related complication is made by the treating physician and does not require approval of the underwriter or policy administrator. The charge for the LODN policy is US$550, with a total benefit of US$250 000.

Since its initiation, four US transplant programmes have elected to purchase this policy for all living kidney donors. The policy is available in all 50 US states, and several individual donors have purchased the policy independently. The coverage is identical regardless of who pays the premium. However, such policies are currently available for only kidney (not liver or pancreatic) donors.

Another worry donors may face is difficulty obtaining life or health insurance after donating; there are numerous anecdotes regarding inability of former donors to obtain coverage.[24] In the USA, several surveys have been performed examining this issue.[25–29] The most recent survey, which included responses from 16 of the 20 largest insurers in the country, found all responding companies (40 of 70 queried) willing to issue policies to healthy donors.[29] Only four expressed concern that donors might be at increased medical risk, and only one would increase rates for donor policies. Thus, most donors should not encounter difficulty in purchasing policies after nephrectomy; those who do

encounter problems are encouraged to seek options with other insurers or agents more experienced in underwriting such coverage.

CONCLUSION

In many countries, financial disincentives remain a reality for live donors, despite the documented cost effectiveness of LDK transplantation. The transplant community should work with government, third-party payers and the society at large to minimize any financial burden associated with organ donation. Moreover, any resulting system should be designed in a way that donors do not have to ask for support and that compensation occurs in a timely fashion. It is very important that seamless lifelong coverage is provided to donors for any complication due to organ donation. Ideally, one institution should provide this coverage (government, insurance company or transplant centre) in order to avoid gaps and shifting responsibility for incurred costs.

There is evidence that the financial burden that donors accept is being addressed. Recently, the State of Wisconsin enacted legislation offering a state income tax deduction to living organ donors in recognition of the benefit to society that living organ donation provides.[30] Unfortunately, this tax deduction is only in effect in one of the 50 US states and does not address US federal income tax.

As a minimum, potential donors should be fully informed regarding financial implications of donation and resources available to assist in the process. There may even be some suggestion that frankly addressing these issues early in the evaluation process may encourage donation in some circumstances.

REFERENCES

1. Levey AS, Beto JA, Coronado BE et al. Controlling the epidemic of cardiovascular disease in chronic renal disease: What do we know? What do we need to learn? Where do we go from here? National Kidney Foundation Task Force on Cardiovascular Disease. *Am J Kidney Dis* 1998; **32**: 853–906.

2. Terasaki PI, Cecka JM, Gjertson DW, Takemoto S. High survival rates of kidney transplants from spousal and living unrelated donors. *N Engl J Med* 1995; **333**: 333–336.

3. United States Renal Data System. *USRDS 1998 Annual Data Report. Transplant: process.* United Renal Data System 2003, 2004: 396–397.

4. Smith PA, Ratner LE, Lynch FC, Corl FM, Fishman EK. Role of CT angiography in the preoperative evaluation for laparoscopic nephrectomy. *Radiographics* 1998; **18**: 589–601.

5. Bachmann A, Dickenmann M, Gurke L et al. Retroperitoneoscopic living donor nephrectomy: a retrospective comparison to the open approach. *Transplantation* 2004; **78**: 168–171.

6. Wadstrom J, Lindstrom P. Hand-assisted retroperitoneoscopic living-donor nephrectomy: initial 10 cases. *Transplantation* 2002; **73**: 1839–1840.

7. Ratner LE, Kavoussi LR, Sroka M et al. Laparoscopic assisted live donor nephrectomy – a comparison with the open approach. *Transplantation* 1997; **63**: 229–233.

8. Smith CR, Woodward RS, Cohen DS et al. Cadaveric versus living donor kidney transplantation: a Medicare payment analysis. *Transplantation* 2000; **69**: 311–314.

9. Section 301, National Organ Transplant Act, 42 U.S.C. 274e, 1984 and Council of Europe Biomedicine Convention.

10. Hiller J, Sroka M, Weber R, Morrison AS, Ratner LE. Identifying donor concerns to increase live organ donation. *J Transpl Coord* 1998; **8**: 51–54.

11. Knotts RS, Finn WF, Armstrong T. Psychosocial factors impacting patients, donors, and nondonors involved in renal transplant evaluation. *National Kidney Foundation Perspectives* 1996; **15**: 11–23.

12. Johnson EM, Anderson JK, Jacobs C et al. Long-term follow-up of living kidney donors: quality of life after donation. *Transplantation* 1999; **67**: 717–721.

13. Smith MD, Kappell DF, Province MA et al. Living-related kidney donors: a multicenter study of donor education, socioeconomic adjustment, and rehabilitation. *Am J Kidney Dis* 1986; **8**: 223–233.

14. Westlie L, Leivestad T, Holdaas H et al. Report from the Norwegian National Hospitals Living Donor Registry: one-year data, January 1, 2002. *Transplant Proc* 2003; **35**: 777–778.

15. Schover LR, Streem SB, Boparai N, Duriak K, Novick AC. The psychosocial impact of donating a kidney: long-term follow-up from a urology based center. *J Urol* 1997; **157**: 1596–1601.

16. Matas AJ, Garvey CA, Jacobs CL, Kahn JP. Nondirected donation of kidneys from living donors. *N Engl J Med* 2000; **343**: 433–436.

17. Peters TG. Selected issues surrounding the current status of living kidney donation. *Contemp Dial Nephrol* 2000; **21**: 33–36.

18. McCune TR, Armata T, Mendez-Picon G et al. The Living Organ Donor Network: a model registry for living kidney donors. *Clin Transpl* 2004; **18**(suppl 12): 33–38.

19. El-Galley R, Hood N, Young CJ, Deierhoi M, Urban DA. Donor nephrectomy: a comparison of techniques and results of open, hand assisted and full laparoscopic nephrectomy. *J Urol* 2004; **171**: 40–43.

20. Matas AJ, Bartlett ST, Leichtman AB, Delmonico FL. Morbidity and mortality after living kidney donation, 1999–2001: survey of United States transplant centers. *Am J Transplant* 2003; **3**: 830–834.

21. Johnson EM, Remucal MJ, Gillingham KJ et al. Complications and risks of living donor nephrectomy. *Transplantation* 1997; **64**: 1124–1128.

22. Abecassis M, Adams M, Adams P et al. Consensus statement on the live organ donor. *JAMA* 2000; **284**: 2919–2926.

23. Wolters HH, Heidenreich S, Senninger N. Living donor kidney transplantation: chance for the recipient-financial risk for the donor? *Transplant Proc* 2003; **35**: 2091–2092.

24. Spital A. More on life insurance for kidney donors. *Transplantation* 1990; **49**: 664.

25. Santiago-Delpin EA. Insurability of kidney donors. *Transplantation* 1997; **64**: 1374.

26. Spital A, Spital M, Spital R. The living kidney donor. Alive and well. *Arch Intern Med* 1986; **146**: 1993–1996.

27. Spital A, Kokmen T. Health insurance for kidney donors: how easy is it to obtain? *Transplantation* 1996; **62**: 1356–1358.

28. Spital A. Life insurance for kidney donors – an update. *Transplantation* 1988; **45**: 819–820.

29. Spital A, Jacobs C. Life insurance for kidney donors: another update. *Transplantation* 2002; **74**: 972–973.

30. Wisconsin Living Donor Tax Deduction Act. 2003 Wisconsin Act 119, signed 30 January 2004 (www.legis.state.wi.us/2003/data/acts; accessed October 2004).

Is it desirable to legitimize paid living donor kidney transplantion programmes?   15

Editorial comment

As noted throughout this volume, recent successes in renal transplantation have created unprecedented demand for transplantable organs and new controversies. Some have looked to commercialization of organ procurement as a potential solution to the donor–recipient imbalance, while others view such practices as anathema. Currently, payment for organs is prohibited in almost all countries and opposed by such bodies as the World Health Organization, the Council of Europe and the Transplantation Society. However, organ sales (both legal and illegal) seem more common and certainly provide the substance for numerous media reports.

Initially, we were inclined to avoid this controversy altogether. However, to remain true to our goal of examining all relevant trends in living donor transplantation, we asked two distinguished colleagues to summarize arguments for and against commercialization of organ procurement. Although unsure ourselves how the argument will ultimately be decided, we hope that the elegant analyses and informed discourse presented here add substance to debates that are likely to continue for the foreseeable future.

An earlier version of this article appeared as 'Feelings and Fudges: the state of argument in the organ selling debate', in the *Medico-Legal Journal*.[1] A much fuller development of many of the arguments given here can be found in 'Nephrarious goings on: kidney sales and moral arguments' in the *Journal of Medicine and Philosophy*.[2]

Part 1: Evidence in favour

Janet Radcliffe Richards

INTRODUCTION

In 1869 John Stuart Mill lamented the hopelessness of trying to achieve political persuasion by rational argument, in contexts where there was 'a mass of feeling to be contended against':

> For if [an opinion] were accepted as a result of argument, the refutation of the argument might shake the solidity of the conviction; but when it rests solely on feeling, the worse it fares in argumentative contest, the more persuaded its adherents are that their feeling must have some deeper ground, which the arguments do not reach; and while the feeling remains, it is always throwing up fresh intrenchments of argument to repair any breach in the old.[3]

Mill was at the time campaigning for legal equality between men and women, and his assaults on conservative argument were so exhaustive, and so decisive, that we now find it hard to understand how his contemporaries could have persisted in their traditional beliefs. But that is probably because our feelings have shifted to Mill's side of the case, rather than because we are better at allowing reason to challenge what is endorsed by feeling. If Mill were to reappear now, in the midst of the simmering debate about kidney sales, he would certainly recognize the same phenomenon. The conviction that selling kidneys for transplantation must be wrong is the fixed point around which a series of defensive arguments has been constructed, and which seems to survive unscathed the refutation of any of them.

The instantaneous outrage that greeted the first revelations of kidney selling by live vendors was not, of course, presented as just a matter of feeling. It was expressed in strong moral language – about the greedy rich and the exploited poor – which made it seem as though the response was immediate only because the moral case was so clear. But if the objectors had really been applying their usual moral principles to this new situation, rather than reacting on the basis of a feeling that organ selling was simply too horrible to countenance, the case would have looked very different. For instance, not many opponents of legalizing sales would deny that human life was of immeasurable value, or that it was right to prevent suffering wherever possible. These are fundamental values – and ones to which the medical profession, in particular, takes itself to be dedicated. They provide a presumption in favour of any procedure that will save lives and prevent suffering; and since kidneys can be obtained by payment that would not otherwise be available, that implies a presumption in favour of any given kidney sale.

Another strong principle, deeply entrenched in our culture since Enlightenment times, is that competent adults should be free to decide what constitutes their own good. In another claim of Mill's, much more familiar than the one quoted above, and widely taken as characterizing modern liberalism:

> The only purpose for which power can be rightfully exercised over any member of a civilized community, against his will, is to prevent harm to others. His own good, either physical or moral, is not a sufficient warrant.[4]

In other words, we can legitimately stop people from harming others, but not from doing what we regard as harm to themselves. The medical profession has been somewhat slower to accept this principle than has the liberal world at large, and the battle of patients against medical paternalism has yet to be won. Nevertheless, the principle of autonomy – according to which doctors provide technical information, but regard competent and informed patients as the appropriate judges of what counts as in their own interests – is now officially accepted by the profession, and increasingly insisted on by patients and the law. From this principle, too, it follows that if an informed and competent individual decides that he needs money more than he needs his spare kidney, that is for him to decide. It also follows, a fortiori, that if two competent adults want to make an exchange they regard as mutually beneficial, there is a presumption in favour of their being allowed to do so.

These considerations do not settle the matter, because any prima facie case may be overturned by further argument. The principle of preventing suffering provides a presumption against sticking needles into people and cutting them open with knives, but doctors do these things all the time because, as most people agree, the presumptive objection is often defeated by the benefits to be achieved. The presumption in favour of allowing the sale of organs may, therefore, be similarly defeasible.

Nevertheless, it is important to start any enquiry into the ethics of organ selling by stressing the presumption in its favour, because it is otherwise likely to be overlooked completely. The likely benefits of any kidney sale were simply not mentioned in the initial outcry against the practice and are still scarcely acknowledged by most proponents of prohibition. When the subject is approached from this direction, the issues look very different from the way they are usually presented.

First, it becomes clear that the burden of proof actually lies on the defenders of prohibition. We should regard organ selling as permissible until good reason is given to think otherwise. Because prohibition is now enshrined in law and professional standards the *political* problem of dislodging it does indeed lie with its opponents, but that does not alter the fact that the *moral* problem lies in the other direction.

Second, the fact that the case in favour of organ sales goes so widely unnoticed provides evidence that the objections are indeed rooted in feeling rather than in reasoning on the basis of established moral standards. Whether or not prohibition can eventually be justified, anyone who had approached the subject by trying to apply our usual standards to a new situation should, at the very least, have agonized over the prospect of legislation that would presumably send many of the 'greedy rich' to their deaths, and many of the 'exploited poor' back to the poverty they had hoped selling a kidney might alleviate. The fact that such considerations were not even mentioned in the headlong rush to what was (in Britain, at least) one of the quickest pieces of legislation on record, is one of many indications that the response was driven by strong emotions.

This is not enough to show that prohibition is wrong. People can reach morally defensible conclusions for morally questionable reasons. It does, however, provide a reason for assessing the arguments in defence of prohibition with considerable care. People who are already passionately committed to some belief are not always the sharpest critics of arguments that seem to support it.

FIRST LINE OF ARGUMENT: THE EXPLOITED VENDOR

If the objection to organ selling does indeed take the rationalizing form described by Mill, the supply of attempted justifications will be limited only by the ingenuity and determination of the rationalizers, and so is potentially endless. However, some illustrations from the most familiar set of arguments – about the need to protect potential kidney vendors – will show the kind of thing that is going on.

The commonest line of argument at the present time starts with distressing reports about the fate of many people who did actually sell kidneys in the expectation of improving their situation, but who found themselves even worse off than they had been before. There is controversy about the authenticity of some of these claims, and also about the extent to which they represent the situation as a whole. But there is no need to go into such questions for the purpose of this debate, because even if the stories are both true and representative, they still do not justify prohibition.

The point here is that the horror stories – about exploitation, shoddy work, unfulfilled contracts, inadequate advice, lack of after care and all the rest – are exactly what you would expect when illegality forces people to resort to black markets. It must be borne in mind that live kidney donation is now so safe that many surgeons encourage it. Losing a kidney is, in itself, the same whether you are giving or selling, which means that anything specially risky about selling must have to do with the surrounding circumstances. The most obvious difference in circumstances is that donation is tightly controlled and supervised, while selling, as long as it is illegal, cannot be controlled at all. Properly regulated selling would be as safe for vendors as for donors. The current abuses are, therefore, among the strongest elements in the case for ending prohibition.

It is, furthermore, irrelevant to reply that no controls would be perfect, and that abuses would continue. That is no doubt true, but it would provide a justification for prohibition only if prohibition could actually succeed in stamping out the practice. As the stories of abuse themselves show, it has not done so. As long as some people are desperate for life-saving operations, and others are in desperate need of money, the two groups will get together by some means or other. A legal market might not succeed in protecting everybody, but until there is one – or a medical advance that removes the need for transplants – we can protect nobody.

Another kind of argument based on concern for potential vendors takes issue with the idea that they can give genuine consent to the procedure. The populations in which people are poor enough to be tempted by kidney selling, it is said, are too uneducated to be competent to understand the risks and therefore to give valid consent.[5,6] This argument is precarious from the start, because no one really believes the premise. A good many people from well-educated populations have said they would sell if they were allowed to, and even the ones from uneducated groups seem to be regarded as competent to consent to other surgical procedures – including kidney donation. If the claim seems plausible, it probably depends on the question-begging assumption that wanting to sell an organ must in itself be proof of non-competence. But even if there were good reason to believe the premise, it would still not support universal prohibition. Nobody thinks, in general, that if some people are incompetent to consent to a procedure, it should be forbidden to everyone. If we apply our usual principles about autonomy and consent to organ selling, they demand our assessing competence on a case-by-case basis and, where non-competence results from ignorance rather than natural incapacity, trying to provide enough information to bring about competence.

A variation on the theme of invalid consent claims that the problem is not so much the vendors' competence as their situation. It is said that they are coerced into organ selling by poverty; and coerced consent is not genuine.[7,8] This time there is indeed a sense in which the premise is likely to be true. Since nobody positively likes the idea of an operation to remove a healthy kidney, most of the people who are likely to choose it will have a relatively limited range of options open to them, and poverty is a severe curtailer of options. But, yet again, the premise cannot support the required conclusion. The coercion-by-poverty claim amounts to saying that someone is being forced into an undesirable option – losing a kidney – because it is

better than anything else available. But if such an unattractive option is the best available, the options left after its removal must be even worse. You cannot improve the situation of someone who has too few choices by taking away what they regard as the best of them.

To this it may be replied that although would-be vendors may think this is their best option, they are really mistaken. The underlying presupposition of all the claims about the need to protect vendors seems to be that – whatever they themselves may think – kidney selling is against their interests, and that even if it means abandoning our usual objections to paternalism, we should prevent their making such a mistake. But even if paternalism is justified, there is still the problem of explaining why a benevolent paternalist should regard a decision to sell as necessarily misguided. As already argued, the experiences of vendors in a black market are not relevant to the question of whether there should be a legal market. There is some minimal risk associated with nephrectomy, as with all surgery, but the worthwhileness of any risk depends on both the nature of the risk and the value of the anticipated reward. Most people will find, if they confront the matter honestly, that there is some level of reward that would be seen as providing a rational basis for taking the minimal risks of nephrectomy, and the poorer you are, the lower that level is likely to be. Even a paternalist should agree that a (properly conducted and rewarded) kidney sale would be strongly in the interests of many of the people who are said to be protected by not being allowed to engage in one.

But, it is said in another change of tack, the poor are, simply in virtue of poverty, vulnerable to exploitation, and we can prevent the exploitation by preventing the selling. Once again the premise is true: poverty does make people exploitable, because when you have hardly any options the offer of a very small improvement in your situation can induce you to go along with the exploiter's wishes. But the very fact that exploitation works by offering marginal improvements to bad situations shows that if you simply abolish some exploitative practice outright, you actually make things worse for the exploited. The only way to prevent exploitation in a way that improves matters for potential vendors – as opposed to just thwarting the exploiters – is to control the trade and make sure they are properly treated and paid.

But surely, it is said, what we should be doing is lifting the poor out of poverty altogether, rather than allowing them to try to alleviate their poverty in this particularly horrible way. No reasonable person could possibly dispute that; but, once again, the admirable premise provides no support at all for the conclusion that organ selling should remain illegal. In fact it implies just the opposite, because if everyone were well enough off to be untempted by organ selling no one would want to sell, and a prohibition would be pointless because it would have nothing to do. Conversely, as long as prohibition has anything to do, there must be people for whom organ selling seems a better option than any other they have, and who are therefore made worse off by prohibition. Concern for the badly off is a good reason for trying to make them better off, but none at all for the prohibition of organ selling.

This collection of arguments does not exhaust even the vendor-protecting arguments for prohibition, and does not even hint at innumerable attempts of other kinds, but they are typical of the field as a whole. They have a superficial plausibility because they invoke attractive-sounding premises in support of a strongly held conclusion; but the premises are often incompatible with their proponents' empirical and moral beliefs in other contexts, and anyway do not support – and frequently even undermine – the case for prohibition.

Once you are on the lookout for these patterns of argument failure, you see them everywhere. Another familiar argument, for instance, is that allowing organ sales is wrong because it gives benefits to the rich that are not available to the poor. But virtually

nobody holds a general principle to the effect that unless everyone can have some benefit, no one should; and it would, anyway, be irrelevant to the issue of organ selling as such, because it would allow – what several people are now suggesting – the purchase of kidneys by public bodies, for distribution on the basis of need. Another familiar claim is that selling cannot be allowed because organ donation must be altruistic. But no one believes as a general principle that if no one is willing to give you something you need, you must do without it – let alone die – rather than be allowed to buy it. And anyway, it still could not explain why principled altruism should (for instance) allow a father to give a kidney to his daughter, but not to sell a kidney to pay for some other treatment she needed.

Both the number and quality of the arguments that are offered show beyond doubt that this is indeed a debate rooted in feeling, and that the arguments are attempted rationalizations of that feeling. As Mill suggests, if your reason for holding a conviction is the one you give, the defeat of the reason should lead you to abandon the conviction, not set off on an anxious hunt for some other justification that might fare better. And, furthermore, the mistakes sketched here are not of an obscure kind, that only a logician could be expected to spot. Nobody would make them in a neutral situation. Such transparently bad reasoning occurs only when people are already convinced of the truth of what they believe, and will snatch at anything that might provide a plausible justification.

A DIFFERENT KIND OF ARGUMENT

However – once again – neither the fact that what is going on is rationalizing rather than reasoning, nor the proliferation of hopelessly bad arguments, is enough to show that the conclusion itself is unjustified. You can have dubious motives for doing what is good, and believe the right thing for the wrong reasons.

The arguments discussed so far, and many others that run into similar difficulties, all try to demonstrate that organ selling is ruled out directly by fundamental moral standards, and they all fail on what are essentially grounds of logic. They run into contradiction and failures of entailment. But there is also in the field a quite different kind of argument, that has the potential to succeed where these other attempts fail outright. It is the kind that works not by claiming that organ selling is bad or wrong in itself, but that it would lead to harms greater than any good it could achieve.

Arguments of this kind are many and various, and range widely in the nature and specificity of the harms they predict. It has been alleged, for instance, that if the sale of organs were allowed, 'mutual respect for all persons [would] be slowly eroded'[9] or that it would '[invite] social and economic corruption... and even criminal dealings in the acquisition of organs for profit'[10] or remove the incentive to overcome resistance to a cadaver programme,[11] or discourage related donors from coming forward.[11,12] The possibilities are endless.

Obviously, there is nothing wrong with the principle of claiming that some proposed course of action should be rejected because the resulting harms would probably outweigh the benefits. And since such arguments depend essentially on empirical claims, they cannot be refuted a priori. Perhaps this is why, now that so many of the early arguments have been exposed as fallacious, arguments of this second kind seem to be increasingly popular. One that recently seems to have gained considerable currency is that allowing a trade in organs would result in a decline in rates of donation and an overall lessening of the supply.

However, although nothing can be said a priori about whether any such argument can succeed or not, there are relevant points that can be made about methodology. There is a radical difference of approach between attempts to rationalize an existing conviction, and a genuine enquiry into whether the presumptive good of allowing organ sales might be outweighed by resultant harms.

First, if you start with a presumption in favour of organ selling, you recognize that you cannot defend prohibition just by raising the possibility of dangers that might ensue. A serious enquiry calls for a careful risk analysis, involving, first, the identification and weighing of possible goods and harms, and then assessing the probability that each would come about. To defeat the presumption in favour would require positive evidence of harm great enough to outweigh the presumptive benefits – not just the possibility of some harm of uncertain extent. And in the absence of such evidence, you should be guided by the presumption in favour, and monitor the situation to see whether harms did ensue. The hypothesis needs to be tested under controlled conditions. Again, the burden of proof is on defenders of prohibition.

Second, the response to real evidence of harm would not be a rush to prohibition, but serious efforts to devise ways of keeping the good while avoiding the bad. Nearly everything we do – including trade of all kinds – carries potential for harm, but it does not usually occur to us to abolish the whole thing rather than just trying to lessen or remove its dangers. When we do have such an impulse, it means that we really regard the activity in question as wrong in itself, and are using the harms as an excuse to oppose it.

Third, it is most unlikely that *any* such evidence could reasonably support a conclusion that prohibition should apply universally: at all times, in all places, and under all circumstances. Whether allowing sales would lead to any particular harm such as a lessening of rates of donation, for instance, might well depend on the attitudes of a particular population or the way the issue was presented.

There is far more evidence now of serious enquiry than there was 10 years ago, as various people make genuine attempts to think of ways to achieve the good while lessening possible harms.[13] But still, most of the arguments adducing harms that might come from allowing organ selling present them as justification for total prohibition, with no suggestion of willingness to experiment or devise ways of limiting harm. They are, furthermore, typically backed up by no evidence at all beyond the strong feelings of their adducers (which, in a context where even the most flagrant logical fallacies are overlooked, are certainly not to be relied on). These are clearly rationalizations, rather than serious attempts to balance goods and harms. Perhaps there are indeed good reasons of these kinds for never allowing organ selling, but at the moment we have no reason to believe it. The feeling that organ selling really must be *wrong in itself* is still lurking in the background, systematically distorting the arguments.

Feelings in ethics

That, however, raises the most fundamental question of all. If the feeling against organ selling really is so strong, and so prevalent, should we not regard that as significant in itself? Some opponents, when they recognize the failure of the usual lines of argument, do move into the position that Mill sees as the final retreat of his non-reasoning opponents: the conviction that their feeling reflects some deeper truth, that argument cannot reach. Many people do want to claim that their strong moral intuitions must take precedence over rational argument.

If the wrongness of organ selling is accepted as moral bedrock, it does not matter that it cannot be justified in terms of other principles. It becomes a fundamental principle in its own right. But anyone tempted to sink with relief into this apparently comfortable position should recognize what it involves. If you want to accept the wrongness of organ selling as a self-standing principle, rather than as derived from other principles, you must accept that there are many possible circumstances in which its implications will actually *conflict* with the implications of those others, and that keeping to it actually involves allowing it to override them. It must be treated as *more* important than saving lives and health, respecting autonomy, increasing options, and preventing the harms done by an inevitable black market.

There is no logical problem about holding the view that selling parts of your body just is wrong, and must not be allowed whatever the costs in other terms. It might, for instance, be defensible in terms of some religious views. But it is clear that most people are not willing to take this line, because if they were they would not engage in endless attempts to justify their opposition to organ selling *in terms of* other values. If they keep saying that organ selling is wrong *because* it is exploitative, or *because* people are not really choosing to do it, or *because* it is too risky, or *because* it will dry up the supply of other organs, that implies an unwillingness to accept that it would be wrong irrespective of such considerations, let alone in spite of conflict with them. Most people, at least in public and in theory, are not willing to recognize the wrongness of organ selling as moral bedrock.

Rationality in ethics is not a matter of disregarding feelings – which must surely lie at the root of any ethics – but in being willing to recognize when feelings conflict with each other, and engage with the question of which should be allowed to prevail. Trusting the strongest feeling at any time, without consideration of whether it is being allowed to override what a little thought would show to be more valuable, may be comfortable, but it has nothing to do with ethics.

CONCLUSION

It remains possible that our present values might justify an outright prohibition of organ selling at particular times and in particular places. But no such case has yet been properly made, and it is hard to imagine any (non-religious) argument that could support a universal and permanent prohibition. Furthermore, it is also clear – from the use of arguments that would be rejected out of hand in contexts where people were trying to reach, as opposed to defend, a conclusion – that there is not even much in the way of serious debate. Serious moral reasoning involves recognizing and confronting conflicts of intuition, not an endless fudging of arguments to smooth those conflicts into an appearance of compatibility.

The situation, then, is this. Although hardly anybody seems willing to say – when forced to confront the question – that the principle of forbidding organ sales *should* be allowed to override familiar values of preserving life, preventing suffering, respecting autonomy, preventing exploitation and malpractice, improving the situation of the badly off, and so on, this is exactly what it is currently being allowed to do. While prohibition remains, defended by spurious arguments and not even seriously discussed, the idea that organ sales must not be tolerated is being allowed in practice the position it is denied in theory: remaining in place *at the cost* of the real interests of the poor and the dying, and of our general principles of freedom and autonomy. An illegal, uncontrollable trade goes on with all its concomitant harms, and people who cannot or will not engage in it – as well as many who do – suffer or die as a result.

For anyone who does not actually believe that the prohibition of organ selling is intrinsically more important than these other matters, this should seem morally appalling. Insisting on the ban amounts to allowing the people who support it – mainly ones who are too rich to need to sell, and unlikely to die for want of a transplant – to indulge their feelings of disgust at the expense of the sick and destitute whose interests are offered as the justification of the policy.

Nobody, probably, thinks that selling is an attractive idea. Everyone, presumably, thinks that there are much better ways of getting organs for transplantation, and that we should be doing all we can to push those forward. But this provides no justification at all for prohibition. To suggest that it does (as many people do) is to make another version of the mistake mentioned earlier, in which the idea that we should be getting people out of poverty is invoked as a justification for prohibition. Once again, if there were enough organs from other sources, no one would want to buy, and prohibition would have

nothing to do. Conversely, as long as anyone does want to buy, the supply is inadequate, and people suffer and die in consequence.

Of course we should be getting organs by other means; of course we should be doing everything we can to alleviate poverty so that no one sells through desperation. But until we achieve those things, the most obvious benefit of prohibition is to keep the desperation and exploitation of both buyers and sellers out of sight of the rich and healthy. As long as people are dying for lack of organs, and both buyers and sellers suffer in the inevitable black market, the current total prohibition is almost certainly unjustified. The issue at least needs serious debate, and serious experiments with this and other unfamiliar approaches to procurement. At the moment much of the debate is not serious at all, and as a result it is – like many other issues in biomedical ethics – in intellectual, and therefore moral, confusion.

REFERENCES

1. Radcliffe Richards J. Feelings and fudges: the state of argument in the organ selling debate. *Med Leg J* 2003; **71**: 119–124.
2. Radcliffe Richards J. Nephrarious goings on: kidney sales and moral arguments. *J Med Philos* 1996; **21**: 375–416.
3. Mill JS. *The Subjection of Women*. Widely reprinted, 1869: 1.
4. Mill JS. *On Liberty* London: Longman, Roberts & Green, 1869.
5. Sells RA. Resolving the conflict in traditional ethics which arises from our demand for organs. *Transplant Proc* 1993; **25**: 2983–2984.
6. Broyer M. Living organ donation; the fight against commercialism. In: Land W, Dossetor JB (eds) *Organ Replacement Therapy: Ethics, Justice, Commerce*. Berlin: Springer-Verlag, 1991: 197–199.
7. Quote from Dossetor JB, Manickavel V. Commercialization: the buying and selling of kidneys. In: Land W, Dossetor JB (eds) *Organ Replacement Therapy: Ethics, Justice, Commerce*. Berlin: Springer-Verlag, 1991: 63 'Surely abject poverty . . . can have no equal when it comes to coercion of individuals to do things – take risks – which their affluent fellow-citizens would not want to take? Can decisions taken under the influence of this terrifying coercion be considered autonomous? Surely not . . .'.
8. Quote from Abouna GM, Sabawi MM, Kumar MSA, Samhan M. The negative impact of paid organ dona-

tion, In: Land W, Dossetor JB (eds) *Organ Replacement Therapy: Ethics, Justice, Commerce.* Berlin: Springer-Verlag, 1991: 166. 'A truly voluntary and noncoerced consent is also unlikely ... the desperate financial need of the donor is an obvious and clear economic coercion'.

9. Dossetor JB, Manickavel V. In: Land W, Dossetor JB (eds) *Organ Replacement Therapy: Ethics, Justice, Commerce.* Berlin: Springer-Verlag, 1991: 66.

10. Abouna GM, Sabawi MM, Kumar MSA, Samhan M. The negative impact of paid organ donation, In: Land W, Dossetor JB (eds) *Organ Replacement*

Therapy: Ethics, Justice, Commerce. Berlin: Springer-Verlag, 1991: 171.

11. Broyer M. In: Land W, Dossetor JB (eds) *Organ Replacement Therapy: Ethics, Justice, Commerce.* Berlin: Springer-Verlag, 1991: 199.

12. Abouna GM, Sabawi MM, Kumar MSA, Samhan M. The negative impact of paid organ donation, In: Land W, Dossetor JB (eds) *Organ Replacement Therapy: Ethics, Justice, Commerce.* Berlin: Springer-Verlag, 1991: 167.

13. Erin CA, Harris J. An ethical market in human organs. *J Med Ethics* 2003; **29**: 137–138.

Is it desirable to legitimize paid living donor kidney transplantation programmes?

15

Part 2: Evidence against

William D Plant

INTRODUCTION

Arguments against paid living donation may be considered in three overlapping strands of discourse – philosophical, political and practical. It is my contention that each of these leads ultimately to the same conclusion. Continued prohibition of paid living donation represents the least worst resolution of the difficult dilemmas posed. For practical purposes the debate will focus predominantly on kidney transplantation, although the same arguments apply when considering other organs.

In many ways, this debate mirrors observations on the development of society expressed by Marx in 1859.[1] In a different context, Marx suggested that material productive forces ('infrastructure') are the drivers of change in prevailing social, political, intellectual and philosophical beliefs ('superstructure'). The social dislocation following the Industrial Revolution thus reflected the tension between the different pace of change in infrastructure (rapid) and superstructure (much slower). Today, advances in biotechnology and medical practice have accelerated at a rate outstripping the ability of ethical, legislative and professional protocols to keep pace. The current debate reflects the tension between the desire to implement relatively novel and apparently beneficial practices ('infrastructure') within an ethical, political and cultural context ('superstructure') that is uncertain as to the legitimacy of the opposing arguments.

In a very short period of time the technology to successfully perform organ transplantation has become routine, and been exported (from its initial location in highly regulated developed economies) to almost all parts of the world. The possibility of saving/enhancing the lives of many patients with previously bleak prospects now exists in a global sense. Unfortunately, there remains a crucial limiting factor in delivering this benefit – the current imbalance between the supply of organs from traditional sources (largely non-directed altruistic cadaveric donation and directed altruistic living donation) and the ever-increasing pool of potential recipients.[2] There is no doubt that organ transplantation is the optimal management for organ failure and that many (particularly in the developing world) will die without such a transplant.[2]

One solution to (or one perspective on) this problem has been to propose that individuals be permitted/encouraged/facilitated to sell selected organs for the benefit of other individuals. A number of models as to how this might be organized have been proposed.[3–5] Other market-based compensation models relate to financial incentives to enhance the donation of organs from cadaveric donors.[6,7] The particular issues that this raises are not within the framework of this discussion. Whatever the proposals for the future, there currently exist extensive illegal and quasi-legal practices of unregulated organ selling and trading.[2,8–10] For many, regulation might seem a better option than continued prohibition with the consequent flourishing of such unsupervised exploitation.

FORMAL OPPOSITION TO PAID LIVING DONATION

It may be fashionable to dismiss the current opposition to paid living donation as emotional, irrational and illogical.[11,12] However, the list of organizations that continue to hold this position is extensive and impressive. A scrutiny of the extensive documentation, consultation and statements relating to this might suggest a more exhaustive, thoughtful and rational process than the polemic from opponents of this stance would suggest. As recently as May 2004, the 57th World Health Assembly[13] (World Health Organization) requested that the Director-General:

> continue examining and collecting global data on the practices, safety, quality, efficacy and epidemiology of allogeneic transplantation and on ethical issues, including living donation, in order to update the Guiding Principles on Human Organ Transplantation.

These Guiding Principles have had considerable influence on practice and it is notable that Items 5, 6, 7 and 8 explicitly prohibit commercial transactions in organ procurement and transplantation.[14] It is acknowledged, however, that some in the field of transplantation are increasingly challenging these principles – prompting the possibility of an update in the near future. It is also important to acknowledge that, as well as ethical issues, issues of safety, efficacy and quality assurance consume considerable time in discussion.

In November 2000, the 52nd World Medical Association General Meeting in Edinburgh adopted an updated Statement[15] on 'Human Organ and Tissue Donation and Transplantation'. Item 34 states that:

> Payment for organs and tissues for donation and transplantation should be prohibited. A financial incentive compromises the voluntariness of the choice and the altruistic basis for organ and tissue donation. Furthermore, access to needed medical treatment based on ability to pay is inconsistent with the principles of justice. Organs suspected to have been obtained through commercial transaction should not be accepted for transplantation. In addition, the advertisement of organs should be prohibited. However, reasonable reimbursement of expenses such as those incurred in procurement, transport, processing, preservation, and implantation is permissible.

In addition, the Statement observes:[15]

> In developing strategy, due consideration should be given to human rights, ethical principles and medical ethics. Ethical, cultural and societal issues arising in connection with ... the subject of donation and transplantation in general, should be resolved, wherever possible, in an open process involving public dialogue and debate informed by sound evidence.

The Transplantation Society, through its ethics committee,[16,17] affirms its continued opposition to the commercialization of organ donation. Meeting in September 2003, the Council of the British Transplant Society identified commercial gain as an unethical justification for organ donation.[18] Articles 21 and 22 of the Convention for the Protection of Human Rights and Dignity of the Human Being with regard to the Application of Biology and Medicine[19] (generally referred to as the Convention on Human Rights and Biomedicine of the Council of Europe) also explicitly prohibit the sale of human organs.

Many professional, political and other groups have also issued agreed statements. The overwhelming consensus supports prohibition of payment for living donation. However, most groups distinguish this from reimbursement of expenses accrued as a consequence of donation. (Whereas there may be an ill-defined boundary between reimbursement and remuneration, the distinction is usually broadly apparent.)

PROPONENTS OF PAID LIVING DONATION

Thus, a formidable edifice of disapproval and prohibition has been constructed over the past two decades. To alter practice would, therefore, require major changes in legislation, in regulatory processes and in codes of professional behaviour. Such changes are very likely to require substantial philosophical, political and medical advocacy to succeed in the face of opposition. I wonder if the advocates of paid donation have thought the thesis all the way through to implementation. Shakespeare may have had this discussion in mind with the following exchange in *Henry IV, Part I*:[20]

| Glendower: | I can call spirits from the vasty deep. |
| Hotspur: | Why, so can I; or so can any man: But will they come, when you do call for them? |

In my opinion, those that advocate permitting paid living donation resemble Glendower – boasting of an ability to deliver remarkable things with ease. I prefer the scepticism of Hotspur, with its implicit caution that that to which we aspire and that which we can achieve may not always be the same.

A standard battery of assertions recur.[4,5,11,12] Prominent is the charge that current position statements derive from an emotional, irrational and (by implication), intellectually shallow analysis of the issues. This suggests that the collective processes for ethical evaluation of large numbers of organizations (including those mentioned above) are all defective, and continue to be defective! This represents a breathtaking degree of arrogance in its dismissive attitude to the intellectual quality of the reflections of others. I do not hold that majority opinion is necessarily correct, but in a pluralistic world it is striking how so many individuals and groups continue to arrive at the same conclusion.

A further assertion is that 'repugnance' has a disproportionately high influence on the views of those that prohibit organ selling. I see nothing unusual or irrational in this. To implement a change in practice requiring a change in public policy will require considerable sensitivity to the 'image' of that activity. I find it incredible that the sordid, exploitative practices[8–10] that currently flourish can be viewed other than with repugnance, and I doubt very much that any democratic political party will ever make state-sponsored or endorsed degradation of its citizenry of this kind a central plank of policy – whatever the demand for organs. It seems to me inevitable that the epidemiology of paid organ donation will be a one-way route: poor to rich, weak to strong, young to old, female to male, black and brown races to white and yellow races, South to North. The potential for negative political fallout is high. Repugnance may be a difficult construct to define philosophically, but it is undoubtedly a powerful motivator of individuals and groups, and its influence on the outcome of this debate cannot be underestimated. Nancy Scheper-Hughes powerfully summarizes:[10]

> Of the many fieldsites in which I have found myself, none compares to the 'world' of transplant surgery for its mythical properties, its codes of secrecy, its impunity, and its exoticism. The 'organs trade' is extensive, lucrative, explicitly illegal in most countries, and unethical according to every governing body of medical professional life. It is therefore covert. In some sites the organs trade links elite surgeons and technicians from the upper strata of bio-medical practice to 'body mafia' from the lowest reaches of the criminal world.

Proponents of paid living donation assert that they wish to abolish the need for practices such as these to exist.[4,5] I would assert that the practical solutions which they have so far proposed ('ethical' markets in selected highly regulated developed societies, with no transborder trade, and 'many safeguards') [4,5] are naïve in the extreme. Once a market is established, its natural development is to become transnational. Once a market is established, its natural development is to encourage competition and seek new opportunities for growth. If prohibition has not controlled the 'body mafia', what chance has regulation? I greatly fear that the only consequence will be a half-tolerated, distasteful, exploitative system (now existing within the law) that the aforementioned 'body mafia' will utilize to greater profit. Having repeatedly referenced the problems of organ shortage in the developing world and the problems posed by illegal organ trading as drivers to change, the only practical changes proposed to date are for nationally regulated markets exclusively in developed nations. This seems logically inconsistent and practically inept. How will this stop organ trading? What kind of signal is this to send to nations with insufficient legislative and cultural resources to operate a regulated system?

The only really consistent point that emerges is the (legitimate and laudable) one that any potential source or organs should be considered for potential harvesting. That alone seems to me to be the motivation of those proposing to allow organ sales. I fear that much of the 'supporting' philosophical discourse is no more that attempts at justification of an already accepted position.

HELPING RECIPIENTS WITHOUT HARMING DONORS

Advocates of a paid donor solution claim that this would greatly increase the pool of donors and, in so doing, reduce/eliminate the waiting list for transplantation. There is some evidence to support this. Iran has experienced a controlled living-unrelated donor (LURD) programme since 1988.[3] This allowed for more than 10 000 transplants (76% from LURDs) to be performed in the 12 years up to 2000, effectively eliminating the waiting list by the end of 1999. In other societies (usually illegal) LURD programmes have provided the bulk of the organs for transplantation.[2,8,9] It would seem to be incontestable that allowing access to paid donors will increase the potential number of transplants. Clearly then, there would need to be additional reasons to oppose paid donation.

Reports on the experience in Iran are very helpful to this debate.[3,21–24] There is no doubt that it has benefited a large number of recipients, but a number of other items of interest emerge. Since 2000, legislation has allowed for the concept of brain death and cadaveric organ donation.[21] However, this still constitutes a very small element of overall activity – in part reflecting cultural and administrative barriers, but also reflecting the success of the existing programme. Similarly, living-related donation (LRD) (the outcome of which is better) activity has also remained low, perhaps for the same reason.[21] It is estimated that 81% of recipients of a kidney from a LURD had had an identified potential LRD.[21] Thus, a controlled paid LURD programme may be diminishing utilization of and access to other sources of organs.

The model in Iran has many of the features proposed by advocates of organ sale. It applies only to Iranian citizens. Recipients are referred to the Dialysis and Transplant Patients Association (DATPA) – an organization of end-stage renal disease patients not receiving remuneration. Volunteers for LURD also apply to DATPA, which functions as a clearing-house for vendor–recipient matching. The government covers medical expenses and is responsible for a financial award made to the donor. Many recipients also give a (limited value) reward to the donor. The Iranian Society of Transplantation oversees the ethical aspects of the programme. It has undoubtedly solved some problems in that country and acted as a bridge to future developments in transplant practice.

What about the donors? Eighty-four per cent of LURDs were classified as 'poor' and 30% had not had education beyond primary school level.[22] Although the recipient group included wealthier and better-educated individuals, some 50% of these were still 'poor' and 38% had had the limited schooling mentioned above. Disturbingly, a study of 300 such LURDs revealed that 68% had sold organs against the wishes of their families – a conflict leading to divorce in 21% and family rejection in 43%.[23] In addition, 79% could not attend for follow-up due to poverty, 65% experienced negative employment consequences and 71% had developed de novo depression post-donation. Many (30–57%) remained preoccupied by the 'loss of a kidney': 85% stated that they would not sell a kidney if given the chance again, and 75% advised that others should not do so. A related study of 100 donors revealed that 51% claimed to 'hate' the recipients and 76% felt that kidney sales should be banned.[24] These findings are extremely disturbing.

The consequences for, and circumstances of, these vendors are not as bad as for those vending in the unregulated trade in India. An important study of 305 LURDs in Chennai, India, revealed that 96% sold organs to pay off debt (not 'to invest in their child's education' or 'to start a small business' or the other fabled motivations attributed to them by the proponents of organ sale).[25] The average payment was about US$1000 (mid-1990s), but 33% of families experienced a decline in income following donation. Three-quarters remained in debt despite vending and 79% would strongly advise others not to donate. Many were in family units in which a spouse also sold an organ.

I suspect that these data are close to identifying the reality of being an organ donor even in a highly regulated developed economy. I accept that it is a current reality of life, but do not accept that organ selling is any way to enhance the autonomy and dignity of these people. It is surprising that the existence of these practices has not politically radicalized these exploited communities, and

this must surely be a possibility if the state decides to facilitate actions of this kind. Political and practical barriers to allowing paid living donation will (should) remain formidable.

PHILOSOPHY

This debate holds a number of perspectives – that of the citizen, the vendor, the patient and the healthcare professionals participating in the act of transplantation. There are different obligations on each.

The ethical framework underpinning Western medicine is characterized by a number of codes of practice and the culture of healthcare workers.[26] Among these are deontological (duty-based) and utilitarian (consequence-based) systems. Both are strongly rational and universalist in tone. However, as all ethical analyses ultimately focus on particular cases, the importance of context may well have been understated in the past. Some current intellectual traditions, notably existentialism, situation ethics, contextualism and post-modernism are less convinced of the existence of general laws/principles that can be applied to particular cases.[27] Rather, they focus on how to solve specific problems as they arise and are open to the insights of other religious, racial, philosophical and cultural traditions. The features in this debate may well be better served by these more relativist approaches.

Deontological traditions, as expressed in the Hippocratic oath and the Declaration of Geneva,[28] stress the duties of practitioners and the rights of patients. Any act should be capable of being expressed as a universal law. Clinicians 'ought' to act in particular ways because this is 'right', often irrespective of the consequences. This tradition stresses the autonomy of the patient and the primacy of the doctor–patient relationship. Individuals should always be viewed as ends, never as means to an end. Utilitarian traditions aspire to acts that lead to 'good' or 'best' outcomes. Maximizing benefit is the primary goal. If the 'right' action does not lead to the 'best' outcome then it should be reviewed or abandoned. In real life, there is a spectrum between cases in which context and situation need to be the dominant consideration and those in which universally derived general principles can be applied. No one tradition or perspective is 'more correct' – each offers different perspectives to problem solving.

Reflection on the four prima facie principles of (i) beneficence, (ii) non-maleficence, (iii) respect for autonomy and (iv) justice, which have traditionally been utilized for this purpose, can further refine our analysis.[26,29,30] The dynamic trade-off between simultaneous adherence to all of these is the central aspect of resolving medical ethical dilemmas. Some authors feel that they represent a dated straitjacket for evaluation,[29] others continue to endorse their utility.[30] Depending on the context (and on whether a deontological or utilitarian approach is favoured), a 'least unsatisfactory' trade-off between principles must be negotiated or achieved.

In any event, an extensive scrutiny of the published literature leads me to conclude that the principal philosophical principle that is invoked by those favouring organ vending is a relatively simple and straightforward question. The question posed is: 'Is it unethical for a person to sell an organ for financial gain and without a sense of altruism?'[11,12,31] Most of the debate has spun upon this particular axis. The further proposition has then been:

> If it cannot be demonstrated *a priori* that it is wrong for an individual to sell an organ for profit, then the current prohibition on this practice is intrinsically illogical . . . and presumably should be abolished.

This is an argument lending itself to many permutations. It also seems to me to be overly simplistic.

Beneficence: doing good

This is the obligation to strive at all times to do good for the patient. Deontologists view this as a universal moral duty, utilitarians as achieving the universally desired best outcome. If this were the only principle of importance, then we should probably seek transplant organs wherever they can be found. A successful transplantation is a clear case of beneficent action – to the recipient. It is more difficult to see how it assists the donor. The externality of an altruistic act is often invoked as beneficent to live donors with a relationship to the recipient. Improvement in family wellbeing/income, etc., may be a more tangible benefit to spouses, partners and family members. Apart from monetary compensation, it is difficult to see a benefit to commercial LURDs – studies cited previously in this chapter repeatedly rebuff the notion that there is much altruism or 'commitment to the common good' as a motivation to donate.[24,25]

Furthermore, it is not actually clear that the outcomes from vending LURDs will be the same as for altruistic LURDs. Central to the argument of those proposing change is that this will be the case; if so, then it will represent an improvement from currently published outcomes,[3,32] which are inferior to altruistic LRD or LURD practice. Undoubtedly it is better to receive a transplant than remain on dialysis; however, increasing the commercial donor pool may not be without unforeseen problems of efficacy and quality assurance.

Non-maleficence: avoiding harm

Since Hippocrates, the principle of *primum non nocere* (first do no harm) has been a central tenet of medical ethics (Hippocrates chose it as his first aphorism).[33] All interventions, however well intentioned, may cause harm. Ensuring an appropriate balance between benefit and harm is an important clinical judgement. With recipients, this is usually straightforward. With donors we enter one of the most difficult areas of medical ethics. Generally it is unethical (and usually illegal) to subject an individual to potential harm unless there is a balanced benefit to the individual himself or herself. For a professional involved in any living donation procedure, this is a unique situation. To justify the potential harm to the donor, there will have to be a compelling case from another principle to balance and justify this action.

Proponents of paid living donation assert that the principle of non-maleficence is violated as much with an altruistic donor as with a commercial donor. This may be so in theory. In practice, the epidemiological data from a range of studies indicate that (in current practice) medical follow-up is less frequent, perceived physical wellbeing is worse, and psychological morbidity more frequent in commercial donors.[23,25] As with the case of beneficence, I have no confidence that regulated commercial donation will produce an equivalent lack of maleficence as currently happens with altruistic live donors.

Respect for autonomy

Individuals should be treated as ends, not as means. Respect for the dignity, integrity and authenticity of the person is a basic human right. Deriving from this is the important issue of consent.[26] Patients with capacity to understand relevant information (explained in broad terms and with simple language), to consider its implications in terms of their own values, and to come to a communicable decision without undue external pressure, are deemed to have decision-making capacity.

Proponents of paid living donation view this principle as representing the strong card in their hand. Surely if an individual has the capacity to consent, then he or she is free to do whatever they wish with their labour, their dignity or their organs? Is not this the essence of freedom?

We need to reflect a little further on models of autonomy. There is a model of absolute autonomy (favoured by neo-liberals and generally hostile to, amongst other things, labour laws, environmental protection and anti-trust legislation), which suggests that all individuals have an inviolable personal autonomy to do as they will without reference to, or without interference from, the state. This model of autonomy ranks the vendor's choice as paramount in the weighing up of important principles. It is hard to oppose this thesis if one accepts that we live within a model of absolute autonomy and if we accept as absolute the dogma that individual choice is the pre-eminent justification of all actions.

As it happens, I do not accept this thesis. Autonomy within society is probably better described by models of *relative autonomy* or *social autonomy*. With the first, an individual has access to advocates and professional advisers; with the second, society is accepted as having a role in protecting the marginalized and implementing policy on the basis of a perceived communal benefit. One may see how close politics comes to philosophy in this analysis. Furthermore, just because exploitation currently flourishes does not make it a universal aspiration. We do know that child labour, prostitution, and dangerous, poorly paid jobs exist. But, unlike in this case, it is rare to hear arguments calling for these to be extended or made more easily accessible to the marginal of society.

Many would argue that if selling an organ appears prominently in the list of choices that an individual may be called upon to make, then that individual is already so constrained in his or her choice that a genuine capacity to consent does not exist! Immanuel Kant himself (the 'high priest' of deontology) distinguished between *rational beings* that act autonomously according to their idea of law and *non-rational beings* whose behaviour is heteronymous − that is, determined by outside causes.[34] It is my fear that the drive to obtain a greater organ donor pool will be justified by an appeal to donor autonomy, when in fact, potential donors are so constrained by economic marginalization that their choices have indeed become heteronymous.

Beneficence to a recipient and respect for the absolute autonomy of a donor might be viewed as sufficient to put to one side concerns regarding deficient application of the principle of non-maleficence to the donor. But, of course, even this will only apply if the processes to provide the donor with full information and adequate compensation (whatever that may be) are in place. Those promoting a respect for autonomy are frequently long on philosophical justification, but short on ensuring that processes will be in place to guarantee that consent is truly genuine – the boast of Owen Glendower is again apposite.[20]

Justice: promoting fairness

We can probably pull all strands of the above discussion together in reflecting on our model of justice. Do the needs of those with organ failure (which may lead to death) outweigh the rights of the marginalized? Maybe it is ethically logical to accept that an individual should be allowed to sell their kidney. But, is it ethically sound to accept that another person should be allowed to buy it? Is it ethically sound that society should organize itself to permit this to happen? Is it ethically sound that healthcare professionals should feel compelled to participate in this kind of activity?

Justice and fairness need to be applied broadly. These principles apply to the individual patient, but also to other patients whose circumstances may be influenced by events relating to that patient. Similarly, we need to be fair to members of the transplant team and to the broader needs of society. Respect is due to the proper application of professional judgement. Respect is due to nation-states trying to improve the lot of their citizens, without having to implement organ trading. Although the plight of those with organ failure is immense, we need to make sure that choices do not create other 'victims'.

A particular point relates to the status of the healthcare professional. To those legitimately zealous as to the plight of those needing transplants, a professional uncomfortable with paid living donation may be labelled as 'paternalistic'. Paternalism is generally an undesirable trait, but its existence is not automatically implied by disagree-

ment with the propositions of others. Similarly, responding uncritically to consumerist demands may also undermine professionalism. Healthcare professionals need to be fair to themselves as well as to others.

We also need to distinguish between 'act utilitarianism' and 'rule utilitarianism'.[26] We may understand and sympathize with a kidney patient in the developing world who uses his resources to purchase a kidney from an unknown other individual. We may even suspect that this was 'right' from his perspective – although the epidemiological evidence already quoted will suggest that it was 'wrong' to the donor. This is an example of 'act utilitarianism'. Our understanding and sympathy is a marker of our humanity. However, this cannot form the basis of public policy that should adopt a 'rule-utilitarian' approach. Policy must be based on practices that are robust, consistent and easily described.

In this debate, it is my thesis that the dangers of changing from current practice exceed the dangers of persisting with it. Only by accepting particular models of society (which are inaccurate, in my opinion) can the philosophical propositions of those promoting change be accepted. The plight of those with organ failure is immense, but paid living donation is not the desired solution to their dilemma. As in all moral dilemmas, whatever judgement we reach is, by definition, not wholly satisfactory. I wish it were otherwise, but we have to make the best decisions as reason, epidemiology and circumstance allow.

PARADIGMS SHIFT (YES, THEY REALLY DO!)

One final perspective on the issue may be the anthropological, as again expressed by Nancy Scheper-Hughes.[10] We do well to recall the short duration in human history during which a shortage of donor organs has been a significant 'problem'. In reality, it is probably such for not more than a decade. Illness and death are normal elements of human culture; advances in technology do not bring instantaneous results and, viewed from an historical-anthropological perspective, John Harris verges on the hysterical with statements such as '*loss of life due to shortage of donor organs is a scandal*' and '*people's lives continue to be put at risk*'.[4] The radical proposal of encouraging the sale of organs may have been entered into without adequate reflection. Scheper-Hughes expands:[10]

> A medically invented, artificial scarcity in human organs for transplantation has generated a kind of panic and a desperate international search for them and for new surgical possibilities. Bearing many similarities to the international market in adoption, those looking for transplant organs are so single minded in their quest that they are sometimes willing to put aside questions about how the organ [or 'the baby' in the case of adoption] was obtained. In both instances the language of 'gifts', 'donations', 'heroic rescues' and 'saving lives' masks the extent to which ethically dubious and even illegal practices are used to obtain the desired 'scarce' commodity, infant or kidney, for which foreigners (or 'better off' nationals) are willing to pay what to ordinary people seems a king's ransom. With desperation built in on both sides of the equation – deathly ill 'buyers' and desperately needy 'sellers' – once seemingly 'timeless' religious beliefs in the sanctity of the body and proscriptions against body mutilation have collapsed over night in some parts of the third world under the weight of these new market's demands.

This seems to me a most eloquent summation of the situation in which we find ourselves. This, of course, does not help those potential recipients desperately hoping for an improvement in quality of life and survival. But, perhaps we are excessively negative in our view of the intermediate future. We should not forget that the capacity to solve this problem in the way we do today did not always exist; that scientific progress remains rapid; that some other solution (xenotransplantation, perhaps) may soon arrive. The paradigm will then shift, and the current debate may hopefully be viewed as an interesting transient sideshow in the ongoing evolution of the ethics of healthcare delivery. Until then we need to drive forward administrative, organizational (particularly in maximizing utilization of cadaveric donors), medical and research endeavours to best help those needing transplants. Better to focus on this than on suggestions that, in the long run, are probably impractical and possibly will soon be redundant.

REFERENCES

1. Marx K. *A Contribution to the Critique of Political Economy* [translated from German by Ryanzanskaya SW; edited and with an introduction by Dobb M] London: Lawrence and Wishart, 1971.
2. Rothman DJ, Rose E, Awaya T et al. The Bellagio Task Force report on transplantation, bodily integrity, and the International Traffic in Organs. *Transplant Proc* 1997; **29**: 2739–2745.
3. Ghods AJ. Renal transplantation in Iran. *Nephrol Dial Transplant* 2002; **17**:222–228.
4. Harris J, Erin C. An ethically defensible market in organs. *BMJ* 2002; **325**: 114–115.
5. Rapoport J, Kagan A, Friedlaender MM. Legalizing the sale of kidneys for transplantation: suggested guidelines. *Isr Med Assoc J* 2002; **4**: 1132–1134.
6. Hansmann H. The economics and ethics of markets for human organs. In: Blumstein JF, Sloan FA (eds) *Organ Transplantation Policy: Issues and Prospects.* Durham: Duke University Press, 1989.
7. Savelescu J. Death, us and our bodies: personal reflections. *J Med Ethics* 2003; **29**: 127–130.
8. Ram V. International traffic in human organs. *Frontline* 2002: 19.
9. Patel T. India kidney sales. *Trade and Environmental Database (TED) Case Studies.* Washington: American University Online Journal, 1996; **5**: 240 (www.american.edu/projects/mandala/TED/kidney.htm).
10. Scheper-Hughes N. The ends of the body: the global commerce in organs for transplant surgery. *Organs Watch.* Online Essay. Berkeley: University of California, 1998.
11. Radcliffe-Richards J, Daar AS, Guttmann RD et al. The case for allowing kidney sales. *Lancet* 1998; **351**: 1950–1952.
12. Richards JR. Nefarious goings on. Kidney sales and moral arguments. *J Med Philos* 1996; **21**: 357–373.

13. 57th World Health Assembly, *Human Organ and Tissue Transplantation*. Geneva: World Health Organization, WHA57.18, 2004.

14. 44th World Health Assembly, *Guiding Principles on Human Organ Transplantation*. Geneva: World Health Organization, WHA44.25, 1991.

15. World Medical Association. *Human Organ & Tissue Donation and Transplantation*. World Medical Association, Edinburgh, UK 2000.

16. www.transplantation-soc.org/policy.php (accessed September 2004).

17. Sheil R. Commercialisation in transplantation: the problems and some guidelines for practice. *Transplant Soc Bull* 1995; **3**: 3.

18. www.bts.org.uk/approvedstatements.htm (accessed September 2004).

19. Council of Europe. Additional Protocol to the Convention on Human Rights and Biomedicine, on Transplantation of Organs and Tissues of Human Origin. Strasbourg, 2002.

20. Shakespeare W. The first part of Henry IV, act III, scene I. In: *The Works of William Shakespeare*, Volume 3. London: William Clowes and Sons: 1934.

21. Ghods AJ, Savaj S, Khosravani P. Adverse effects of a controlled living-unrelated donor renal transplant program on living-related and cadaveric kidney donation. *Transplant Proc* 2000; **32**: 541.

22. Ghods AJ, Ossareh S, Khosravani P. Comparison of some socioeconomic characteristics of donors and recipients in a controlled living unrelated donor renal transplant program. *Transplant Proc* 2001; **33**: 2626–2627.

23. Zargooshi J. Quality of life of Iranian kidney 'donors'. *J Urol* 2001; **166**: 1790–1799.

24. Zargooshi J. Iranian kidney donors: motivations and relations with recipients. *J Urol* 2001; **165**: 386–392.

25. Goyal M, Mehta RL, Schneiderman LJ, Sehgal AR. Economic and health consequences of selling a kidney in India. *JAMA* 2002; **288**: 1589–1593.

26. Plant WD, Akyol MA, Rudge CA. The ethical dimension to organ transplantation. In: Forsythe JLR (ed,) *Transplantation Surgery: Current Dilemmas*, 2nd edn. London: WB Saunders, 2001: 1–24.

27. Blackburn S. *The Oxford Dictionary of Philosophy*. Oxford: Oxford University Press, 1994.

28. World Medical Association. *Declaration of Geneva*. World Medical Association, Stockholm, Sweden 1994.

29. Harris J. In praise of unprincipled ethics. *J Med Ethics* 2003; **29**: 303–306.

30. Gillon R. Ethics needs principles – four can encompass the rest – and respect for autonomy should be first among equals. *J Med Ethics* 2003; **29**: 307–312.

31. Savelescu J. Is the sale of body parts wrong? *J Med Ethics* 2003; **29**: 138–139.

32. Sever MS, Kazancioglu R, Yildiz A et al. Outcome of living unrelated (commercial) renal transplantation. *Kidney Int* 2001; **60**: 1477–1483.

33. Hippocrates. *Hippocratic Writings* [translated from Greek by Chadwick J, Mann WN; edited with an introduction by Lloyd GER]. New York: Penguin, 1978.

34. Kant I. Groundwork of the metaphysics of morals. In: Paton HJ (ed) *The Moral Law*. London: Hutchinson University Library, 1964: 80.

Index